Primary Care
Radiology

Primary Care Radiology

FRED A. METTLER, JR., M.D., M.P.H.
Professor and Chair
Department of Radiology and Nuclear Medicine
University of New Mexico Health Sciences Center
Albuquerque, New Mexico

MILTON J. GUIBERTEAU, M.D.
Professor of Clinical Radiology
University of Texas Medical School at Houston
Chairman, Department of Radiology
St. Joseph's Hospital
Houston, Texas

CAROLYN M. VOSS, M.D.
Associate Professor
Department of Internal Medicine
University of New Mexico Health Sciences Center
Albuquerque, New Mexico

CHRISTOPHER E. URBINA, M.D., M.P.H.
Associate Professor
Department of Family and Community Medicine
University of New Mexico Health Sciences Center
Albuquerque, New Mexico

W.B. SAUNDERS COMPANY
A Harcourt Health Sciences Company
Philadelphia   London   New York   St. Louis   Sydney   Toronto

W.B. SAUNDERS COMPANY
A Harcourt Health Sciences Company

The Curtis Center
Independence Square West
Philadelphia, Pennsylvania 19106

Library of Congress Cataloging-in-Publication Data

Primary care radiology/Fred A. Mettler Jr. . . . [et al.].—1st ed.

p.; cm.

ISBN 0–7216–8333–9

1. Radiography, Medical.   2. Primary care (Medicine)   I. Mettler, Fred A.
[DNLM: 1. Diagnostic Imaging—methods.   2. Primary Health Care—methods.
WN 180 P952 2000]

RC78.P77   2000
616.07′572—dc21   99-057427

Acquisitions Editor: Lisette Bralow
Manuscript Editor: Judith Gandy
Production Manager: Shelley Hampton
Illustration Specialist: Walter Verbitski

PRIMARY CARE RADIOLOGY   ISBN 0–7216–8333–9

Some illustrations and tables for this text are used with permission from Mettler FA Jr: Essentials of Radiology. Philadelphia, WB Saunders Company, 1996.

Printed in the United States of America.

Last digit is the print number: 9   8   7   6   5   4   3   2   1

PREFACE

This book is intended to be a practical text on appropriate use and interpretation of imaging for primary care practitioners. In the era of managed care, primary care practitioners have assumed a leadership role in the management of their patients. As a result, many more expensive and detailed imaging studies are being ordered by primary care practitioners.

The education of primary care providers has traditionally been directed at the indications and interpretation of common studies such as chest and skeletal radiographs, with little training in the appropriate use of complex imaging procedures. Primary care practitioners now must understand the imaging work-up of various conditions. It is at least as important to know what not to order as what to order.

As a basis for this book, we began by researching the most common inpatient and outpatient diagnoses made by primary care providers at the University of New Mexico Hospital. We have included some images and material from the book *Essentials of Radiology* (by Mettler), published by WB Saunders in 1996. The entire direction of the text has been changed, however, with a major emphasis on the appropriate ordering and indications for various imaging procedures. To do this we also examined the extensive literature on "guidelines" and algorithms for appropriate imaging, although we could not include the thousands of detailed references that exist. Individual references are not included, but we have chosen to include what we believe to be the general consensus in medicine today. We have also reviewed summaries and publications of various organizations and companies, which often used expert panels and reviewed and analyzed the extensive scientific literature. Many of the recommendations are quite similar or overlap substantially. We have found certain major reviews to be particularly valuable, however, and the reader may want to pursue those. They are as follows:

National Cancer Institute, PDQ, Screening and Prevention. 1-800-422-6237 or http://cancernet.nci .nih.gov/pdqfull.htm

American College of Radiology, Appropriateness Criteria for Imaging and Treatment Decisions. 1-800-ACR-Line or http://www.acr.org

American College of Emergency Physicians, Cost Effective Diagnostic Testing in Emergency Medicine, Guidelines for Appropriate Utilization of Clinical Laboratory and Radiology Studies

InterQual, Indications for Imaging. 1-800-582-1738 or iq@interqual.com or http://www.interqual.com

Quality First, Institute for Health Care Quality, Health Risk Management Inc. 1-800-241-4270 or http://www.hrmi.com

The book is organized by anatomic system and then by suspected clinical problem or symptom. The text explains the imaging work-up of common clinical problems. For reference, we have included normal anatomy and normal variants. We have also included images of the most common radiologic diagnoses. As a rule, we did not include images of complicated procedures that usually require a radiologist for interpretation.

Fred A. Mettler, Jr., M.D., M.P.H
Milton J. Guiberteau, M.D.
Carolyn M. Voss, M.D.
Christopher E. Urbina, M.D., M.P.H.

CONTENTS

1

INTRODUCTION

ORDERING TESTS

The first step in the efficient and effective use of medical imaging is to obtain an appropriate history and to examine the patient. Only after this step can one decide which imaging study is the most appropriate or perhaps that an imaging study is not needed at all. Knowing what not to order is as important as knowing what to order. Imaging is only one way to make a diagnosis, and imaging does not stand alone but should be integrated in clinical pathways with other types of testing.

If imaging is warranted, the appropriate imaging study is dependent on circumstances of the individual patient. For example, the symptom of low back pain does not provide enough knowledge to make an informed decision regarding imaging. If the patient has recurrent low back pain that he or she has had many times before, the correct action may be to suggest specific therapy rather than order any imaging studies. If there is back pain with radicular symptoms and neurologic deficit, a magnetic resonance (MR) scan is appropriate. In many circumstances, even if the clinical scenario is specified in detail, a number of algorithms or guidelines may be available without sufficient evidence to allow definite consensus on the right one. One reason for this is that a number of imaging modalities have similar sensitivities and specificities.

In this text, we provide guidelines that are generally accepted for the primary care provider to use as a starting point. These guidelines should not be construed as the only correct courses of action. The actual imaging test ordered depends on a number of factors, such as availability of equipment, expertise of personnel, and acuteness of the clinical situation. One should also realize that many hospitals have instituted site-specific guidelines, and by moving from one practice to another, he or she may be expected to work-up and treat the same clinical condition in a different manner.

What should be expected from an imaging examination? Typically, one expects to find the exact location of a problem and hopes to discern its etiology. This is often easier said than done. Although some diseases present a characteristic picture, most can appear in a variety of forms, depending on their stage. As a result, image interpretation often yields a differential diagnosis that must be placed in the context of the clinical findings.

BASIC PRINCIPLES ABOUT INTERPRETATION OF IMAGING STUDIES

Regardless of issues surrounding who should interpret imaging studies, many times the primary care provider is faced with an imaging study, and no radiologist is available to render a definitive interpretation. Under these circumstances, one must be able to identify common entities, normal variants, and, especially, life-threatening abnormalities.

Although it may appear simple, examination of images requires a logical approach. First, one must be oriented to the technique employed, as well as the type of image produced, and be cautious of the limitations of that technique. For example, it may be useful to begin by mentally stating, "I am looking at a coronal computed tomography (CT) scan of the head done with intravenous contrast material." This is important because intravenous contrast material can be confused with fresh blood in the brain. Second, look at the name and age on the film label. This keeps one from mixing up patients, and it allows one to make a differential diagnosis that applies to a patient of that particular age and sex.

The next step is to decide what are the abnormal findings on the image. This means that one needs to know the normal anatomy and variants of that particular part of the body as well as their appearance on the imaging technique used. After this step, the abnormal areas must be described. This needs to be done because it mentally assists one in assembling a differential diagnosis. The most common mistake is to look at an abnormal image and immediately name a disease. When this is done, the mind may be locked on that diagnosis (perhaps the wrong one). It is better to say something such as, "I am going to give a differential diagnosis of generalized cardiac enlargement with normal pulmonary vasculature in a 40-year-old man," rather than to blurt out viral cardiomyopathy in a patient who really has a pericardial effusion.

After practicing for a number of years, a provider knows where pathology is most commonly visualized. Throughout this text, we point out the high yield areas to scrutinize on different examinations. Although there are no absolute rules, knowing the pathology and natural history of different diseases helps. For example, some tumors typically cause large round lung metastases, whereas others cause a myriad of small nodules.

After reviewing common causes of the x-ray findings that the primary care provider has observed, he or she should reorder the etiologies in view of the clinical findings. At this point, one probably thinks that he or she is done. Not so. Often there is a plethora of information contained in the patient's film jacket. This comes in the form of previous findings and histories supplied for the patient's other imaging examinations. Reviewing the old reports directs one to areas of pathology on the current film that would have been missed. A simple example is a pneumonia that has almost but not completely resolved or a pulmonary nodule that, because of inspiratory difference, is hiding behind a rib on the current examination.

As a final step, remember that there may be a number of entities, which have not yet been considered, that could cause the findings on the image. After looking at a case, it is useful to try to go through a set sequence of categories in search of other differential possibilities. Example categories are congenital, physical and chemical, infectious, neoplastic, metabolic, circulatory, and miscellaneous.

CONSULTING WITH RADIOLOGISTS

The radiologist is a consultant physician. The consulting role includes helping the primary care provider select the correct view or examination in complicated situations. Primary care providers are now more frequently faced with taking care of patients formerly managed by specialists and are simultaneously sorting through a rapidly expanding array of imaging technology. It is the radiologist who knows the different indications, sensitivities, specificities, and protocols for each study. In fact, imaging is so complex that one radiologist often does not have all the information the primary care provider may need. A consultation with a neuroradiologist in some circumstances and a nuclear medicine specialist in other cases may be necessary.

In most settings, the radiologist also provides definitive interpretation of imaging studies and advises additional imaging tests if necessary. Because the clinical context is so important for the most accurate interpretation of the examination, providing as much clinical information as possible is not only practicing good medicine but is also appreciated by the radiologist. Unfortunately, current computer systems often limit the allowable space for clinical information on the computer-generated request, and clerks may put in unrecognizable abbreviations.

Accurate and comprehensive clinical information is especially important for expensive, technically complex, and invasive examinations. As an example, quite a number of protocols are used to perform a CT scan of the chest. They each give varied information. The evaluation protocols are quite different for a potential dissecting aortic aneurysm than for a potential lung cancer. If the wrong history is provided, the information necessary to make the diagnosis may not be obtained from the examination if the appropriate protocol has not been selected.

Consulting with the radiologist should not end when a printed report is received. If the findings do not match the primary care provider's clinical impression, he or she may want to ask the radiologist why this might be. In addition, the radiologist may use unfamiliar terms or acronyms that have not been encountered by the provider before. This is a good opportunity to expand one's knowledge base.

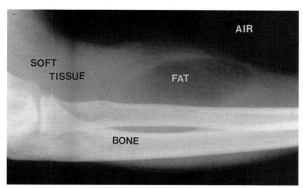

FIGURE 1–1. **The four basic densities on a radiograph.** A lateral view of the forearm shows that the bone is the most dense and therefore white; soft tissue is gray; fat is somewhat dark; and air is quite dark. The abnormality in this case is the fat in the soft tissue of the forearm, which is due to a lipoma.

■ **PLAIN RADIOGRAPHS**

Regular x-ray examinations, or plain radiography, account for more than 80% of imaging examinations. X-ray films (plain radiographs) are made by an x-ray beam passing through the patient and thereby producing an x-ray shadow on film. The x-rays are absorbed in different amounts by the various tissues or materials in the body. A percentage of the radiation beam entering the patient exits the other side of the patient and strikes a fluorescent screen, which produces light that exposes the film.

There are four basic densities or shades visible on plain films. These are air, fat, water (blood and soft tissue), and bone. Obviously, air does not absorb much radiation. As a result, in the area of the lungs on a chest radiograph, more of the beam passes through the patient and strikes the fluorescent screen, exposing the film more and causing it to be dark. On radiographs, fat is generally gray and

darker than muscle or blood (Fig. 1–1). Bone and calcium appear almost white. Items that contain metal (such as prosthetic hips) and contrast materials also appear white. The contrast agents generally used are barium for most gastrointestinal studies and iodine for most intravenously administered agents.

It should be remembered that standard or plain radiographs are a two-dimensional presentation of three-dimensional information. That is why frontal and lateral views are often needed. Without these, mistakes can easily be made. An object visualized on one view is somewhere in the path of the x-ray beam (not necessarily in the patient) (Fig. 1–2). Each additional view needed to make a diagnosis requires an additional x-ray exposure and therefore adds to the patient's radiation dose.

The terminology used to describe plain radiographs is usually quite straightforward. Chest and abdominal films are referred to as *upright* or *supine* depending on the position of the patient. In addition, chest radiographs are usually described as *posteroanterior* (PA) or *anteroposterior* (AP) (Fig. 1–3). These terms indicate the direction in which the x-ray beam traversed the patient on its way to the film. PA means that the x-ray beam entered the posterior aspect of the patient and exited anteriorly. AP means that the beam direction through the patient was anterior to posterior. A left lateral decubitus view is one taken with the patient's left side down.

Position is important because it can affect magnification, organ position, and blood flow; therefore, it significantly affects image interpretation. For example, the heart appears larger on AP than on PA films. This is because on an AP film the heart is farther from the film and is magnified more by the diverging x-ray beam. It also appears larger on

FIGURE 1–2. **Spatial localization on a radiograph.** On both anteroposterior and lateral projections, the square and round objects are seen projecting within the view of the chest, even though the square object is, in fact, located outside the chest wall. If an object (the triangle), projects outside the chest wall on at least one view it is, in fact, outside the chest. However, if an object looks as though it is inside the chest on both views, it may be either inside or outside.

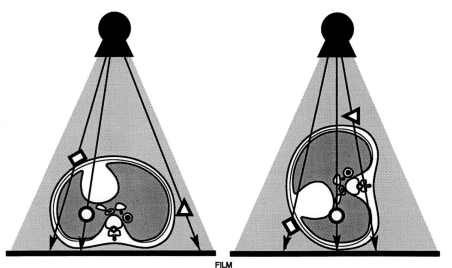

FILM

ANTERIOR-POSTERIOR   **LATERAL**

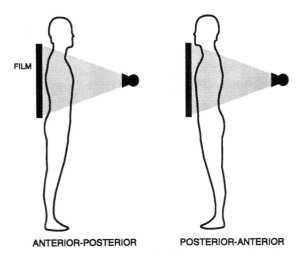

FILM

ANTERIOR-POSTERIOR   POSTERIOR-ANTERIOR

FIGURE 1–3. **Typical x-ray projections.** X-ray projections are typically listed as anteroposterior or posteroanterior. This designation depends on whether the x-ray beam passes into the patient from anterior to posterior or the reverse. Lateral and oblique views are also commonly obtained.

supine than on upright films because the hemidiaphragms are pushed up, making the heart appear wider. A portable film is taken with the tube closer to the patient than on standard upright films, and this also magnifies the heart. Pulmonary blood flow is another example of more flow to the upper lungs when the patient is in the supine position.

Use of contrast agents permits visualization of anatomic structures that are normally not seen. For example, intravenous or intra-arterially injected agents allow visualization of blood vessels (Fig. 1–4). If imaging is done with a standard format, the blood vessels appear white. Newer imaging technology using computers may show the vessels as black.

Contrast agents are used to fill either a hollow viscus (such as the stomach) or anatomic tubular structures that can be accessed in some way (such as blood vessels, ureter, and common bile duct). Contrast agents instilled orally, rectally, or retrograde into the ureter or bladder have little or no risk unless there is aspiration or perforation. With intravenously or intra-arterially administered agents, there is a small but real risk of contrast material reaction. About 5% of patients experience an immediate mild reaction, such as a metallic taste or a feeling of warmth; some patients experience nausea and vomiting or wheezing or may get hives as a result of these contrast agents. Because many contrast agents also reduce renal function, they should not be used routinely in patients with compromised renal function or multiple myeloma. To avoid lactic acidosis, patients receiving metformin therapy should have it discontinued at the time of a procedure requiring intravenous contrast material and for 48 hours thereafter.

A small number (about 1 in 1000) of patients have a severe reaction to intravenous contrast material. Such reactions include vasovagal syncope, laryngeal edema, severe hypotension, anaphylactic-type reaction, or cardiac arrest. The risk of death from a study using intravenously administered ionic contrast agents is about 1 in 40,000. There are newer (and more expensive) nonionic contrast agents that reduce the risk of severe, but not of less severe, reactions. Many hospitals now use nonionic contrast agents for most intravenous studies.

■ COMPUTED TOMOGRAPHY

CT is accomplished by passing a rotating fan beam of x-rays through the patient and measuring the transmission through the patient at thousands of points. The data are handled by a computer that calculates exactly what the x-ray absorption by the patient was at any given spot. The data can be manipulated in a number of ways, displayed on a screen, and photographed. Because the data points are in the computer memory, it is possible to window the image and obtain a number of different filmed images that highlight various structures and tissues without additional radiation exposure (Fig. 1–5). Compared with plain radiographs, a patient undergoing CT receives about 10 to 100 times more radiation. This is due to the rotational geometry needed for CT and the decreased sensitivity of the CT detector systems compared with that of standard x-ray systems.

CT scans are presented as a series of slices of a body part. The method is similar in principle to slicing a loaf of bread and pulling up one slice at a time to examine it. Thus, CT is a two-dimensional display of two-dimensional information, and objects appear where they really are in space. The transverse (axial) scans or slices are shown as if you are viewing the patient from the foot of the bed. Thus, the individual's right side is on your left (Fig. 1–6). This is also the convention used for the transverse images of ultrasonography and magnetic resonance imaging.

Contrast agents, frequently employed in CT scans, are usually the same water-soluble oral, rectal, or intravenous-iodinated agents used in other imaging studies. Intravenous contrast agents are used in 50 to 75% of all CT studies and carry the risk of contrast material reactions discussed previously.

The appeal of CT is that a large number of structures are visualized simultaneously. In a patient with abdominal pain, one CT examination shows the liver, adrenal glands, kidneys, spleen, aorta, pancreas, and other structures. This allows the clinician to quickly identify macroscopic pathology.

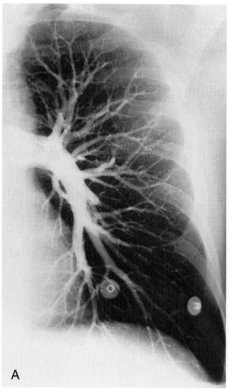
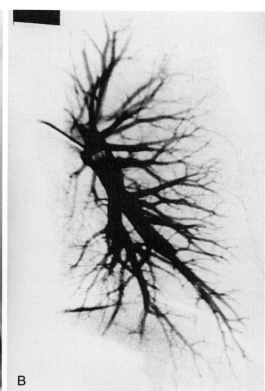

FIGURE 1–4. **Pulmonary angiogram.** A conventional view (A) of blood vessels can be obtained by injecting iodinated contrast material into the vessels. On these images, the vessels and the bones appear white. A digital subtraction technique using computers may show the vessels as either black (B) or white, but the bones are subtracted from the image.

A

B

ULTRASONOGRAPHY

Ultrasonography uses high-frequency sound waves to make images. The technology is that of sonar or a glorified fish-finder used by fishermen. The image is made by sending high-frequency sound into the patient and assessing the strength and time of returning echoes. Echoes are the result of interfaces or changes in density between tissues. Typically, a cyst has few, if any, echoes because it is mostly water. Tissues such as that of the liver or spleen result in a picture with rather homogeneous small echoes because of fibrous interstitial tissue (Fig. 1–7). High intensity echoes are caused by calcification, fat, and air.

The technology of ultrasonography is attractive because it does not use ionizing radiation and because the machines employed are relatively inexpensive. For these reasons, ultrasonography has found widespread use in obstetrics. The use of so-called real-time ultrasonography allows the images to be seen in sequential frames just like a movie. This capability has proved popular for imaging rapidly moving structures, such as the heart. Unfortunately, the quality with which ultrasound images are generated is dependent on the expertise of the person performing the study. In addition, the field of view within the patient is limited. Thus, unless clear labels indicate the description of the image orientation, the study can be difficult or impossible for the novice to interpret. Ultrasound images are usually presented as white echoes on a black background.

In addition to using echoes to generate images, returning echo frequencies can also be analyzed. This so-called Doppler analysis allows the identification of moving blood as well as the assessment of its direction and magnitude of flow. One example of the use of this technique is the identification and quantitation of stenoses in the carotid arteries.

NUCLEAR MEDICINE

Nuclear medicine images are made by giving the patient a short-lived radioactive material. The most commonly used radionuclides decay rapidly and have half-lives of only hours. Most materials administered are not detectable within a day or so after administration. By attaching a radionuclide (such as technetium 99m) to specific carrier compounds, there can be concentration of the radioactivity in a chosen organ, tissue, or pathologic process such as the thyroid, bone, lung, heart, abscess, or tumor. There are essentially no significant patient reactions to radiopharmaceuticals used for diagnosis.

Nuclear medicine images are made by a gamma camera that records radiation emanating from the patient and produces an image of the distribution of the radioactive material (Fig. 1–8). The radiation dose to the patient is determined by the amount of radioactive material initially injected into the body.

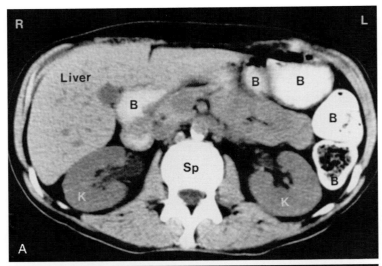

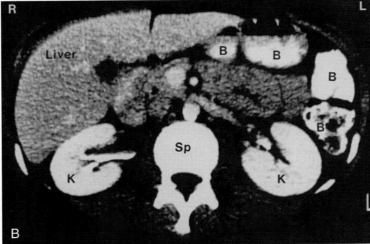

FIGURE 1–5. **Computed tomography.** Images of the abdomen are presented here. *A*, The image is done using relatively wide windows during filming, and no intravenous contrast material is used. *B*, The windows are narrowed, producing a rather grainy image, and intravenous contrast material is administered so that you can see enhancement of the aorta, abdominal vessels, and both kidneys (K). In both images, contrast material is used in the bowel (B) to differentiate the bowel from solid organs and structures. Sp = spleen.

FIGURE 1–6. **Orientation of computed tomography (CT) and magnetic resonance (MR) images.** CT and MR usually present images as transverse (axial) slices of the body. The orientation of most slices is the same as viewing a patient from the foot of the bed.

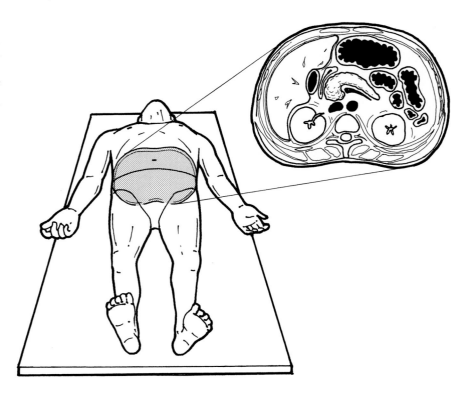

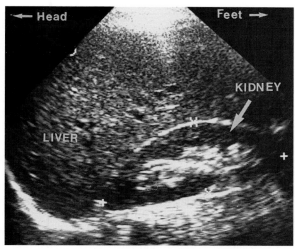

FIGURE 1–7. **Ultrasonography of the liver and kidney.** This is a longitudinal image essentially looking at the patient from the side. The patient's head is to the reader's left. The liver has rather homogeneous echoes, and the kidney is easily seen as a bean-shaped organ posterior to the right lobe of the liver.

Therefore, once the dose has been given, additional images can be obtained without increasing the radiation exposure. Images are usually obtained as planar images, which, as in plain radiographs, display three-dimensional data in two dimensions. These images are labeled as anterior, lateral, and so forth. Computer technology (similar to CT) applied to nuclear medicine displays images of slices of the tissue of interest. This single photon emission computed tomography (SPECT) technology is commonly applied to brain, cardiac, and bone imaging.

The major advantage of nuclear medicine is its ability to obtain an image of physiologic function. For example, there is virtually no other imaging technique that can assess regional pulmonary ventilation or hepatic function.

■ MAGNETIC RESONANCE

MR generates images by applying a varying magnetic field to the body. The magnetic field aligns atoms. When the field is released, radio waves are generated. The frequency of the emitted radio waves is related to the chemical environment of the atoms. With computer analysis of these data, MR images (which are essentially hydrogen maps) can be generated.

Although there are many MR techniques, there are two basic types of images, T1 and T2 weighted. T1-weighted images show fat as a white or bright signal, whereas water (or cerebrospinal fluid [CSF]) is dark. On a T2-weighted image, fat is dark, and blood, edema, and CSF appear white (Fig. 1–9). Unfortunately, calcium and bone are difficult to see

on MR images. What appears to be bone is really the visualization of fat in the marrow. Computer manipulation of MR images allows the display of slices similar to the technique used in CT. An intravenous contrast agent (gadolinium) is often used in conjunction with brain imaging. This contrast agent is quite expensive, adding about $100 to $200 to the cost of the examination. There are few significant patient reactions to this agent.

The primary advantage of MR is that it obtains exquisite images of the central nervous system and stationary soft tissues (such as the knee joint). It also does not use ionizing radiation. Recent developments have allowed images of blood vessels to be generated without the need to inject contrast material into the patient (Fig. 1–10).

Disadvantages of MR have been the visualization of artifacts due to patient motion, the inability to bring ferrous objects near the magnet, and the high cost. The major safety problem with these magnets is because they are so strong, if a ferromagnetic

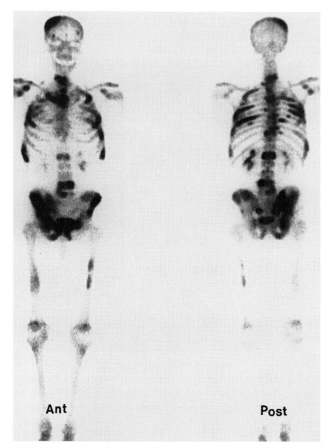

FIGURE 1–8. **Nuclear medicine bone scan.** Radioactivity is introduced intravenously and localizes in specific organs. In this case, a tracer has been given that makes the radioactivity localize in the bone and the kidneys. Nuclear medicine can obtain images of a number of organs, including lungs, heart, and liver. The extremely dark areas in the bones are due to metastatic prostate carcinoma.

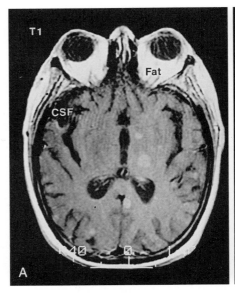 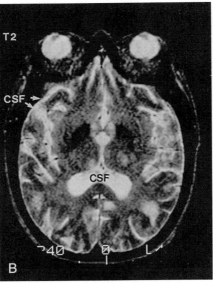

FIGURE 1–9. **Magnetic resonance (MR) images of the brain.** There are a wide variety of imaging parameters that can make tissues appear quite different. The two most common presentations are T1-weighted images *(A)*, in which fat appears white, water and cerebrospinal fluid appear black, and brain and muscle appear gray. In almost all MR images, bone gives off no signal and appears black. With T2-weighted imaging *(B)*, fat is dark, and water and cerebrospinal fluid have a high signal and appear bright or white. The brain and soft tissues still appear gray.

object (such as a wrench) is brought into the room containing the magnet, the object can quickly accelerate to 150 miles per hour. If a patient is in the machine at the time, there could be lethal consequences. Physicians should be aware that some sandbags used for neck stabilization actually contain small BBs that can destroy magnets. Contraindications to having an MR scan include cardiac pacemakers, defibrillators, spinal cord stimulators, and most aneurysm clips. Titanium wire, prosthetic valves, and orthopedic hardware such as plates and screws are safe, although they cause degrading artifacts on the images.

GENERAL SUGGESTED READINGS

General Radiology

Juhl JH, Crummy AB, Kuhlman JE (eds): Paul and Juhl's Essentials of Radiologic Imaging, 7th ed. Philadelphia, Lippincott-Raven, 1998.

Keats T: Atlas of Normal Roentgen Variants That May Simulate Disease, 4th ed. Chicago, Year Book Medical, 1988.

Wiest P, Roth P: Fundamentals of Emergency Radiology. Philadelphia, WB Saunders, 1996.

Computed Tomography and Magnetic Resonance

Lee J, Sagel S, Stanley R, Heiken J: Computed Body Tomography With MRI Correlation, 3rd ed. Philadelphia, Lippincott-Raven, 1998.

Ultrasonography

Williamson M: Essentials of Ultrasound. Philadelphia, WB Saunders, 1996.

Nuclear Medicine

Mettler F, Guiberteau M: Essentials of Nuclear Medicine Imaging, 4th ed. Philadelphia, WB Saunders, 1998.

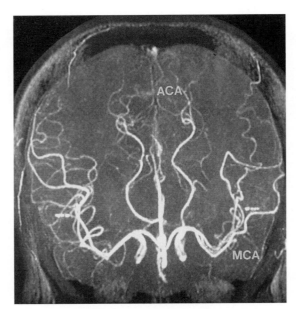

FIGURE 1–10. **Magnetic resonance angiogram.** An anterior view of the head showing intracerebral vessels, including the anterior cerebral artery (ACA) and the middle cerebral artery (MCA). These images were obtained without injection of any contrast agent.

2

HEAD AND NECK

▓ IMAGING OF THE CRANIUM AND ITS CONTENTS

Definitive imaging of the skull and brain is best done by either computed tomography (CT) or magnetic resonance imaging (MRI). CT is the procedure of choice when there are questions of bone integrity, penetrating injury, or hemorrhage. MRI is used to answer most other questions. If there is a contraindication to an MRI (see Chapter 1) or if an MRI scanner is not available, CT can often give useful information. Contrast angiography is usually performed if surgery or embolization is contemplated. Table 2–1 lists the initial imaging study of choice for a number of clinical problems. In addition to CT and MRI, plain skull films play a limited role in skull and brain evaluation as well.

Normal anatomy of the brain in standard x-ray projections is shown in Figure 2–1. The most common problem on plain skull films is distinguishing cranial sutures from vascular grooves and fractures. The main sutures are coronal, sagittal, and lambdoid. A suture also runs in a rainbow shape over the ear (the squamosal suture). In adults, sutures are symmetric, are wiggly, and have sclerotic (extremely white) edges. Vascular grooves are usually best seen on the lateral view and extend posteriorly and superiorly from just in front of the ear. They do not have sclerotic edges, are not perfectly straight, and frequently have branching.

There are a few common variants on skull films. Hyperostosis frontalis interna is a benign condition

of females in which thickening of the bone and sclerosis or increased density is seen in the frontal region. It typically spares the midline. A number of benign intracranial calcifications can be seen on skull films. A vertical linear calcification seen in the midline on the frontal film is almost always due to calcification of the falx cerebri. A punctate central calcification is usually due to benign pineal or habenular calcification, and symmetric bilateral calcification of the choroid plexus can occasionally be seen. None of these findings is of clinical importance. Large, asymmetric, or amorphous focal intracranial calcification is always suggestive of a benign or malignant neoplasm.

Occasionally, areas of lucency (dark areas) can be seen, which indicate that the bone is thinned. The most common normal variants that cause this are vascular lakes or biparietal foramina. Asymmetric round or ill-defined holes should be suggestive of metastatic disease. Normal anatomy of the brain on CT and MRI is shown in Figures 2–2 and 2–3.

Headache

Headaches can be due to a myriad of causes and should be characterized by location, duration, type of pain, provoking factors, and age and sex of the patient. In the primary care population, only less than 0.5% of acute headaches are the result of serious intracranial pathology. Simple headaches, tension headaches, migraine headaches, and cluster headaches do not warrant imaging studies. A good

Text continued on page 17

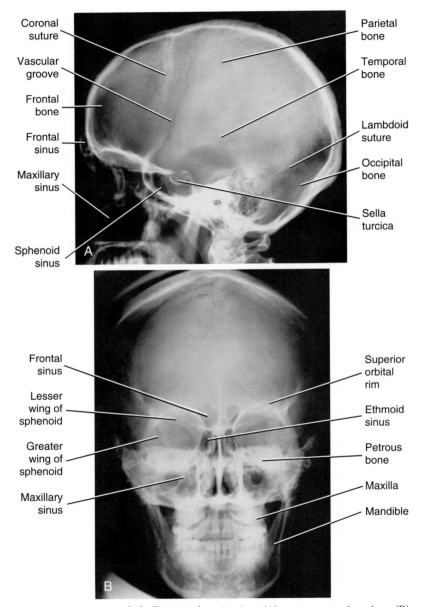

FIGURE 2–1. **Normal skull.** Lateral projection *(A)*, anteroposterior view *(B)*.

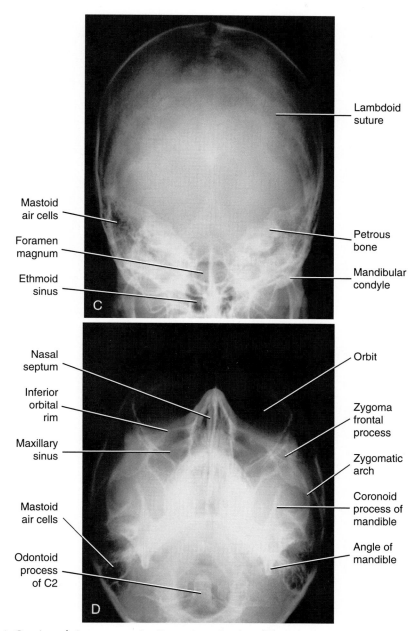

Lambdoid
suture

Mastoid
air cells

Foramen
magnum

Ethmoid
sinus

C

Petrous
bone

Mandibular
condyle

Nasal
septum

Inferior
orbital
rim

Maxillary
sinus

Mastoid
air cells

Odontoid
process
of C2

D

Orbit

Zygoma
frontal
process

Zygomatic
arch

Coronoid
process of
mandible

Angle of
mandible

FIGURE 2–1 *Continued.* Anteroposterior Towne's projection *(C)*, and anteroposterior Waters' view *(D)*.

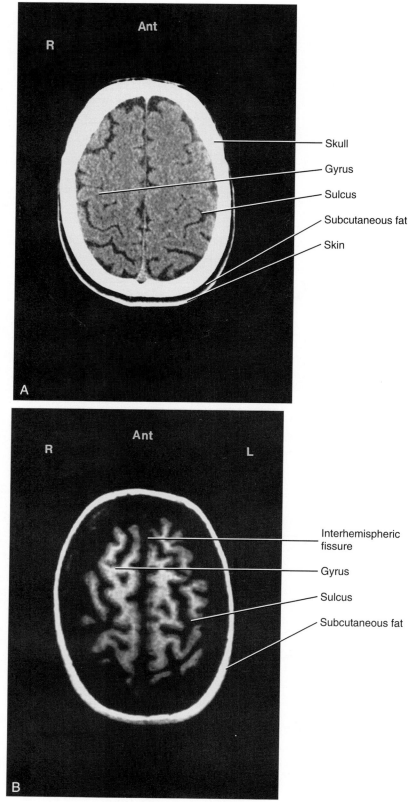

FIGURE 2–2. **Normal anatomy of the brain in transverse (axial) images.** *A* to *H,* Noncontrasted computed tomography scans and T1-weighted magnetic resonance images are shown for the same levels.

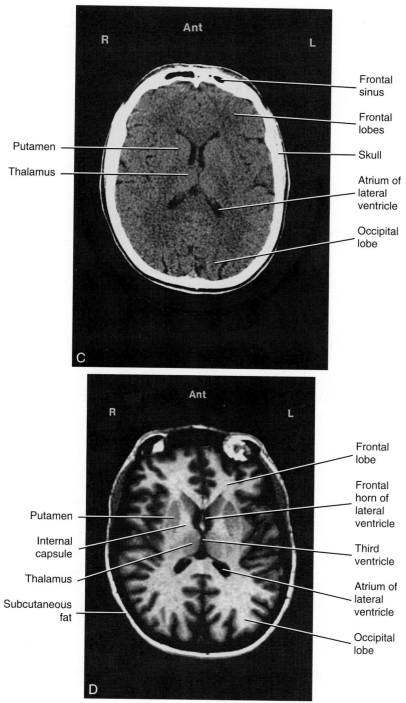

Figure 2–2 *Continued*
Illustration continued on following page

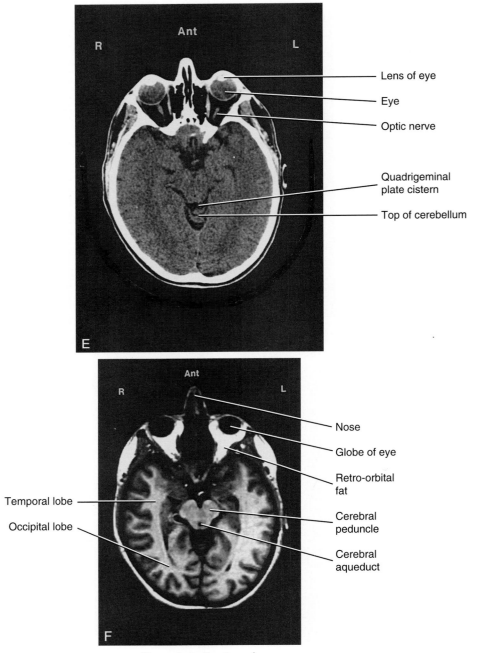

Figure 2–2 *Continued*

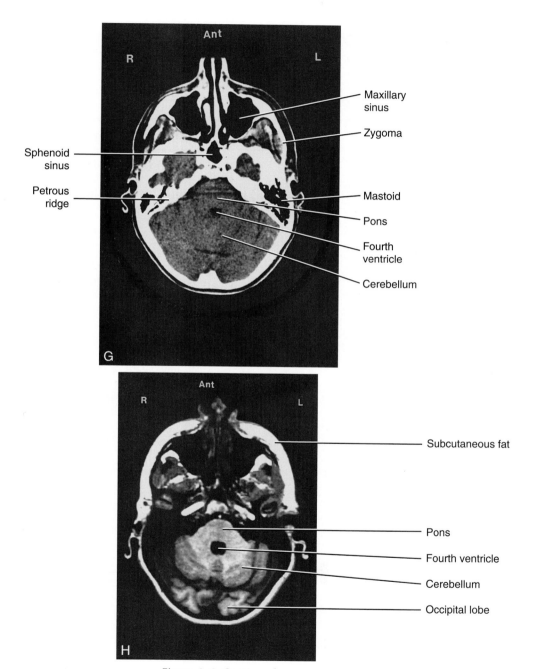

Figure 2–2 *Continued*

TABLE 2–1 Imaging Modalities for Cranial Problems

Suspected Cranial Problem	Initial Imaging Study
Skull fracture (depressed)	CT brain scan including bone windows
Major head trauma	CT (neurologically unstable); MRI (neurologically stable)
Mild head trauma	Observe; CT (if persistent headache)
Acute hemorrhage	Noncontrasted CT
Suspected intracerebral aneurysm or arteriovenous malformations	MRI
Hydrocephalus	Noncontrasted CT
Transient ischemic attack	Noncontrasted CT, MRI if vertebrobasilar findings; consider carotid ultrasonography if bruit present
Acute transient or persistent CNS symptoms or findings	See Table 2–3
Acute stroke (suspected hemorrhagic)	Noncontrasted CT
Acute stroke (suspected nonhemorrhagic)	MRI
Multiple sclerosis	MRI of the brain
Tumor or metastases	MRI
Aneurysm (chronic history)	MR angiogram or contrasted CT
Abscess	Contrasted CT or MRI
Preoperative for cranial surgery	Contrast angiography
Meningitis	Lumbar tap; CT (only to exclude complications)
Seizure (new onset or poor therapeutic response)	MRI
Seizure (febrile or alcohol withdrawal without neurologic deficit)	Imaging not indicated
Neurologic deficit with known primary tumor elsewhere	MRI if associated sensorineural findings
Vertigo (if suspect acoustic neuroma or posterior fossa tumor)	MRI or contrasted CT
Headache	See Table 2–2
Dementia	Nothing, or MRI
Alzheimer's disease	Nuclear medicine SPECT scan
Sinusitis	See Table 2–5

CNS = central nervous system; CT = computed tomography; MRI = magnetic resonance imaging; SPECT = single photon emission computed tomography.

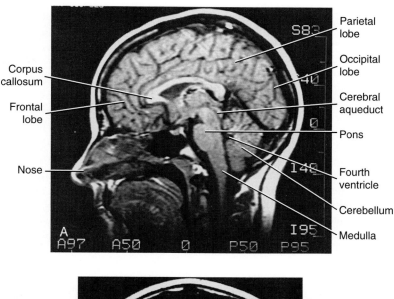

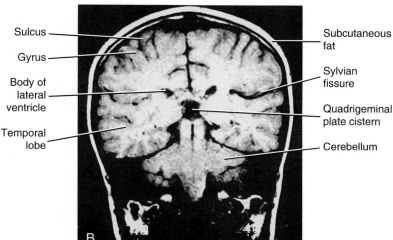

FIGURE 2–3. *A and B,* **Normal magnetic resonance anatomy of the brain in coronal and sagittal projections.**

physical examination is essential, including evaluation of the blood pressure, urine, eyes (for papilledema), temporal arteries, sinuses, ears, neurologic system, and neck. In a patient with a febrile illness, headache, and stiff neck, a lumbar puncture should be performed. However, there are only a few circumstances in which imaging is indicated.

In general, imaging is indicated when a headache is accompanied by neurologic findings, syncope, confusion, seizure, and mental status changes or after major trauma. Sudden onset of "the worst headache of one's life" (thunderclap headache) should raise a question of subarachnoid hemorrhage. Sudden onset of a unilateral headache with a suspected carotid or vertebral dissection or ipsilateral Horner's syndrome should prompt an MRI and possibly a magnetic resonance angiogram. Other indications for MRI or CT are shown in Tables 2–2 and 2–3.

Sinus headaches can usually be differentiated from other etiologies because they worsen when leaning forward or with application of pressure over the affected sinus. Indications for CT use are discussed in the sinus section later in this chapter.

Head Trauma

On a plain skull film, fractures are dark lines that have sharp edges and tend to be extremely straight (Fig. 2–4). If there is a fracture over the middle meningeal artery area, an associated epidural hematoma may be present. If there is a depressed fracture, the lucent fracture lines can be stellate or semicircular (Fig. 2–5). In either of these cases, there can also be substantial brain injury, and a CT scan including bone windows is indicated. In general, skull films are ordered too frequently. Skull fracture without a history of loss of consciousness is quite rare, and significant brain injury may result without a skull fracture.

The patient must be examined clinically to decide whether physical findings and medical history indicate mild, moderate, or severe head injury. CT, MRI, or skull radiography is not needed for low risk patients, defined as those who are asymptomatic or have only dizziness, mild headache, scalp laceration or hematoma, and scalp contusion or abrasion; are

TABLE 2–2 Imaging Indications for Headaches

MRI is indicated for the following:
- Sudden onset of the "worst headache of one's life" (thunderclap headache)
- A headache that
    worsens with exertion
    is associated with a decrease in alertness
    is positionally related
    awakens one from sleep
    changes in pattern over time
- A new headache in an HIV-positive individual
- Associated with papilledema
- Associated with focal neurologic deficit
- Associated with mental status changes

For most of the above indications, CT is acceptable if an MRI is not feasible or available. MRI is usually not indicated for sinus headaches. See Table 2–5 for CT indications in sinus disease.

MRI = magnetic resonance imaging; HIV = human immunodeficiency virus; CT = computed tomography.

older than 2 years of age; and have no moderate or high risk findings.

Patients at moderate risk are those who have any of the following conditions: history of change in the level of consciousness at any time after the injury, progressive or severe headache, post-traumatic seizure, persistent vomiting, multiple trauma, serious facial injury, signs of basilar skull fracture (hemotympanum, "raccoon eyes," cerebrospinal fluid [CSF] rhinorrhea or otorrhea), suspected child abuse, bleeding disorder, or age younger than 2 years (unless the injury is trivial).

High risk patients are those presenting with any of the following conditions: focal neurologic findings, a Glasgow Coma Scale score of 8 or less, definite skull penetration, metabolic derangement, postictal

TABLE 2–3 Imaging Indications With a New Neurologic Deficit

Acute onset or persistence of the following neurologic deficits are an indication for computed tomography or magnetic resonance imaging:
- New vision loss
- Aphasia
- Mental status change (memory loss, confusion, impaired level of consciousness)
- Sensory abnormalities (hemianesthesia/hypesthesia including single limb)
- Motor paralysis (hemiparesis or single limb)
- Vertigo with headache, diplopia, motor or sensory deficit, ataxia, dysarthria, or dysmetria

state, or decreased or depressed level of consciousness (unrelated to drugs, alcohol, other central nervous system [CNS] depressants).

If there is moderate or severe injury or the patient is neurologically unstable, a CT scan should be done as the initial examination to exclude hemorrhage. If the patient is neurologically stable or if there is suspected child abuse, an MRI scan is preferable to look for parenchymal shearing injuries. An MRI scan may also be indicated if there is a significant discrepancy between clinical and CT

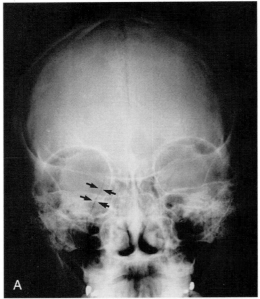

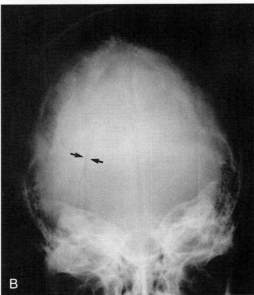

FIGURE 2–4. **Linear skull fracture.** Skull fractures (arrows) are usually dark lines that are sharply defined and do not have white margins. On the anteroposterior view (A), one cannot tell whether the fracture is in the front or the back of the skull. With Towne's view (B), however, in which the neck is flexed and the occiput is raised, the fracture (arrows) can clearly be localized to the occipital bone.

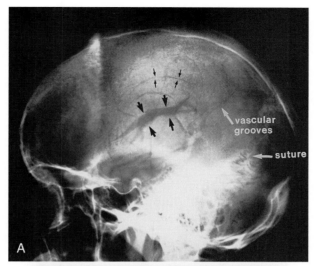

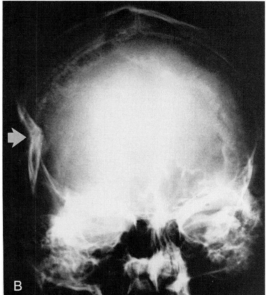

FIGURE 2–5. **Depressed skull fracture.** This patient was hit in the head with a hammer. The lateral view (*A*) shows the central portion of the fracture, which is stellate (*large arrows*), and the surrounding concentric fracture line (*small arrows*). Note the wiggly posterior suture lines and the normally radiating vascular grooves. The anteroposterior view (*B*) shows the amount of depression of the fracture, although this is usually much better seen on a computed tomography scan.

findings. In patients with a subacute closed head injury and late neurologic deterioration, either CT or MRI is appropriate.

Suspected Intracranial Hemorrhage

Intraparenchymal hemorrhage can result from a ruptured aneurysm, a stroke, trauma, or a tumor and is a common complication of hypertension. A suspected stroke in a patient with hypertension or a patient on anticoagulant therapy accompanied by headache symptoms should raise the possibility of

intracranial hemorrhage. The major finding of acute hemorrhage on a noncontrasted CT scan is increased density in the parenchyma (Fig. 2–6). There can be an associated mass effect with compression of the ventricles or midline shift. Grave prognostic factors are large amount of hemorrhage or brainstem location. Most hypertensive bleeds (80%) occur in the basal ganglia; 10% occur in the pons and 10% in the cerebellum. In patients with hypertension, an intracerebral hematoma may be due to a ruptured aneurysm, and an angiogram is indicated.

The study of choice in this situation is a CT scan done without intravenous contrast agent. The reason for doing the scan without contrast agent is that acute hemorrhage appears as a white area on a CT scan and so does contrast material. Hemorrhage into the ventricles is usually seen in the posterior horns of the lateral ventricles. Blood is denser than CSF and therefore settles dependently. A CT scan may be nondiagnostic in a small percentage of cases. Thus, if the CT scan is negative but there is CSF blood by lumbar puncture, an angiogram is indicated.

Subdural hematomas are seen as crescent-shaped abnormalities between the brain and the

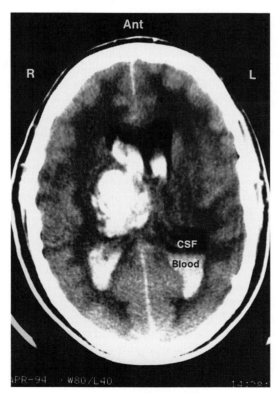

FIGURE 2–6. **Intracerebral hemorrhage.** In this hypertensive patient with an acute severe headache, the noncontrasted computed tomography scan shows a large area of fresh blood in the region of the right thalamus. Blood is also seen in the anterior and posterior horns of the lateral ventricles. Because blood is denser than cerebrospinal fluid (CSF), it is layered dependently.

skull. They can cross suture lines, but they do not cross the tentorium or falx. In some cases, subdural hematomas can be quite difficult to see because acute blood in a subdural hematoma appears denser or whiter than brain tissue (Fig. 2–7A), but as the blood ages (more than several weeks), it becomes less dense than brain (see Fig. 2–7B). There is a subacute phase during which the blood is the same density (isodense) as the brain. In this stage, sometimes the only clue that a subdural hematoma is present is effacement of the gyral pattern on the affected side, a midline shift away from the affected side, or ventricular compression on the affected side.

Epidural hematomas follow the same changing pattern of density as subdural hematomas. The major difference from an imaging viewpoint is that epidural hematomas are lenticular (biconvex) rather than crescentic (Fig. 2–8), and they tend not to cross suture lines of the skull. Epidural hematomas are often (but not always) associated with temporal bone fractures that have resulted in a tear of the middle meningeal artery.

Subarachnoid hemorrhage is usually the result of trauma or a ruptured aneurysm. It is most often accompanied by a severe sudden-onset headache, occasionally preceded by hours or days of a "sentinel" headache. Subarachnoid hemorrhage can really be visualized only in the acute stage, when the blood is radiographically denser (whiter) than the CSF. The most common appearance is increased density in the region around the brainstem (CSF cisterns), in a pattern sometimes referred to as a "Texaco star" (Fig. 2–9). Increased density due to blood can also be seen as a white line in the sylvian fissure, the anterior interhemispheric fissure, or the region of the tentorium. When these findings are present in the absence of trauma, a ruptured aneurysm should be suspected, and an angiogram is indicated.

Pneumocephalus

Air within the cranial vault is almost always the result of trauma. Even tiny amounts of air are easily seen on CT as decreased density (black). It is preferable to do a CT scan instead of an MRI examination because of the superior ability of CT to localize skull fractures and fresh hemorrhage. It is also easier to manage an unstable patient in a CT scanner than in an MRI machine.

Suspected Hydrocephalus

Dilatation of the ventricles can be either obstructive or nonobstructive. The ventricles are easily

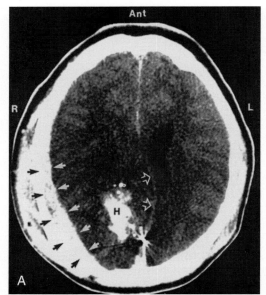
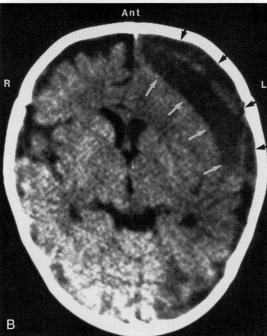

FIGURE 2–7. **Subdural hematomas.** A noncontrasted computed tomography scan of an acute subdural hematoma *(A)* shows a crescentic area of increased density in the right posterior parietal region between the brain and the skull *(black and white arrows)*. An area of intraparenchymal hemorrhage (H) is also seen; in addition, there is mass effect causing a midline shift to the left *(open arrows)*. A chronic subdural hematoma is seen in a different patient *(B)*. There is an area of decreased density in the left frontoparietal region *(arrows)* effacing the sulci, compressing the anterior horn of the left lateral ventricle, and shifting the midline somewhat to the right.

seen on a noncontrasted CT or MRI study. If the cause is obstructive, both modalities have a good chance of finding the site of obstruction. In a patient who has a ventricular shunt and increasing ventric-

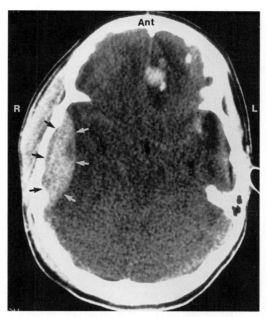

FIGURE 2–8. **Epidural hematoma.** In this patient who was in a motor vehicle accident, a lenticular area of increased density is seen on a noncontrasted axial computed tomography scan in the right parietal region *(arrows)*. These typically occur over the groove of the middle meningeal artery. Areas of hemorrhage are also seen in the left frontal lobe.

ular size, a nuclear medicine shunt study may be necessary to determine the site of any shunt obstruction.

Transient Ischemic Attack

A transient ischemic attack (TIA) is defined as a neurologic deficit that has an abrupt onset and from which there is rapid recovery, often within minutes but always within 24 hours. A TIA indicates that the patient may be at high risk for stroke. In the acute setting the initial test of choice is a CT scan to differentiate an ischemic from a hemorrhagic event. A second CT can be obtained in 24 to 72 hours if the diagnosis is in doubt, but MRI is more sensitive in identifying early ischemic damage and may establish the cause of the TIA. If there are initial vertebrobasilar findings, an MRI study provides better evaluation of the posterior fossa than a CT scan. Regardless of whether a carotid bruit is present in this setting, a duplex Doppler ultrasound examination of the carotid arteries is indicated if the patient would be a surgical candidate for endarterectomy. Magnetic resonance angiography can be used to visualize carotid stenosis, but many vascular surgeons want a true arteriogram (because of better spatial resolution) before surgery.

Stroke

A stroke may be ischemic or associated with hemorrhage. Hemorrhagic strokes are more common in hypertensive or anticoagulated patients. An acute hemorrhagic stroke is most easily visualized on a noncontrasted CT scan, because the fresh blood is quite dense (white). A diagnosis of stroke cannot be excluded even with normal results on a CT scan if the scan is done within 12 hours of a suspected

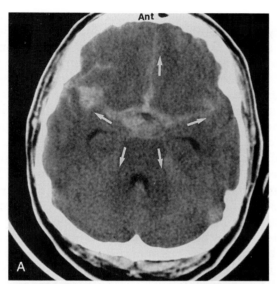

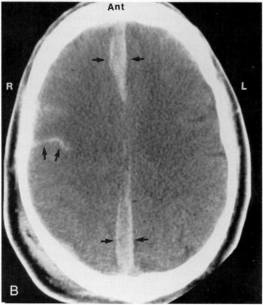

FIGURE 2–9. **Acute subarachnoid hemorrhage.** A noncontrasted axial computed tomography scan shows the blood as areas of increased density. A transverse view *(A)* near the base of the brain shows blood in the "Texaco star" pattern, formed by blood radiating *(arrows)* from the suprasellar cistern into the sylvian fissure and the anterior interhemispheric fissure. A higher cut *(B)* shows blood as an area of increased density in the anterior and posterior interhemispheric fissures as well as in the sulci on the right (arrows).

stroke. A purely ischemic acute stroke is difficult to visualize on a CT scan unless there is mass effect. This is noted as compression of the lateral ventricle, possible midline shift, and effacement of the sulci on the affected side. One key to identification of most strokes is that they are usually confined to one vascular territory (such as the middle cerebral artery). An acute ischemic stroke is quite easy to see on an MRI study, because the edema (increased water) can be identified as a bright area on T2-weighted images. In spite of this, an MRI scan is not needed in a patient with an acute stroke. If anticoagulant therapy is being contemplated, a noncontrasted CT scan should be obtained to exclude hemorrhage (which would be a contraindication to such therapy).

If a stroke is in the carotid distribution by physical examination (weakness, paralysis, numbness, or paresthesia of the contralateral extremities or face), a carotid duplex ultrasound examination is indicated.

After about 24 hours, the edema associated with a stroke can be seen on a CT scan as an area of low density (darker than normal brain). If a contrasted CT scan is done one to several days after a stroke, there may be enhancement (increased density or whiteness) at the edges of the area (so-called luxury perfusion). During the months after a stroke, atrophy of the brain can be seen as a widened sulci and a focally dilated lateral ventricle on the affected side (Fig. 2–10). Follow-up imaging of strokes is usually not necessary on a routine basis but is indicated if CNS symptoms worsen or new ones develop.

Suspected Intracranial Aneurysm

Intracranial aneurysms occur in about 2 to 4% of the population and are a cause of intracranial hemorrhage. Most aneurysms occur in the anterior communicating artery or near the base of the brain. They can sometimes be seen on plain radiographs if they have eggshell-like calcification. The best initial way to visualize intracranial aneurysms is with CT or MRI.

In a patient with an acute headache and suspected acute intracranial bleeding, a noncontrasted CT study should be done; if negative, it is followed by a contrasted CT or MRI scan. The noncontrasted CT study shows extravascular acute hemorrhage as denser (whiter) than the normal brain. If this is seen, an angiogram is done, and the contrasted CT scan is not needed. A completely thrombosed aneurysm is frequently seen as a hypodense region with a surrounding thin ring of calcium. On the contrasted study, a large nonthrombosed aneurysm is generally filled with contrast material. There may

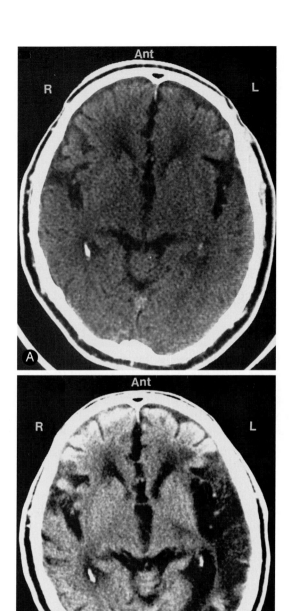

FIGURE 2–10. **Acute and chronic stroke.** An axial computed tomography scan performed on a patient with an acute stroke *(A)* has little, if any, definable abnormality within the first several hours. At an advanced time, there may be some low density and mass effect as a result of edema. Another scan, approximately 2 years later *(B),* shows an area of atrophy and scarring as low density in the region of the distribution of the left middle cerebral artery.

be only partial filling in situations in which a thrombus does not completely fill the aneurysm sac. With MRI, the aneurysm may be seen as an area signal void (black) on the T1-weighted images. If gadolinium is used as the contrast agent, the aneurysm may fill and have an increased signal (white).

In the acute setting, CT or MRI is usually followed by a conventional contrast arteriogram before surgery. This is done because of the high spatial resolution of the conventional arteriogram. Some CT and magnetic resonance machines can give angiographic images, but many surgeons still require a regular angiogram. Patients who have an acute bleeding episode as the result of a ruptured aneurysm may have associated spasm (occurring after a day or so and lasting up to a week). This can make the aneurysm difficult or impossible to see on an arteriogram. For this reason, if subarachnoid hemorrhage is present and an aneurysm is not seen, the angiogram is often repeated a week or so later. For patients who have a long history of headaches or a familial history of aneurysms, and intracranial bleeding is not suggested, a noninvasive magnetic resonance arteriogram is the procedure of choice.

Primary Brain Tumors and Metastases

There are a variety of brain tumors. For essentially all CNS neoplasms, MRI is the imaging method of choice except perhaps for meningiomas (Fig. 2–11). Astrocytomas can be high or low grade and typically occur within the brain substance. Low-grade tumors may contain some calcium, but they are low density (dark) on a noncontrasted CT scan and have minimal surrounding low density edema. The more edema that is present and the more enhancement that occurs after administration of intravenous contrast agent, the more malignant the lesion is likely to be. On MRI scans, these tumors are usually low signal (dark) in T1-weighted images and high signal (bright) on T2-weighted images. They can also show enhancement when intravenously administered gadolinium is used as a contrast agent. Other intracranial tumors, such as pinealomas, papillomas, lipomas, epidermoids, lymphomas, pituitary tumors, and others, have variable appearances on MRI.

Periodic assessment in a patient with a brain tumor is done only if initial imaging was positive; it should be done no more frequently than every two cycles of chemotherapy. It is indicated at the end of radiotherapy if the initial scan was positive. If there is a question of subsequent radiation necrosis vs. recurrent tumor, a nuclear medicine perfusion and thallium scan is indicated.

Metastases to the skull can be seen on plain skull films (Fig. 2–12), CT with bone windows, or nuclear medicine bone scan. Metastatic disease to the brain is best identified by MRI using intravenous gadolinium (Fig. 2–13). A contrasted CT scan can be used, but it is not as sensitive as MRI. Most metastases enhance with contrast agents. The reason for ordering any study should be carefully considered to determine if the findings affect the treatment. There may be little reason to do a cranial MRI or CT scan on a patient who has known metastases elsewhere. If there is a question of tumor seeding of the meninges or impingement of the spinal cord by tumor, MRI is the imaging method of choice. Pretreatment

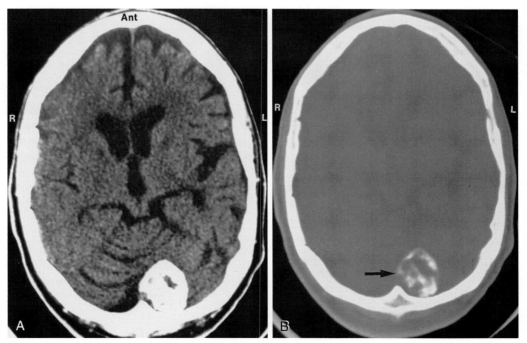

FIGURE 2–11. **Meningioma.** A noncontrasted computed tomography scan *(A)* shows an extremely dense, peripherally based lesion in the left cerebellar area. A bone window image *(B)* obtained at the same level shows that the density is due to calcification within this lesion *(arrow).*

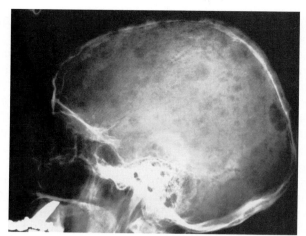

FIGURE 2–12. **Multiple myeloma.** Multiple asymmetric holes in the skull are seen only with metastatic disease. Metastatic lung or breast carcinoma can look exactly the same as this case of multiple myeloma.

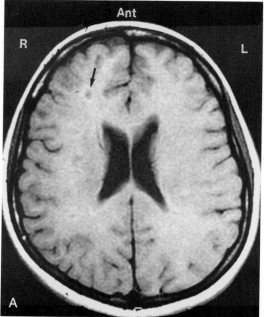

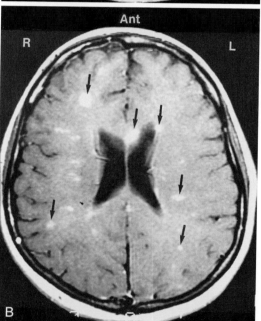

FIGURE 2–14. **Multiple sclerosis.** The noncontrasted T1-weighted magnetic resonance scan (A) is generally unremarkable with the exception of one lesion (arrow) in the right frontal lobe. A gadolinium-enhanced scan (B) is much better and shows many enhancing lesions, only some of which are indicated (arrows).

evaluation to exclude CNS metastases is indicated for staging of sarcoma, melanoma, and small cell lung cancer.

Multiple Sclerosis

Multiple sclerosis is effectively imaged only by MRI. There are often small high signal (bright) lesions in the white matter seen on either T1- or T2-weighted images (Fig. 2–14). MRI of the brain should be done as the initial study rather than an MRI study of the spine. Multiple sclerosis plaques

can have contrast enhancement to varying degrees in the same patient. Whether the enhancement is related to activity of disease remains a matter of debate.

Dementia and Slow-Onset Mental Changes

Dementias may be due to a wide variety of conditions, many of which do not have an effective ther-

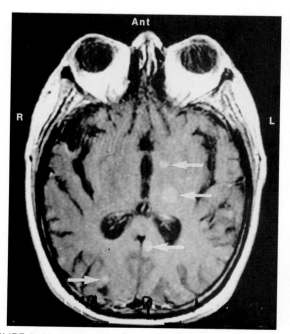

FIGURE 2–13. **Metastatic disease to the brain.** A gadolinium-enhanced T1-weighted image shows multiple metastases as areas of increased signal (arrows).

apy. About 2 to 5% of dementias are potentially treatable conditions. These include thyroid dysfunction, congestive heart failure, occult infections or neoplasm, CNS metastases, hydrocephalus, chronic subdural hematomas, and multi-infarct dementia. After a general medical work-up, a chest radiograph and perhaps a lumbar puncture are done, and an MRI scan may be indicated to exclude some treatable conditions. A CT scan can be ordered, but it is usually inappropriate because if it is found to be negative it is usually followed by an MRI scan.

It is possible to do a nuclear medicine tomographic brain scan (single photon emission computed tomography [SPECT] of the brain) using radioactive substances that are extracted on the first pass through the cerebral circulation. These scans show bilateral reduced blood flow to the temporoparietal areas in Alzheimer's disease and scattered areas of reduced perfusion in multi-infarct dementias. Although helping in obtaining a diagnosis, such studies may not be cost-effective until effective therapy for these entities is available.

Vertigo and Dizziness

Sometimes vertigo and dizziness are confused. Symptoms of vertigo are quite specific and occur in only a small subset of patients who complain of dizziness. Nystagmus almost always accompanies true vertigo but is usually absent between episodes. The work-up of most patients with vertigo rarely involves the use of imaging procedures. If the patient does not respond to conservative measures, imaging studies should be considered in consultation with an ear, nose, and throat specialist. If the patient has vertigo with sensorineural hearing loss or a suspected acoustic neuroma or posterior fossa tumor, a noncontrasted MRI is indicated. If there is conductive hearing loss and vertigo, a noncontrasted CT scan of the petrous bone may be indicated. Other types of dizziness may have a wide number of etiologies ranging from postural hypotension to TIAs. There are few, if any, imaging tests indicated for dizziness until the underlying etiology becomes clear.

Suspected Intracranial Infection

Most, if not all, suspected intracranial infections are best imaged by MRI. Probably the only exception to this is when a sinus infection is suspected, and then a CT should be ordered. It should be remembered that the primary method for diagnosis of meningitis is lumbar puncture.

Seizures

Examination of a patient with a seizure should include a thorough medical history, physical examination, and blood and urine evaluation. Particularly pertinent history includes information regarding seizures (personally or in the family), drug abuse, and trauma.

Unenhanced MRI is the imaging procedure of choice although enhanced CT scanning may be used. Imaging is usually done for persons who are otherwise healthy with a new onset of seizures, those who have epilepsy and a poor therapeutic response, alcoholics with a new onset of seizures, or seizure patients with a neurologic deficit or abnormal electroencephalogram (EEG). Noncontrasted CT scanning is usually used in patients with seizures and acute head trauma or other emergent pathology. Imaging is not usually needed in children who have a suspected febrile seizure, in otherwise healthy children with seizures, and in adults without neurologic deficits who are in chemical withdrawal or have metabolic abnormalities.

Psychiatric Disorders

Imaging studies on most psychiatric patients usually have a low yield of useful diagnostic information. One must remember, however, that a number of CNS abnormalities may present with apparent psychiatric symptoms particularly in the elderly. For example, common conditions that may be mistaken for a depressive disorder include infections, malignancies, and stroke. Patients treated for chronic alcoholism may have unrecognized subdural hematomas. Obtaining a thorough history and performing a careful physical examination are essential. If there are associated neurologic findings or disparities between the psychiatric findings and common diagnoses, imaging may be in order. In such circumstances an MRI scan is probably the initial study of choice.

Some authors have suggested that neuroimaging studies are unnecessary if the mental status examination, neurologic examination, and EEG are normal. If the patient is younger than 40 years of age, has no history of head injury, has normal mental status and neurologic examinations, but abnormal EEG, the neuroimaging examination is not likely to give additional diagnostic information.

■ IMAGING THE FACIAL REGION

Appropriate imaging studies for a number of face and neck problems are shown in Table 2–4.

TABLE 2–4 Indicated Imaging for Face and Neck Problems

Suspected Face and Neck Problem	Initial Imaging Study
Unilateral proptosis, periorbital swelling or mass	CT or MRI
Facial fracture	Plain radiographs, CT for complicated cases
Mandibular fracture	Panorex
Carotid bruit (see text)	Duplex ultrasound
Epiglottitis	Lateral soft tissue radiograph of neck
Foreign body	Plain radiograph if calcified or metallic (fish bones not visible)
Retropharyngeal abscess	Lateral soft tissue x-ray film; if positive, CT to determine extent
Lymphadenopathy fixed, nontender (or no decrease in size over 4 weeks)	CT (preferred) or MRI
Hyperthyroidism	Serum TSH and free T_4 (no imaging needed)
Suspected goiter or ectopic thyroid	Nuclear medicine thyroid scan
Thyroid nodule (palpable)	Fine needle aspiration (no imaging needed)
Known thyroid cancer (postoperative)	Nuclear medicine whole body radioiodine scan
Exclude recurrent thyroid tumor	Serum thyroglobulin
Suspected hyperparathyroidism	CT or nuclear medicine scan

CT = computed tomography; MRI = magnetic resonance imaging; TSH = thyroid-stimulating hormone; T_4 = thyroxine.

Sinuses and Sinusitis

The frontal skull film is best used to evaluate the frontal and ethmoid sinuses. The frontal Waters' view (done with the head tipped back) is used to evaluate the maxillary sinuses (Fig. 2–15). Sinus series need not be ordered to rule out sinusitis on initial presentation but may be helpful if there is no response to antibiotic therapy. Sinuses are not developed or well pneumatized until children are 3 to 4 years old.

Most patients with suspected sinusitis do not need sinus films for clinical management. Sinusitis is most common in the maxillary sinuses. Acute sinusitis is diagnosed radiographically if there is an air-fluid level in the sinus (Fig. 2–16) or complete opacification. After trauma, hemorrhage can also cause an air-fluid level. With chronic sinusitis, mucosal thickening and indistinctness of the sinus walls occur. CT is vastly superior to plain radiography and MRI for evaluation of the paranasal sinuses, the mastoid sinuses, and the adjacent bone. Limited coronal sections are often the most cost-effective. The indications are shown in Table 2–5.

Malignancy should be suspected if there are recurrent episodes of unilateral epistaxis with no visible bleeding site, constant facial pain, anosmia, recurrent unilateral otitis media, a soft tissue mass, or bone destruction on a sinus or dental radiograph.

TABLE 2–5 Indications for Computed Tomography (CT) in Sinus Disease

CT scanning is indicated in acute complicated sinusitis if the patient has
- Sinus pain/discharge and
- Fever and
- A complicating factor such as
  mental status change
  facial or orbital cellulitis
  meningitis by lumbar puncture
  focal neurologic findings
  intractable pain after 48 hours of intravenous antibiotic therapy
  immunocompromised host
- Three or more episodes of acute sinusitis within 1 year in which the patient has signs of infection

CT scanning is indicated in chronic sinusitis if there is no improvement after 4 weeks of antibiotic therapy based on culture or if there is no improvement after 4 weeks of intranasal steroid spray.

CT scanning is also indicated in cases of suspected sinus malignancy.

Facial Fractures

About 5% of patients with head injuries have associated facial fractures. Many facial fractures can be visualized with plain radiography, and this is the initial procedure of choice. In cases of multiple facial fractures and possible reconstructive surgery, CT scanning is usually necessary.

Zygoma. Fractures of the zygoma can result from a direct blow to the arch or to the zygomatic process. The arch and the skull form a rigid bony ring. Just like a pretzel, it cannot be broken in only

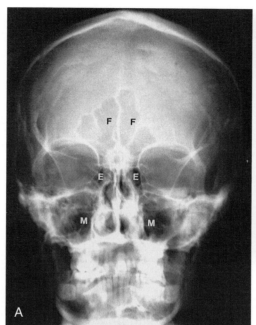

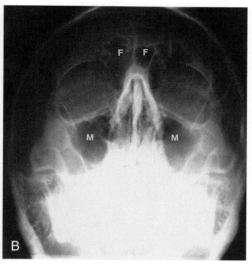

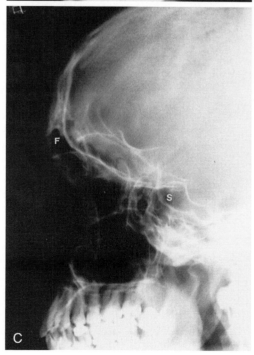

FIGURE 2–15. **Normal x-ray anatomy of the sinuses.** Typical radiographic projections are anteroposterior *(A)*, Waters' *(B)*, and lateral *(C)* views of the face. F = frontal; E = ethmoid; M = maxillary; S = sphenoid.

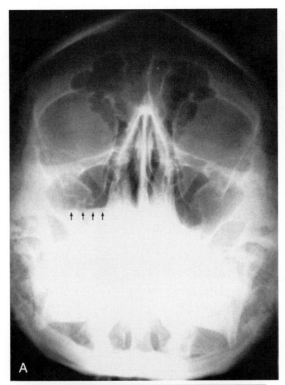

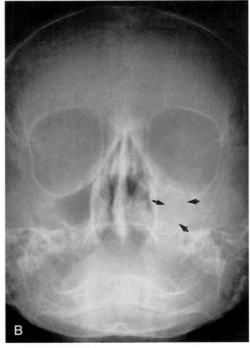

FIGURE 2–16. **Sinusitis.** A Waters view taken in the upright position *(A)* may show an air-fluid interface *(arrows)* in acute sinusitis. In another patient *(B)*, a child, opacification of the left maxillary antrum *(arrows)* is present, which may represent either acute or chronic sinusitis.

one place. The view that should be ordered if an arch fracture is suspected is called the jug handle view. If only one fracture is seen in the arch, then films of the facial bones should be obtained to exclude a so-called tripod fracture. The tripod fracture results from a direct blow to the zygomatic process. It actually consists of four fractures, not three as the name suggests. The fractures are of the zygomatic arch, the lateral orbital rim, the inferior orbital rim, and the lateral wall of the maxillary sinus (Fig. 2–17).

Nasal. Nasal films are only useful to look for depressed fractures or lateral deviation. The latter is often clinically obvious. On the lateral view, the nasal bone has normal lucent lines that are often mistaken for fractures. If the lines follow along the length of the nose, however, they are not fractures. Fractures are seen as dark lines that are perpendicular or sharply oblique to the length of the nose (Fig. 2–18). Difficulty or absence of the ability to smell (dysosmia or anosmia) should raise the possibility of a neoplasm, and a CT scan is indicated.

Orbit. Blowout fractures occur from a direct blow to the globe of the eye. Most often this is due to trauma from a small object, such as a racquet ball or fist. The pressure on the eyeball fractures the weak medial or inferior walls of the orbit. The usual blowout fracture is down through the orbital floor. Waters' view provides the best image to look for this

characteristic. The findings that may be present are discontinuity of the orbital floor, a soft tissue mass hanging down into the maxillary antrum (Fig. 2–19), fluid in the maxillary antrum, and, rarely, air in the orbit (coming up from the sinus). Blowout fractures can also occur medially into the ethmoid sinus seen on the frontal skull view only as opacification (whiteness) in the affected ethmoid sinus.

Le Fort's Fractures of the Face. These rare injuries are produced by massive facial trauma. They are associated with many other smaller fractures. A Le Fort I fracture is a fracture through the maxilla, usually caused by being hit in the upper mouth with something like a baseball bat. A Le Fort II fracture involves the maxilla, nose, and inferior and medial orbital walls. A Le Fort III fracture is a *facial-cranial dissociation,* or a separation between the face and the skull. Owing to the massive trauma required for the Le Fort III fracture, there is a high fatality rate from the associated brain injury.

Mandible. Mandibular fractures should be suspected especially if there is malocclusion after trauma. Occasionally, temporomandibular joint dislocation is present. The easiest way to visualize these entities is to order a Panorex view of the mandible. This displays the mandible as if it were flattened out. If a Panorex machine is not available, standard oblique views of the mandible are satisfac-

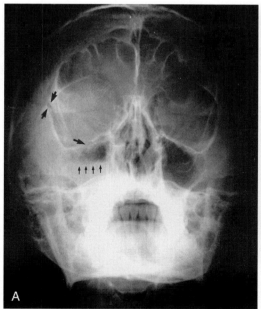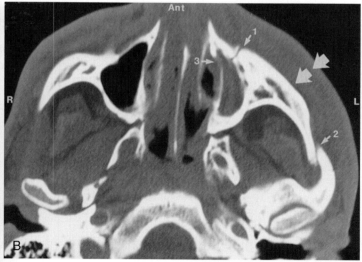

FIGURE 2–17. **Tripod (zygomatic) fracture.** In this patient who had a direct blow to the zygomatic process, Waters' anteroposterior view of the skull obtained in the upright position *(A)* shows an air-fluid level *(small arrows)* (as a result of hemorrhage) in the right maxillary antrum. There is also discontinuity of the inferior and right lateral orbital walls, representing a fracture *(large arrows).* A transverse computed tomography view in a different patient *(B)* shows a tripod fracture on the left caused by a direct blow in the direction indicated by the *large arrows.* Fractures of the anterior (1) and posterior (2) zygoma as well as the medial wall of the left maxillary sinus (3) are seen.

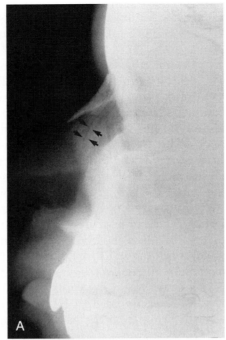

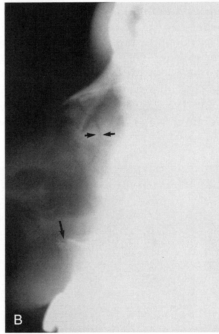

FIGURE 2–18. **Normal and fractured nasal bones.** A normal lateral view *(A)* of the nose shows normal dark longitudinal lines in the nasal bone *(arrows)*. A nasal fracture *(B)* is seen as a lucent line that is not in the long axis of the nose *(arrows)*. A fracture *(single arrow)* of the anterior maxillary spine is also seen in this patient.

tory but harder to interpret. For evaluation of temporomandibular joint dysfunction, an MRI scan should be obtained.

Eye, Ear, and Nasopharynx Disorders

Few imaging studies are useful in the initial evaluation of most eye or ear disorders. The excep-

tion to this general rule is that patients who have an obvious traumatic insult should undergo facial radiography. CT is useful in selected cases, for example, when tumor or infection is suspected as a result of unilateral proptosis, when there is an orbital or periorbital mass, or when there is constant unilateral facial pain of more than one-month duration.

■ IMAGING THE SOFT TISSUES OF THE NECK

For a discussion of work-up of carotid bruit see Chapter 5. For neck pain, radiculopathy, cervical fractures, and dislocation, the reader is referred to Chapter 8. Imaging is not usually used for patients with disorders such as sleep apnea and uncomplicated tonsillitis or tonsillar hypertrophy.

Foreign Bodies

Typical foreign bodies that get stuck in the neck include chicken bones, fish bones, and coins. Lateral projection plain radiographs of the soft tissues of the neck are sometimes helpful; however, they do not detect fish bones because they are composed of cartilage. Plastic objects are also not usually visualized on x-ray examination. Often endoscopy is necessary to make the diagnosis and remove the offending item.

Epiglottitis

Epiglottitis is usually thought of as a childhood disease, but it can occur in adults as well. The best

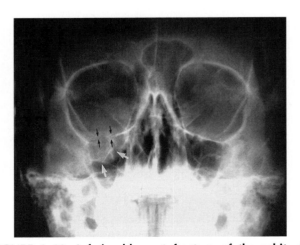

FIGURE 2–19. **Inferior blowout fracture of the orbit.** An anteroposterior view of the face shows air in the orbit, discontinuity of the floor of the right orbit *(black arrows)*, a soft tissue mass hanging down from the orbit into the maxillary antrum *(white arrows)*, and blood in the dependent part of the sinus.

initial imaging modality for upper airway obstruction (as with a suspected foreign body) is a lateral soft tissue view of the neck. This is essentially an underexposed lateral cervical spine view, and the airway is usually well seen. With epiglottitis, swelling of the epiglottis is seen easily on the lateral view. The affected epiglottis looks somewhat like a thumb rather than its normal thin delicate curved shape (Fig. 2–20). For a discussion of croup and pediatric epiglottitis the reader is referred to Chapter 9.

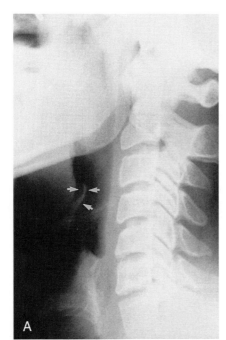

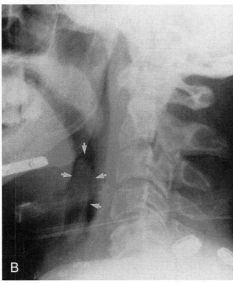

FIGURE 2–20. **Normal epiglottis and epiglottitis.** The normal epiglottis is well seen on the lateral soft tissue view of the neck (A) as a delicate curved structure (arrows). In a patient with epiglottitis (B), the epiglottis is swollen (arrows) and significantly reduces the diameter of the airway.

Retropharyngeal Abscess

This is another cause of upper airway obstruction and dysphagia. The soft tissue lateral radiograph is the initial imaging procedure of choice. There is usually prevertebral soft tissue swelling. There may or may not be air within these swollen soft tissues (Fig. 2–21). An intravenously contrasted CT scan or an MRI is often of great value to help discern the lateral and inferior margins of the abscess and the location of the great vessels of the neck. Retropharyngeal abscesses can extend inferiorly into the mediastinum or laterally into the neck in the region of the carotid artery and jugular vein.

Subcutaneous Emphysema

On a plain radiograph of the neck, dark vertical lines of air within the anterior and lateral soft tissues of the neck may represent air tracking up from a pneumothorax or mediastinal emphysema. These are both potentially life-threatening abnormalities, and a chest x-ray examination should be ordered. (See Chapter 3 for a full description of these entities.)

Thyroid

The thyroid is a symmetric gland that lies lateral and anterior to the trachea, just above the thoracic inlet. Large goiters can compress the trachea in a symmetric fashion, although this is unusual. More commonly, there is asymmetric enlargement, and the trachea is deviated to one side or the other. Before diagnosing tracheal deviation be sure that the patient is not rotated. On a well-positioned posteroanterior or anteroposterior film, the medial aspect of the clavicles is equidistant from the posterior spinous processes (Fig. 2–22).

A number of patients will present with hyperthyroidism and a smoothly enlarged gland (Graves' disease) or a lumpy enlarged gland (multinodular goiter). The most appropriate imaging study for these patients is a nuclear medicine thyroid scan done after administration of a radioactive material that concentrates in the thyroid gland (such as technetium-99m pertechnetate or iodine 123). Radioactive iodine 131 is often given orally to treat both hyperthyroidism and thyroid cancer (after initial thyroidectomy).

Imaging is not usually necessary of a solitary thyroid nodule or a multinodular goiter. Neither nuclear medicine nor ultrasound is reliable in differentiation of cancer from benign nodules, other than simple cysts. Fine needle aspiration should be

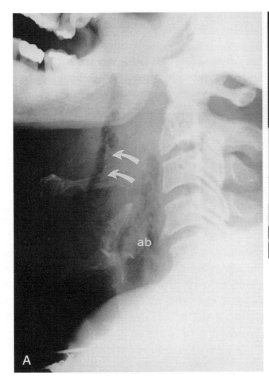

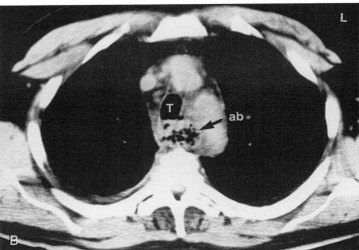

FIGURE 2–21. **Retropharyngeal abscess.** On a lateral soft tissue view of the neck *(A)*, the normal air column is displaced forward *(curved arrows)*. A large amount of soft tissue swelling in front of the cervical spine is present. Gas, which represents an abscess (ab), is seen in the lower portion. A computed tomography scan through the upper thorax in the same patient *(B)* shows extension of the abscess (ab) down into the mediastinum between the trachea (T) and the spine.

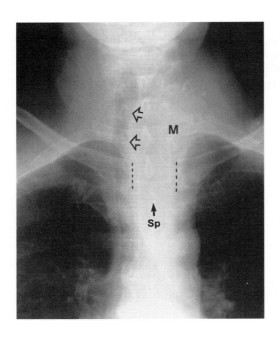

FIGURE 2–22. **Thyroid mass.** A large thyroid adenoma has displaced the trachea to the right *(open arrows)*. This pattern can be simulated if the patient is rotated slightly when the radiograph is taken. In this case, however, the medial aspects of the clavicles *(dotted lines)* can be seen to be centered over the posterior spinous processes (Sp), indicating that the patient was not rotated and a mass (M) is truly present.

performed if a nodule is suspected of being malignant.

Parathyroid

The most common parathyroid problem requiring imaging is hypercalcemia secondary to a parathyroid adenoma (80%) or to hyperplasia (20%). In the setting of hyperparathyroidism, imaging is useful before surgery because adenomas can be quite difficult to locate. A nuclear medicine scan using radioactive compounds that accumulate in the thyroid and parathyroid is performed. The resulting images are quite accurate in localizing the adenomas. At this point, there is little reason to perform CT, MRI, or ultrasonography for these lesions.

GENERAL SUGGESTED READINGS

Hart B, Benzel E, Ford C: Fundamentals of Neuroradiology. Philadelphia, WB Saunders, 1996.
Osborne A: Diagnostic Neuroradiology. St. Louis, Mosby, 1993.
Ramsey RG: Neuroradiology, 3rd ed. Philadelphia, WB Saunders, 1994.

3

CHEST IMAGING

This chapter contains information on imaging the lungs, the mediastinum, and thoracic soft tissues. Important examination steps in the evaluation of a chest radiograph are given in Table 3-1. The appropriate imaging studies to order in various clinical situations are shown in Table 3-2. Circumstances in which a chest radiograph is not indicated are given in Table 3-3. Details on the heart, the great vessels, and pulmonary embolism are presented in Chapter 5.

■ TECHNICAL CONSIDERATIONS AND THE NORMAL CHEST RADIOGRAPH

Exposure. A correctly exposed film should allow visualization of vessels to at least the peripheral

---

TABLE 3-1 How to Look at a Chest Radiograph

Determine the age, sex, and history of the patient	Pleural effusions, blunting of costophrenic angles
Identify the projection and technique used:	Rib, clavicle, and spine fractures or other lesions
AP, PA, lateral, portable, or standard distance	Check tube placement
Identify the position of the patient:	Recheck what you thought was normal anatomy and look at
Upright, supine, decubitus, lordotic	typical blind spots
Look at the inspiratory effort:	Behind the heart
Adequate, hypoinflated, hyperinflated	Behind the hemidiaphragms
Identify the obvious and common abnormalities:	In the lung apices
Heart size, large or normal	Pneumothorax present?
Heart shape, specific chamber enlargement	Costophrenic angles
Upper mediastinal contours	Chest wall
Examine airway, tracheal deviation	Lytic rib lesions
Lung symmetry	Shoulders
Any mediastinal shift?	Look for old films, not just the last one
Hilar position	Decide what the findings are and their location
Lung infiltrates, masses, or nodules	Give a common differential diagnosis correlated with the
Pulmonary vascularity	clinical history
Increased, decreased, or normal	
Lower greater than upper	

AP = anteroposterior; PA = posteroanterior.

34

TABLE 3–2 Suggested Imaging Procedures for Various Chest Problems

Clinical Problem	Imaging Study
Pneumonia (diagnosed clinically)	Chest radiograph (confirmatory)
COPD (with acute exacerbation)	Chest radiograph
CHF (new or worsening)	Chest radiograph, echocardiogram
Trauma	Chest radiograph, CT
Chest pain (in adults older than 40 years or positive physical examination)	Chest radiograph (additional studies depend on suspected cause)
Shortness of breath (severe or long duration or in adults age 40 years or older)	Chest radiograph
Asthma (suspected superimposed disease or resistant to therapy)	Chest radiograph
Interstitial lung disease	Chest radiograph, pulmonary function studies
Immunosuppressed patient (with fever, cough, or dyspnea)	Chest radiograph
Foreign body	Inspiration/expiration chest radiograph
Aspiration pneumonia	Chest radiograph
Mediastinal mass	Contrasted CT
Solitary pulmonary nodule	PA and lateral chest radiograph (possibly with nipple markers), High-resolution CT of nodule, regular CT of chest, CT of chest to include adrenals
Lung tumor	Chest radiograph and CT or bronchoscopy
Pleural mass or fluid	CT
Localization of pleural effusion for thoracentesis	Stethoscope, ultrasound
Suspected pneumothorax	Chest radiograph (possibly expiration view as well)
Hemoptysis	Chest radiograph / bronchoscopy
Pericardial effusion	Cardiac ultrasound
Myocardial thickness	Cardiac ultrasound
Cardiac wall motion	Cardiac ultrasound
Cardiac ejection fraction	Nuclear medicine (gated blood pool study) or ultrasound
Pulmonary embolism	Chest radiograph, nuclear medicine (ventilation/perfusion scan), pulmonary arteriogram
Coronary ischemia	Stress ECG, stress nuclear medicine (myocardial perfusion scan) or stress echocardiogram, coronary angiogram
Aortic aneurysm	Contrasted CT or transesophageal ultrasound
Aortic tear	CT or angiogram
Aortic dissection	Contrasted CT or transesophageal ultrasound

COPD = chronic obstructive pulmonary disease; CHF = congestive heart failure; CT = computed tomography; ECG = electrocardiogram; PA = posteroanterior.

one third of the lung and, at the same time, allow visualization of the left hemidiaphragm behind the heart. Overexposure causes a film to be dark. Under these circumstances, the thoracic spine, mediastinal structures, retrocardiac areas, and nasogastric (NG) and endotracheal (ET) tubes are well seen, but small nodules and fine structures in the lung cannot be seen (Fig. 3–1A).

Underexposure causes the film to be extremely white. This is a major problem for adequate interpretation because it makes the small pulmonary blood vessels appear prominent and may suggest generalized infiltrates when none are really present. Underexposure also makes it impossible to see the detail of the mediastinal, retrocardiac, or spinal anatomy (see Fig. 3–1B).

Male vs. Female Chest Radiographs. The major distinction between male and female chest radiographs is caused by differences in the amount of breast tissue. This is only relevant in the interpretation of a posteroanterior (PA) or an anteroposterior (AP) film. Breast tissue absorbs some of the x-ray beam, causing relative underexposure of the tissues in the path. This results in the lung behind the breasts appearing whiter and the pulmonary vascular pattern in the same area to appear more prominent. If the breasts are pendulous, the overlying tissue can simulate bilateral basilar lung infiltrates. A unilateral mastectomy makes the lung on the side of the mastectomy appear darker than the lung on the opposite side (Fig. 3–2).

Visualization of a single well-defined nodule in

TABLE 3–3 Circumstances In Which a Chest
Radiograph Is Not Indicated

Prenatal chest radiograph
Routine admission or preoperative (no cardiac or chest
    problem) in a patient <65 years
Routine pre-employment
Screening for occult lung cancer
Screening for tuberculosis
Uncomplicated asthmatic attack
Chronic obstructive pulmonary disease without acute
    exacerbation
Dyspnea of short duration and intensity in an adult <40
    years
Chest pain in an adult <40 years with a normal physical
    examination and no history of trauma
Uncomplicated hypertension
Chronic bronchitis
Acute respiratory illness in an adult <40 years with a
    negative physical examination and no other symptoms or
    risk factors

the lower lung zone only on a PA or an AP chest radiograph should suggest a nipple shadow simulating a real pulmonary nodule. The first thing to do is to look at the opposite lung and see if there is a comparable density. If there remains a question, a small metallic BB can be taped over the nipples and the single PA view repeated.

PA vs. AP Chest Radiographs. Chest radiographs on ambulatory patients are usually done with the patient's chest up against the film holder. The x-ray tube is behind the patient, and the x-ray beam passes in from the back and exits the front of the chest. This is referred to as a *PA projection*. If the patient is lying down, it is standard practice to take the image with the x-ray beam entering the front of the chest and to have the film behind the patient. This is called an *AP projection*. For interpretive purposes, the main difference is that the heart is more magnified on the AP projection (Fig. 3–3).

Upright vs. Supine Chest Radiographs. Patients who are able to stand or sit usually have their chest x-ray examinations done in the upright position for a number of reasons. In this position, the amount of inspiration is greater, spreading the pulmonary vessels and allowing clearer visualization of the lungs. Another reason for preferring an upright examination is that small pleural effusions tend to run down into the normally sharp costophrenic angles, allowing relatively small effusions to be identified. Small pneumothoraces tend to go to the lung apex and can be relatively easy to see on an upright chest radiograph. Conversely, small effu-

sions and pneumothoraces may be present but impossible to see on a supine film.

Another problem with supine chest radiographs is that the patient cannot take a full inspiration; the result is that the pulmonary vessels are crowded, and the blood flow to the upper lungs is essentially equal to that in the lower lobes. This may mimic congestive heart failure (CHF). An addi-

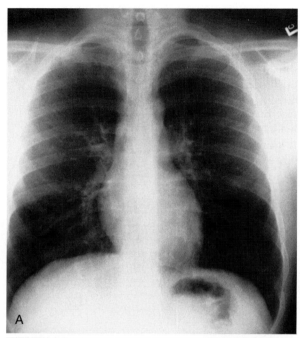

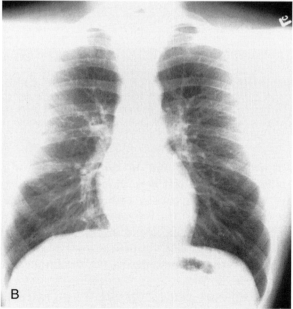

FIGURE 3–1. **Effect of overexposure and underexposure on a chest radiograph.** Overexposure *(A)* makes it easy to see behind the heart and the regions of the clavicles and thoracic spine, but the peripheral pulmonary vessels are impossible to see. Underexposure *(B)* accentuates the pulmonary vascularity, but pathology behind the heart or behind the hemidiaphragms is missed.

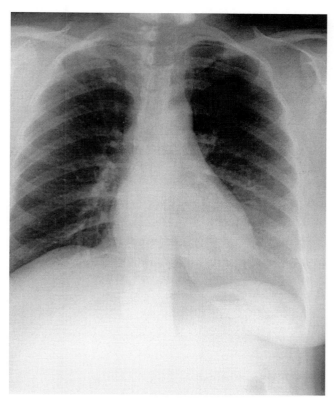

FIGURE 3–2. **Right mastectomy.** The remaining left breast causes the pulmonary vessels at the base of the left lung to be accentuated, and this can be mistaken for a left lower lobe infiltrate. In contrast, the right lung appears darker than the left. Notice also that it is easier to see the left lateral ribs and the right axillary region, because the right breast has been removed.

tional limitation of a supine film is that the AP projection combined with the cephalic push of the abdominal contents, elevating the diaphragm, can make a normal heart appear enlarged.

Inspiration vs. Expiration Chest Radiographs. When standing, most adults can easily take an inspiration that brings the domes of the hemidiaphragms down to the level of the 10th ribs posteriorly. If the radiograph has the domes of the diaphragms at the seventh ribs posteriorly or higher, the chest should be considered hypoinflated, and caution should be exercised before diagnosing basilar pneumonia or cardiomegaly.

Expiration films do have occasional constructive uses. If a small pneumothorax is present, an expiration view makes the lung smaller and denser and the pneumothorax relatively larger and easier to see. In the case of a foreign body (e.g., a peanut) lodged in a major bronchus, inspiration and expiration films should be ordered to look for either postobstructive atelectasis or a ball-valve phenomenon. In the latter case, the air can get in past the object during inspiration, but during expiration (as the bronchus gets smaller), the air cannot get out

around the object. As a result, air trapping in the affected lung with a shift of the mediastinum toward the normal side is evident on the expiration film.

Normal Anatomy and Variants

Normal anatomy, as visualized on a chest radiograph, is important to understand. The major structures are shown in Figure 3–4.

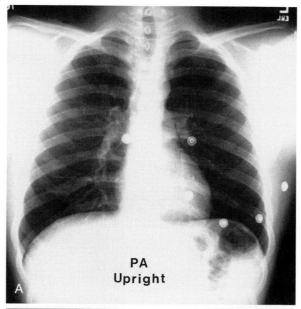

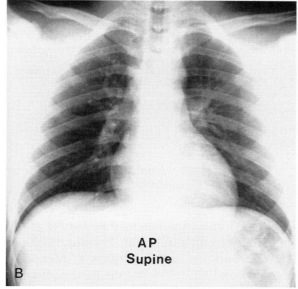

FIGURE 3–3. **Effect of position on the chest radiograph.** A posteroanterior (PA) upright view *(A)* allows for fuller inspiration than does a supine view. The small round objects over the left lower chest are snaps on the patient's clothing. In an anteroposterior (AP) supine view *(B)*, the abdominal contents are pushing the hemidiaphragms up, and the chest appears hypoinflated. This projection also magnifies the heart relative to a PA view.

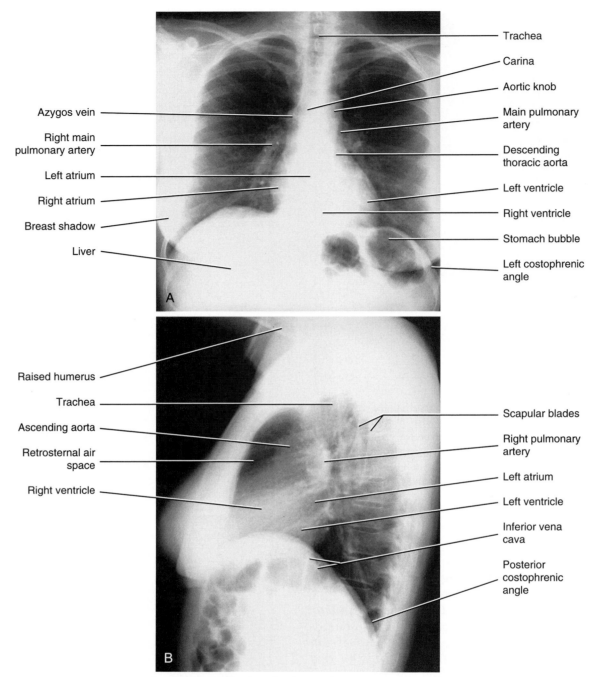

Trachea

Carina

Aortic knob

Main pulmonary artery

Descending thoracic aorta

Left ventricle

Right ventricle

Stomach bubble

Left costophrenic angle

Azygos vein

Right main pulmonary artery

Left atrium

Right atrium

Breast shadow

Liver

A

Raised humerus

Trachea

Ascending aorta

Retrosternal air space

Right ventricle

Scapular blades

Right pulmonary artery

Left atrium

Left ventricle

Inferior vena cava

Posterior costophrenic angle

B

FIGURE 3–4. Normal anatomy on the female chest radiograph in the upright posteroanterior (A) projection and the lateral (B) projection.

On the PA view, the left cardiac border is much more prominent than the right. The heart chambers are rotated relative to the AP axis of the body. On both the PA and lateral views, the cardiac chambers mostly overlie each other, with the right ventricle being anterior to the left. Cardiomegaly is determined by finding the farthest right and left portions of the cardiac silhouette. Often these are not at the same horizontal level. On an upright PA chest radiograph, the greatest width of the heart should be less than half the width of the thoracic cavity at its widest point (Fig. 3–5).

HILA AND LUNGS

The hila are made up of the main pulmonary arteries and major bronchi. The right hilum is usually somewhat lower than the left; it should not be at the same level or higher. The pulmonary veins are usually more difficult to see than the arteries. They converge on the atria at a level 1 to 3 inches below the pulmonary arteries. Lymph nodes are normally not seen on a chest radiograph in either the hilar regions or the mediastinum.

The lungs are mostly composed of air; therefore,

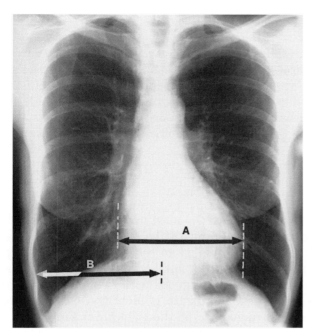

FIGURE 3–5. **Measurement of cardiomegaly.** The width of the normal heart from its most lateral borders *(A)* should not exceed the width of half of the hemithorax measured from the middle of the spine to the widest portion of the inner ribs *(B)*.

there is normally not much to see other than blood vessels. These should be distinct and remain that way as they are traced back to the hila. If you cannot see them clearly near the hila, there may be a perihilar infiltrate or fluid (such as from CHF). Normal hila are sometimes indistinct on portable radiographs because the portable exposure takes longer and the vessels are blurred by motion.

The blood vessels in the lung are usually clearly seen out to within 2 to 3 cm of the chest wall. Lines located within 2 cm of the chest wall are abnormal and probably represent interstitial abnormalities such as edema, fibrosis, or metastatic disease. Secondary bronchi are not normally visualized except near the hilum, where they can sometimes be seen end-on. The walls of the visualized bronchi should not be thicker than a fine pencil point.

On a PA or an AP chest radiograph, 40% of the lung area and 25% of the lung volume is partially obscured by the heart and the mediastinum. It is important to look carefully in these areas to not miss significant pulmonary pathology.

DIAPHRAGMS

The diaphragms are typically dome-shaped, although many people have polyarcuate diaphragms that look like several domes rather than one. This is an important normal variant and should not be mistaken for a pleural or diaphragmatic tumor (Fig.

3–6). The edges of both hemidiaphragms form acute angles with the chest wall, and blunting of these angles is suggestive of pleural fluid.

Most people have trouble distinguishing the right from the left hemidiaphragm on the lateral view. The right hemidiaphragm is usually higher than the left and can be seen extending from the anterior chest wall to the posterior ribs. The left hemidiaphragm can usually be seen only from the posterior aspect of the heart to the posterior ribs. It is the side most likely to have a gas bubble (stomach or colon) immediately beneath it.

BONY STRUCTURES

Skeletal structures of interest on a chest radiograph include the ribs, sternum, spine, and shoulder girdle. Only the upper ribs are completely seen on a PA chest radiograph. Ribs are difficult to evaluate on the lateral view owing to superimposition of the right and left ribs. Evaluation should include searches for cervical ribs, fractures, deformities, missing ribs (from surgery), and lytic (destructive) lesions. The upper margin of the ribs is usually well seen because here the rib is rounded. The lower edge of the ribs is usually quite thin, and the inferior cortical margin can be difficult to appreciate. If they are bilaterally symmetric, they are usually normal. At the anterior ends of the ribs, cartilage connects to the sternum. In older individuals, significant calcification of this cartilage is a normal finding.

The sternum is well seen only on the lateral view of the chest. On this view, one can look for pectus deformities, fractures, and lytic lesions. A pectus excavation deformity can cause apparent cardiomegaly on a PA chest radiograph. This is because the sternum is depressed and compresses the heart

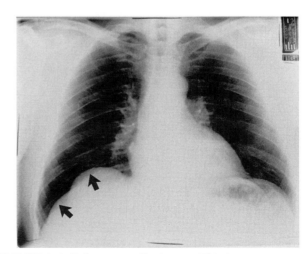

FIGURE 3–6. **Polyarcuate diaphragm.** This is a common normal variant in which the diaphragm has several small domes *(arrows)* instead of one large one.

against the spine. The clavicles and shoulders should also be routinely examined. There is often a scalloped appearance to the inferior and medial portion of the clavicle. This is called a *rhomboid fossa*, and it is bilateral. It should not be mistaken for a pathologic bone lesion.

There normally should not be much soft tissue or water density between the peripheral aerated lung and the ribs. The pleura is normally not seen at the lung margins. In some adults, a collection of fat along the chest wall between the lung and the ribs accrues. This is extrapleural fat, which is usually seen only on the PA view of the chest and almost always in the upper outer portion of the thoracic cavity (Fig. 3–7). The biggest pitfall is mistaking this for bilateral pleural effusions. If there is no other sign of effusion (e.g., costophrenic angle blunting) and if the finding is bilateral, is seen near the upper lateral lung zones, and does not exceed 3 to 4 mm in thickness, it is almost certainly extrapleural fat rather than pleural fluid.

The thoracic spine is only incompletely seen on a standard chest radiograph. This is because the frontal view is obscured by the heart and the mediastinal structures. In older people, there can be substantial degenerative changes or bone spurs extending laterally from the vertebral bodies. These can often be seen on the PA view. On the lateral

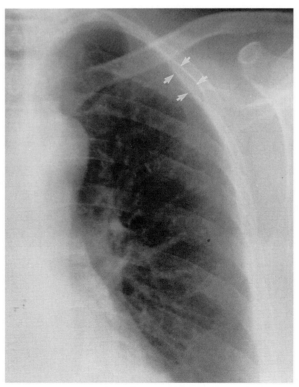

FIGURE 3–7. **Extrapleural fat.** This is a normal finding *(arrows)* in the upper and lateral hemithorax. It is symmetric between right and left and should not be mistaken for a pleural effusion.

view, the spurs can look like pulmonary nodules. A key to differentiating bony spurs from nodules is that spurs project over the vertebral disks on the lateral view and do not look like round nodules on the frontal chest radiograph. A common confusing artifact can be caused by hair (especially braids). If the hair is oily and braided, strange artifacts that may be mistaken for apical lung infiltrates can be seen.

■ SILHOUETTE SIGN

This is perhaps the most useful sign in interpreting chest radiographs. It helps determine the location of an abnormality in relation to normal structures. Loss of a normal border occurs if there is an abnormality contiguous with that structure. For example, if an infiltrate is identified on an AP or PA chest radiograph in the right lower lung zone, it could be in either the right middle lobe or the lower lobe. If there is loss of the right cardiac border, the infiltrate must abut the heart and must be in the medial segment of the right middle lobe. If, however, there is loss of the outline of the right hemidiaphragm, the infiltrate must abut the diaphragm and be in the right lower lobe. The silhouette sign can also be used in the reverse fashion. If, on a PA chest radiograph, there is a mass projecting over the aortic knob and the aortic knob is clearly visible, the mass must be either in front of, or behind, the aortic knob.

■ COMPUTED TOMOGRAPHY AND ANATOMY

Most standard computed tomography (CT) techniques provide image slices that are 8 or 10 mm thick. In the evaluation of a lung nodule, thinner slices should be used, and intravenous contrast material is not needed. For evaluation of a potential dissecting aortic aneurysm, a bolus of intravenous contrast material is essential. If available, spiral CT is often done because the entire chest can be scanned in several seconds while the patient holds his or her breath. After the scan is done, the technologist films the computer data using both mediastinal windows and pulmonary parenchymal windows. This affords a good look at the pulmonary parenchyma and still allows differentiation of mediastinal structures (Fig. 3–8).

Under special circumstances, when a look at the fine detail of the lung is needed, high-resolution CT is used. The slices that are obtained are 1 to 2 mm thick. This cannot be done for the whole lung because it would involve too many images and is not necessary to make most diagnoses. For this reason,

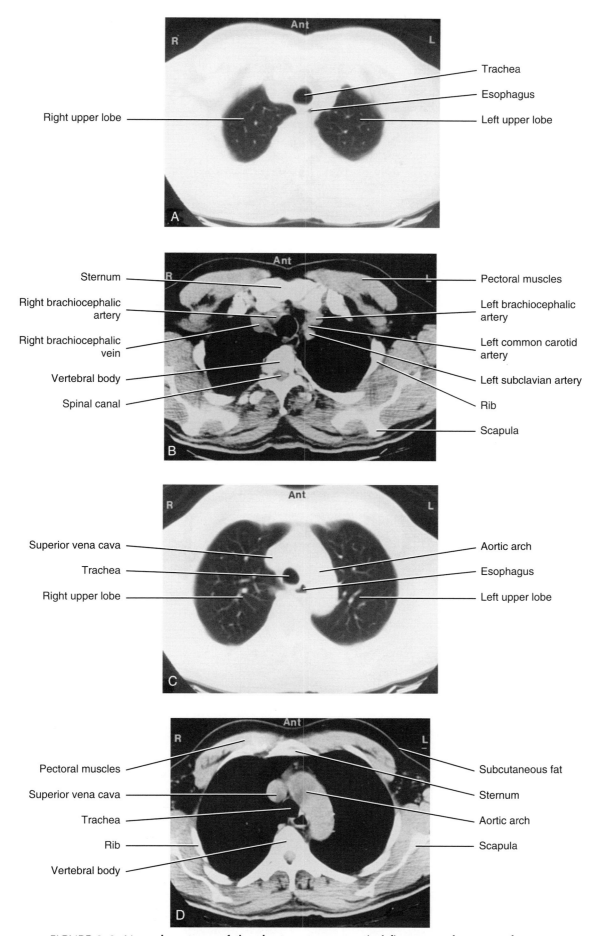

Trachea

Esophagus

Right upper lobe

Left upper lobe

A

Sternum

Pectoral muscles

Right brachiocephalic
artery

Left brachiocephalic
artery

Right brachiocephalic
vein

Left common carotid
artery

Vertebral body

Left subclavian artery

Spinal canal

Rib

Scapula

B

Superior vena cava

Aortic arch

Trachea

Esophagus

Right upper lobe

Left upper lobe

C

Pectoral muscles

Subcutaneous fat

Superior vena cava

Sternum

Trachea

Aortic arch

Rib

Scapula

Vertebral body

D

FIGURE 3–8. **Normal anatomy of the chest on transverse (axial) computed tomography scans.**
Identical levels have been filmed using pulmonary parenchymal windows and soft tissue windows.

Illustration continued on following page

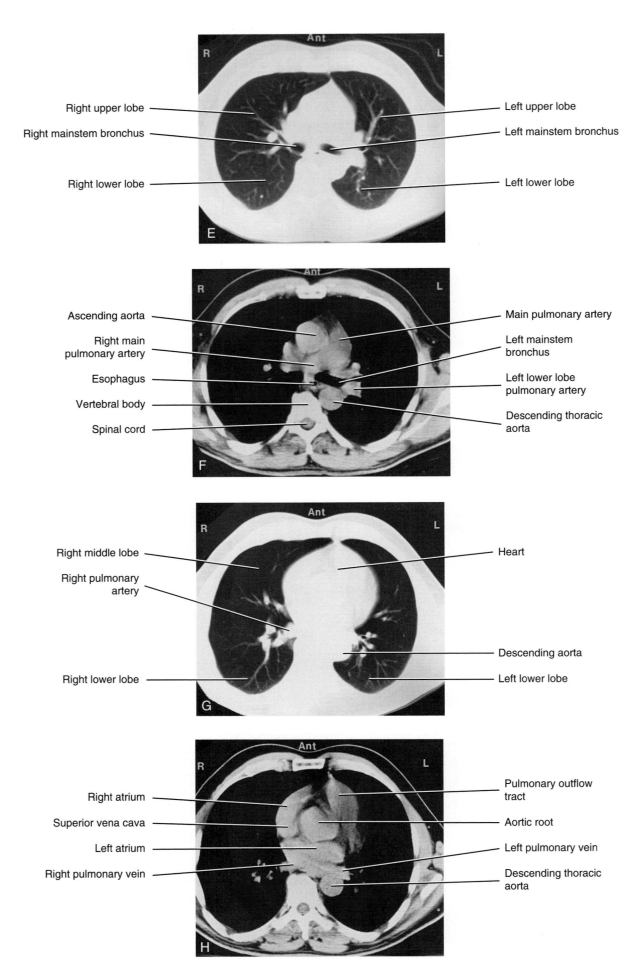

Right upper lobe

Right mainstem bronchus

Right lower lobe

Left upper lobe

Left mainstem bronchus

Left lower lobe

E

Ascending aorta

Right main pulmonary artery

Esophagus

Vertebral body

Spinal cord

Main pulmonary artery

Left mainstem bronchus

Left lower lobe pulmonary artery

Descending thoracic aorta

F

Right middle lobe

Right pulmonary artery

Right lower lobe

Heart

Descending aorta

Left lower lobe

G

Right atrium

Superior vena cava

Left atrium

Right pulmonary vein

Pulmonary outflow tract

Aortic root

Left pulmonary vein

Descending thoracic aorta

H

FIGURE 3–8 *Continued*

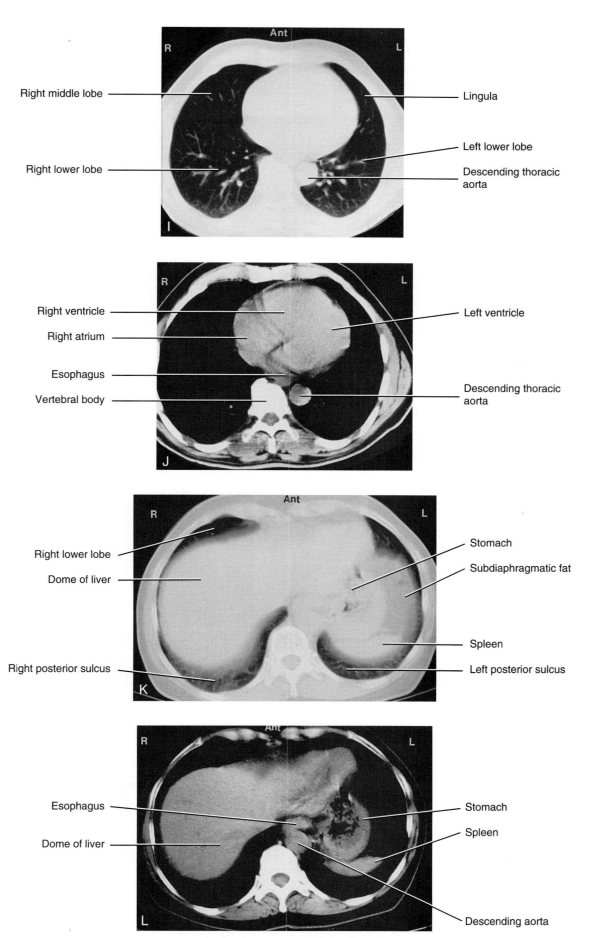

FIGURE 3-8 *Continued*

a regular CT scan of the entire lungs is often done with thin high-resolution cuts at selected levels.

▨ TUBES AND WIRES

ET Tubes. This is probably the easiest item to identify because it is within the air shadow of the trachea. The ET tip should be at least 1 cm (preferably slightly more) above the carina. A tube in a lower position can obstruct air flow to one side and cause atelectasis (collapse) of a lung or a portion of a lung. An ET tube in low position usually goes into the right mainstem bronchus because it is more vertically oriented than the left mainstem bronchus (Fig. 3–9). At its highest, an ET tube tip should be midway between the level of the suprasternal notch (which is midway between the proximal clavicles) and T1.

NG Tubes. An NG tube should follow the expected course of the esophagus on the frontal chest radiograph; on the lateral view, it passes behind the trachea and then along the posterior aspect of the heart (Fig. 3–10). The tip position can often be determined by clinical means without resorting to a chest radiograph. The most common method is to put air into the tube and listen over the stomach with a stethoscope.

NG tubes have two favorite abnormal positions. The most common is with the NG tube only partly down the esophagus or coiled in the esophagus. In this position, fluid placed down the tube can reflux and be aspirated into the lungs. Less commonly, the NG tube can pass into the trachea instead of going into the esophagus during insertion. When this happens, it tends to go down the right mainstem bron-

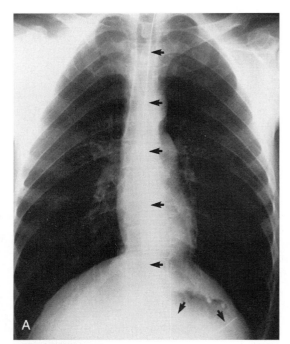

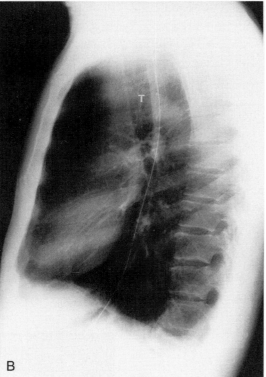

FIGURE 3–10. **Normal course of a nasogastric tube.** In the posteroanterior projection of the chest *(A)*, the nasogastric tube passes directly behind the trachea *(arrows)* until it gets past the carina and then curves slightly to the left at the gastroesophageal junction. On the lateral view *(B)*, the nasogastric tube can be seen behind the trachea (T) and going down behind the heart.

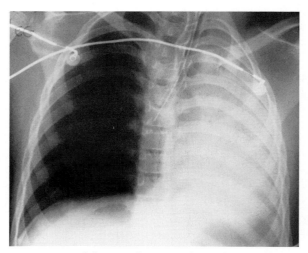

FIGURE 3–9. **Left lung atelectasis.** The endotracheal tube is down too far, and the tip is located in the right mainstem bronchus. The left mainstem bronchus has become totally obstructed, the air in the left lung has been resorbed, and there is volume loss of the left lung with shift of the mediastinum to the left.

chus (just like ET tubes that are advanced too far). Because NG tubes can be stiff and have a rigid end, if pushed hard enough they can perforate the lung and go out into the pleural space (Fig. 3–11). Ali-

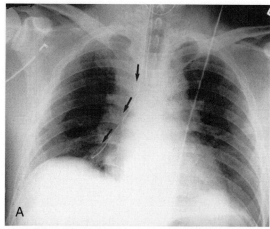

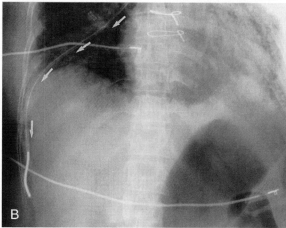

FIGURE 3–11. **Nasogastric tube in right mainstem bronchus.** *A,* If the nasogastric tube gets into the trachea, it usually goes down the right mainstem bronchus *(black arrows). B,* These tubes are quite rigid and if pushed, can perforate the lung and go out into the pleural space *(white arrows).*

mentation via enteric feeding tube works best if the tube tip is in the distal duodenal loop.

Short Jugular or Subclavian Venous Line. After central venous lines and other supporting tubes have been placed in the emergency room or intensive care unit, a routine radiograph is indicated to assure proper tip placement and the absence of complications such as a pneumothorax. There has been increased use of both ultrasonography and C-arm fluoroscopy at the time of tube placement. When this is done, a routine postprocedure chest radiograph is not indicated.

The tip of a central venous catheter should optimally be placed in the superior vena cava (SVC). On the frontal chest radiograph, the catheter tip should be about 1 to 4 cm below the medial aspect of the right clavicle (Fig. 3–12). The favorite abnormal positions of subclavian catheter tips are those that have turned up into the jugular vein rather than down into the SVC and those that have crossed the midline and extended into the opposite subclavian vein (Fig. 3–13).

Swan-Ganz or Pulmonary Arterial Catheter. The normal course is almost circular: down the SVC, through the right atrium and right ventricle, and out into the main pulmonary arteries. The most common natural course that the catheter tends to follow is into the right rather than the left main pulmonary artery (Fig. 3–14). A central venous catheter placed too far out into a pulmonary artery obstructs blood flow and can result in pulmonary infarction. For this reason, the tip of a central venous pressure line should not extend more than halfway between the hilum and the lung periphery.

Pleural Tubes. One common question about these tubes concerns the location of the tip and side port. The tip should not abut the mediastinum. The side port can be seen as a discontinuity in the radiodense marker line, and it should be inside the chest cavity and not out in the soft tissues of the chest.

Cardiac Pacers. Pacers are usually obvious. Unipolar pacers have the tip in the apex of the right ventricle (Fig. 3–15), whereas bipolar pacers have a second wire with the tip in the right atrium.

Overlying Electrocardiography Wires and Tubes. Electrocardiography leads are metallic wires and are therefore more dense than most tubes and catheters. They can also be recognized because they usually have a button or snap on the end, are usually over the upper chest, and do not follow any reasonable internal anatomic pathway (such as venous structures).

■ PORTABLE CHEST RADIOGRAPHS IN THE INTENSIVE CARE UNIT

Much has been written about the utility or overutilization of chest radiographs in intensive care units. Standing or routine orders for chest radiographs should be avoided in general. However, by definition, patients in intensive care units are very sick, are usually lying supine all day, and are not ventilating normally. Almost all these patients have supporting tubes and lines that are changed or repositioned frequently. Daily chest radiographs are indicated on patients with an ET tube or recently placed tracheostomy tube. In such patients, about 60% of daily radiographs do not disclose either new major or minor findings, and about 20% have new minor findings. However, about 20% of the time new major findings are clinically unsuspected and only discovered by chest radiography. Chest radiographs are also indicated after a chest tube or central line has been placed to assess the position and potential presence of a pneumothorax.

■ ADMISSION, PREOPERATIVE, AND PRENATAL CHEST RADIOGRAPHS

Routine admission chest radiographs have a low yield and are therefore not indicated. If a patient is

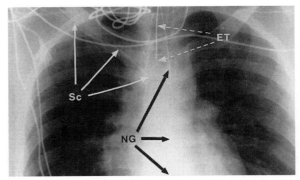

FIGURE 3–12. **Normal subclavian catheter course.** The subclavian catheter (Sc) should progress medially and then inferiorly to the medial clavicle, with the tip being located in the superior vena cava. An endotracheal (ET) tube and nasogastric (NG) tube are also present. The remainder of overlying and coiled wires are electrocardiogram leads.

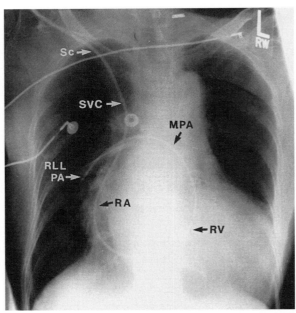

FIGURE 3–14. **Normal course of a Swan-Ganz catheter.** A Swan-Ganz catheter inserted on the right goes into the subclavian vein (Sc), into the superior vena cava (SVC), right atrium (RA), right ventricle (RV), main pulmonary artery (MPA), and in this case, the right lower lobe pulmonary artery (RLL PA).

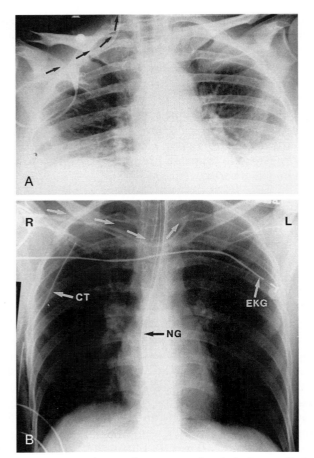

FIGURE 3–13. **Abnormal courses of subclavian catheter.** Common abnormal courses include *(A)* the tip of the catheter going up the jugular vein *(black arrows)* or *(B)* across the brachiocephalic vein into the opposite subclavian vein *(white arrows)*. Nasogastric (NG) tube and electrocardiogram leads are also seen. A chest tube (CT) is seen on the right. Note the discontinuity in the radiodense line of the pleural tube just outside the ribs. This discontinuity represents a tube port, indicating that the CT has not been inserted far enough.

being admitted with a cardiothoracic problem, cancer, or a febrile illness, a chest radiograph is appropriately obtained. In a similar fashion, routine preoperative chest radiographs are not indicated (e.g., before foot or knee surgery). However, they are indicated in patients undergoing neck or chest surgery and those who have a history of respiratory or cardiac problems; are febrile; are immunocompromised; have an altered mental status, an acute abdomen, a known cancer; or are older than 65 years. A chest radiograph is also appropriate for children who are admitted to a pediatric intensive care unit for any reason. Management of persons with positive purified protein derivative (PPD) tuberculin skin tests is discussed later in the section on tuberculosis.

■ CHEST X-RAY EXAMINATIONS IN OCCUPATIONAL MEDICINE

Pre-employment and preplacement chest radiographs should only be done selectively based on pertinent factors in the medical history, clinical examination, and proposed work assignment. Surveillance of persons who work with or may be exposed to substances that adversely affect pulmonary function or cause pulmonary disease should be done if this is the diagnostic procedure with the greatest accuracy and earliest detection. The periodicity of

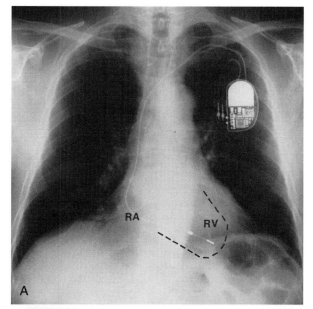

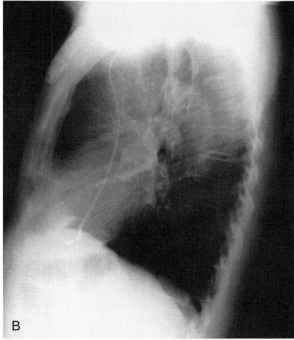

FIGURE 3–15. **Cardiac pacer.** On the posteroanterior view *(A)*, the control portion is underneath the skin and is seen projecting over the right lung apex. It extends into the brachiocephalic vein and down into the right atrium (RA) and has the tip in the right ventricle (RV). On the lateral view *(B)*, the course can be clearly identified.

such testing would vary with the particular circumstance.

▪ TRAUMA

A plain chest radiograph is all that is needed to look for a pneumothorax, atelectasis, or a pleural fluid collection; it should be obtained as soon as possible after emergency department admission for trauma (Table 3–4). With major chest trauma, consideration of spine and sternal injuries may require additional x-ray examinations. A widened mediastinum raises the question of vascular injury and either CT or aortography is indicated. Plain radiographs often underestimate the extent of soft tissue injury. As a result, many trauma surgeons order a chest, abdominal, and pelvic CT scan after major trauma. Although this is expensive, it often identifies life-threatening soft tissue injuries that require prompt surgical intervention.

Often if there is minor chest trauma, rib films are ordered in addition to a chest radiograph. These are usually not indicated because there is no change in treatment as a result of an uncomplicated rib fracture.

Pulmonary infiltrates are common after lung trauma. Pulmonary contusions can occur without rib fractures and are seen within hours of an accident. About 50% of patients have hemoptysis. Contusions are seen radiographically as ill-defined pulmonary parenchymal infiltrates caused by hemorrhage and edema. If uncomplicated, they normally resolve over 4 to 5 days. Pulmonary hematomas are caused by bleeding as a result of shearing injuries of the lung parenchyma. These can present as nodules or masses, and they may cavitate. They

TABLE 3–4 Abnormalities to Look for on a Postsurgical or Post-traumatic Chest X-ray Examination

Position of the endotracheal tube, pleural tubes, venous catheters
Upper mediastinal widening
Left apical pleural cap
Ill-defined aortic knob or anteroposterior window (signs of aortic tear)
Pneumothorax
  Apical
  Loculated or basilar
Mediastinal emphysema
Subcutaneous emphysema
Infiltrates (? changing)
Mediastinal shift
Atelectasis
  Lobar
  Focal
Pleural fluid collection
Rib or sternal fractures
Spine fractures (including paraspinous soft tissue widening)
Shoulder fractures and dislocations
Free air under the diaphragms

take weeks to resolve. Pneumomediastinum or sub-cutaneous emphysema should also be identified. The latter indicates a high probability of rib fracture, pneumothorax, or penetrating injury.

▪ OBSTRUCTIVE PULMONARY DISEASE

Obstructive lung disease includes a heterogenous group of entities including asthma, bronchiectasis, chronic bronchitis, chronic obstructive pulmonary disease (COPD), and obstructing masses.

Asthma

An acute asthma attack can result in a pneumomediastinum but rarely a pneumothorax. Patients with recurrent asthmatic attacks may have a prominent interstitial pattern caused by scarring, and they may have slightly thickened bronchial walls (Fig. 3–16).

Imaging studies are usually not necessary in an uncomplicated asthmatic attack; however, it is important to exclude (by history) possible aspiration of a foreign body. A chest radiograph is only ordered if there is suspicion of superimposed disease or if the attack is resistant to therapy. Even in these circumstances, the examination is usually of low yield.

Bronchiectasis

Diffuse or focal dilatation of the bronchi is usually the result of chronic or childhood infection and subsequent cartilage damage. It is also seen in patients with rare entities such as cystic fibrosis and allergic bronchopulmonary aspergillosis. Symptoms are chronic cough, purulent sputum, and sometimes hemoptysis. Bronchiectasis typically involves the medial aspects of both right and left lower lobes. This is visualized on a plain chest radiograph by the associated bronchial wall thickening, which is the result of infection (Fig. 3–17).

Early bronchiectasis may be associated with a normal chest radiograph, although in later stages the bronchial wall thickening causes the appearance of a stringy or honeycomb (coarse mesh-like) infiltrate at both lung bases. In addition, sometimes tram-tracking can be seen. This refers to two parallel linear densities seen as white lines that represent the thickened bronchial walls (see Fig. 3–17). Late bronchiectasis is seen as cavities or as a honeycomb appearance at the lung bases. Although it is difficult to see bronchiectasis on a plain chest radiograph, it is quite easy to identify using thin-slice or high-resolution CT scanning.

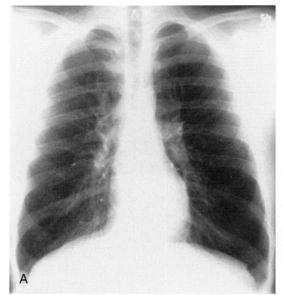

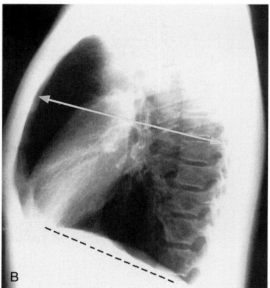

FIGURE 3–16. **Asthma.** During a severe asthma attack, hyperinflation, similar to that seen in chronic obstructive pulmonary disease, can be seen. On the posteroanterior view *(A)*, there is hyperinflation with the superior aspect of the hemidiaphragms located at the level of the posterior 11th ribs. On the lateral view *(B)*, there is an increase in the anteroposterior diameter *(arrow)* and some flattening of the hemidiaphragm *(dotted line)*. The patient does not have the barrel-shaped chest seen in chronic obstructive pulmonary disease (see Fig. 3–18). Most patients with asthma have normal chest radiographs.

Chronic Bronchitis, Emphysema, and Chronic Obstructive Pulmonary Disease

The diagnosis of chronic bronchitis is made clinically in patients who have at least 3 consecutive months of productive cough for 2 consecutive years. On a chest radiograph, there is usually increased or indistinct bronchovascular markings especially at the lung bases. There may also be bronchial wall

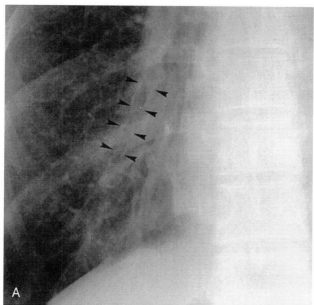

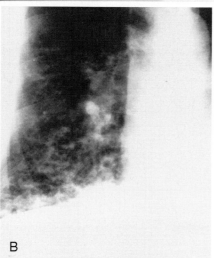

FIGURE 3–17. **Bronchiectasis.** A posteroanterior chest radiograph in a patient with bronchiectasis demonstrates bronchial wall thickening, which is most pronounced at the lung bases *(A)*. This is often referred to as *tram-tracking* or linear parallel lines that represent thickened bronchial walls *(arrows)*. In advanced bronchiectasis *(B)*, coarse basilar lung infiltrates may appear cavitary.

thickening with tram-tracking as seen in bronchiectasis. These findings are neither sensitive nor specific. Chest radiographs and high-resolution CT are usually not indicated.

A chest radiograph can detect only moderate or advanced COPD. In early stages, the chest radiograph is normal, and one must rely on clinical findings and pulmonary function tests to make this diagnosis. Chest radiographs are not indicated in patients with COPD unless there is an acute exacerbation, a suspected pneumonia, or a weight loss.

In advanced stages, obvious signs of hyperinflation occur. On the PA radiograph, the superior por-

tions of the hemidiaphragms may be down to the level of the posterior 12th ribs, and there is often blunting of the costophrenic angles. There is also an increase in the AP diameter of the chest on the lateral view, a large anterior clear space between the sternum and ascending aorta, and marked flattening or even inversion of the hemidiaphragms (Fig. 3–18). An associated finding may be the presence of bullae or large air cavities within the lungs as a result of destruction of alveoli. Because most COPD is associated with smoking, using a chest radiograph to screen for an occult lung cancer may seem like a good idea, but early cancer detection of lung cancer does not appear to significantly decrease mortality.

Atelectasis

Atelectasis refers to collapse of a lung or a portion of the lung with resorption of air from the alveoli. This can result from an obstructing bronchial lesion, extrinsic compression (from pleural effusions, tumor, or bullae), fibrosis, or a loss of surface tension in the alveoli (as in hyaline membrane disease). Atelectasis can involve a small subsegmental region of a lung or the entire lung.

Linear (discoid or plate-like) atelectasis is almost always seen in the middle or lower lung zones as a horizontal or near-horizonal line of increased density (whiteness). This minimal form of subsegmental collapse is most commonly seen in patients who have difficulty breathing (e.g., after recent surgery or rib fractures). Atelectasis may appear quickly (within hours) and can disappear just as quickly after the patient has been encouraged to breathe deeply or after respiratory therapy (Fig. 3–19).

Collapse of entire lung segments, occurs typically as a result of a mucous plug, tumor, or malplacement of ET tubes. Early lobar atelectasis is seen as a hazy density. As air is resorbed, there is increasing density and decreasing volume. During this process, the minor and major fissures move, the trachea can be pulled toward the affected side, and the hila can be pulled up or down depending on the location of the atelectasis. Examples of atelectasis are shown in Figures 3–20 and 3–21. Entire lung atelectasis, atelectasis of a lobe of more than 2 days' duration, and segmental atelectasis of more than 2 weeks' duration are indications for further evaluation with either bronchoscopy or CT to determine the cause of obstruction.

Blebs and Bullae

Both these terms refer to a portion of lung in which there is an air space without alveoli. Most

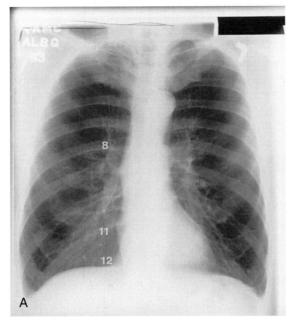

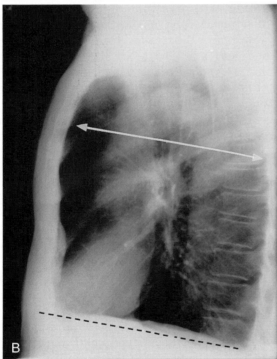

FIGURE 3–18. **Chronic obstructive pulmonary disease (COPD).** The posteroanterior view *(A)* shows that the superior aspect of the hemidiaphragms is at the same level as the posterior aspect of the 12th ribs. Hyperinflation is also seen on the lateral view *(B)* as an increase in the anteroposterior diameter and flattening of the hemidiaphragms.

people consider a bleb to be a relatively small air cavity, usually on the order of 1 cm or less. A bulla is greater than 1 cm and often significantly larger, measuring several inches in diameter. Both a bleb and a bulla should have walls that are thin and well defined (if they can be seen at all) (Fig. 3–22). If a thick wall is present, an inflammatory or neo-

plastic cavitary lesion should be at the top of the differential. Because the walls of blebs and bullae are so thin, the sensitivity of a chest radiograph for detection of these lesions is quite poor, although they are easily seen on a CT scan. The presence of a bulla can sometimes be inferred on a chest radiograph by noting a region of lung that does not seem to have pulmonary vessels.

■ AIR SPACE PATHOLOGY

Types of Infiltrates

For appropriate differential diagnosis of a patchy or diffusely increased density in the lungs, one

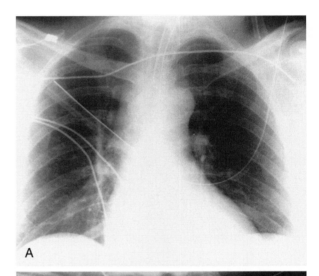

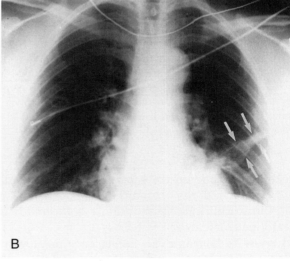

FIGURE 3–19. **Linear atelectasis.** An immediate postoperative anteroposterior chest radiograph *(A)* is unremarkable with the exception of an endotracheal tube being present and overlying tubes and electrocardiogram leads. A chest radiograph obtained several hours after the patient had been extubated *(B)* shows an area of linear atelectasis *(arrows)*. This can clear up quickly if the patient is given appropriate respiratory therapy.

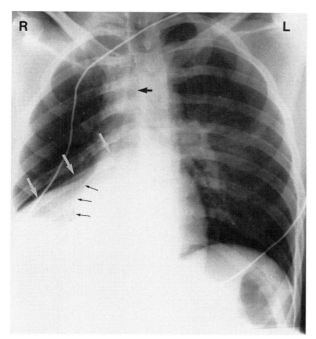

FIGURE 3–20. **Right lower lobe atelectasis.** Complete collapse of the right lower lobe with volume loss evidenced by shift of the trachea and cardiac border to the right side *(black arrows)*. Air in the right lower lobe has been resorbed, resulting in a diffuse infiltrate *(white arrows)*.

needs to characterize the radiographic appearance and correlate this with the clinical history. Most radiologists report an infiltrate as alveolar, interstitial, nodular, or mixed, and whether it is focal or diffuse. The terms *alveolar* and *interstitial* are often difficult for both the novice and the expert radiologist to differentiate and agree on.

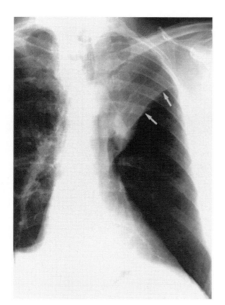

FIGURE 3–21. **Left upper lobe atelectasis.** Right or left upper lobe atelectasis is often seen as a diffuse increase in density with upward bowing of the minor fissure. The volume loss also elevates the hilum on the affected side *(arrows)*.

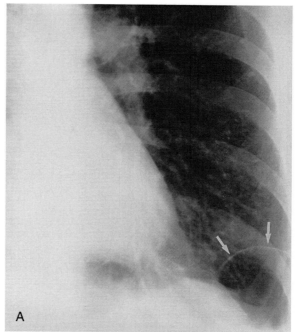

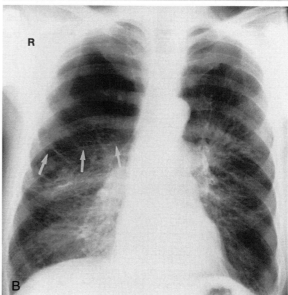

FIGURE 3–22. **Bullae.** Sometimes small bullae can be seen on a chest radiograph *(A)* owing to the fact that their thin wall *(arrows)* can be visualized. Larger bullae *(B)* are sometimes identified only by the fact that there is an area on the chest radiograph that does not appear to have any pulmonary vessels *(arrows)*, and at the periphery, there may be crowding of the normal lung and vessels.

An *alveolar infiltrate* simply means that the alveolar spaces are filled with some material such as pus, blood, fluid, or cells. Given this, it is not possible radiographically to tell whether an alveolar infiltrate is due to a pneumonia (pus), pulmonary hemorrhage (blood), pulmonary edema (fluid), or alveolar tumor (cells) (Fig. 3–23). Most alveolar infiltrates either are somewhat fluffy or represent areas of complete consolidation. As filling of the

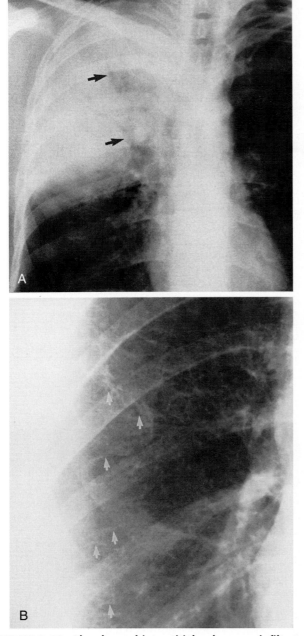

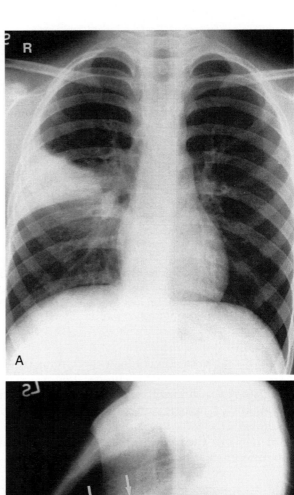

the alveoli. Interstitial processes are usually diffuse and are seen as thin white lines. Occasionally, they may be somewhat honeycombed in appearance, and the differential diagnosis of these processes often

FIGURE 3–23. **Alveolar and interstitial pulmonary infiltrates.** Alveolar lung infiltrates are seen initially as patchy densities, but as they become more confluent and the process fills the alveolar spaces *(A)* the only air that remains is in the bronchi. This results in what is termed an *air bronchogram (arrows)*. An interstitial infiltrate is seen on the chest radiograph of a different patient as multiple, extremely white, thin lines *(B)*. Pulmonary vessels are not normally seen at the very periphery of the lung, and, therefore, the lines shown here by the *white arrows* represent an interstitial process.

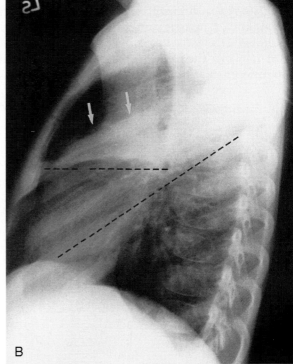

alveoli progresses, the only entities left with air in them are the bronchi, and thus "air bronchograms" can be seen. A bronchus filled with air and outlined by increased density indicates an alveolar process.

Interstitial infiltrates are caused by a wide variety of disease processes that affect tissues outside

FIGURE 3–24. **Right upper lobe pneumonia.** On the posteroanterior chest radiograph *(A)*, note that the right cardiac border is well seen. The alveolar infiltrate is seen in the right midlung. Localization is quite easy on the lateral view *(B)* by noting where the major and minor fissures should be. The infiltrate *(arrows)* can be seen above the minor fissure, indicating that it is in the upper lobe.

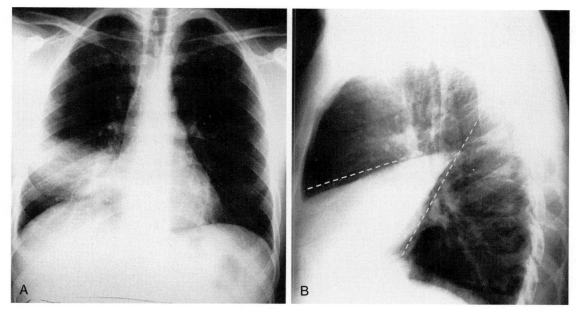

FIGURE 3–25. **Right middle lobe pneumonia.** On the posteroanterior chest radiograph *(A)*, the alveolar infiltrate obscures the right cardiac border. This silhouette sign means that the pathologic process is up against the right cardiac border and, therefore, must be in the middle lobe. This is confirmed on the lateral view *(B)* by noting that the consolidation is anterior to the major fissure but below the minor fissure.

depends on whether the interstitial infiltrate is acute or chronic. The finding of an interstitial infiltrate is nonspecific. Increased fluid in the interstitium and interlobular septa can be seen in CHF, lymphangitic spread of tumor, idiopathic pulmonary fibrosis, collagen vascular diseases, and other conditions. Both interstitial and alveolar signs can be present on the same chest radiograph because many processes, such as CHF, can cause both types of infiltrates.

Community-Acquired Pneumonia in Adults

The diagnosis of pneumonia should be made clinically, based on fever, cough, dyspnea, pleuritic chest pain, rales, localized diminished breath sounds, percussion dullness, or egophony on auscultation. The chest radiograph is confirmatory. A chest radiograph also helps differentiate pneumonia from other conditions that may have similar symptoms (e.g., bronchial obstruction) and may demonstrate findings that suggest a complicated course or prolonged recovery, such as multilobar distribution and pleural effusions.

Most bacterial pneumonias produce lobar, segmental, or patchy alveolar infiltrates. The alveolar filling and consolidation are usually not enough to be able to see distinct air bronchograms. Accurate localization of a pneumonia to a segment of the lung usually requires both PA and lateral chest radiographs. When the consolidation is fairly dense, the infiltrate is quite easy to localize. A right or left upper lobe infiltrate is usually seen as increased density in the upper portions of the lung on the AP

or PA view. The lateral film is generally unnecessary for this diagnosis (Fig. 3–24).

A right middle lobe infiltrate or pneumonia can be in the medial segment, the lateral segment, or both. An infiltrate in the medial segment of the right middle lobe may obscure the right heart border on the frontal view and on the lateral view is seen as a triangular density radiating from the hilum toward the anterior and lower part of the chest (Fig. 3–25).

Right and left lower lobe infiltrates can be visualized by one of three methods. They may obscure the right or left hemidiaphragm on the frontal view. Remember, on an AP or a PA chest radiograph, one should normally be able to see the course of the hemidiaphragms from the lateral costophrenic angles almost all the way to the spine (even behind the heart) (Fig. 3–26A). On the lateral view, lower lobe infiltrates can be identified as being behind the location of the major fissure (see Fig. 3–26B); alternatively, they can be identified by utilizing the "spine sign" on a lateral projection; the vertebral bodies of the thoracic spine usually get darker as you proceed lower in the chest. If the vertebral bodies get darker down to about the midportion of the thoracic spine and then get whiter or lighter inferiorly, you should suspect a lower lobe infiltrate (see Fig. 3–26C). Determining whether this is on the right or left requires correlation with the frontal chest radiograph.

Pneumonias need not always be segmental or lobar; they can be round or diffuse. Round pneumonias can simulate mass lesions, such as a neoplasm,

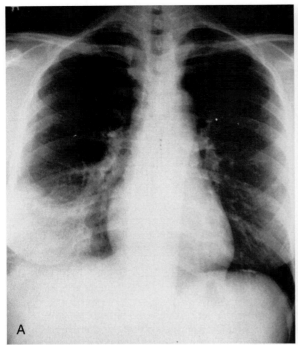

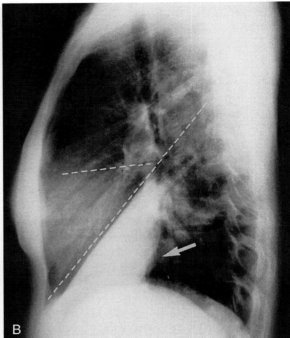

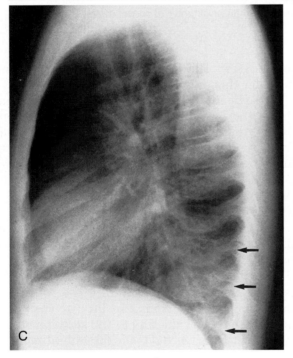

FIGURE 3–26. **Right lower lobe pneumonia.** On the posteroanterior chest radiograph *(A)*, an alveolar infiltrate can easily be seen at the right lung base. The fact that the right heart border is clearly identified suggests that this is not in the right middle lobe but is probably in the lower lobe. The lateral view *(B)* shows that the infiltrate is behind the major fissure and is in the anterior segment of the right lower lobe. The lateral view in a different patient *(C)* also shows a right lower lobe infiltrate. In this case, the "spine sign" is used to detect an early infiltrate. The vertebral bodies of the spine should become darker as one goes from upper to lower thoracic spine, but the ones marked with black arrows are getting whiter rather than darker, indicating that there is an overlying infiltrate.

although the clinical presentation is quite different. Round pneumonias occur more commonly in children than in adults.

Pneumonias that are interstitial and symmetrically diffuse throughout both lungs are often atypical pneumonias. These include pneumonias caused by *Mycoplasma*, viruses, and *Pneumocystis*. The most likely cause of an interstitial pneumonia in a nonimmunocompromised adult is mycoplasmal infection.

CT is not indicated for pneumonias unless re-

peated chest radiography after 2 weeks does not show improvement, or there is no improvement after two separate trials of antibiotic therapy based on Gram stain sputum and blood cultures. CT is indicated in a patient with recurrent pneumonia at the same site within 6 months.

Immunocompromised Patients

In immunocompromised patients with a fever, chest radiography is indicated. If the radiograph is positive, the patient is treated and followed clinically. If the chest radiograph is negative and the patient is symptomatic or hypoxic and the rest of the examination is negative, a CT scan may be indicated but bronchoscopy usually provides sufficient information for diagnosis and management. In patients with acquired immunodeficiency syndrome (AIDS), it is best to characterize the air space disease as diffuse, localized, or multiple nodules.

Lobar or segmental infiltrates in immunocompromised adults are most likely bacterial or fungal in origin (Fig. 3–27), although a patient who has *Pneumocystis carinii* pneumonia (PCP) can have a relatively normal chest radiograph. Diffuse air space disease in immunocompromised patients is usually due to PCP with or without cytomegalovirus infection. Early *Pneumocystis* infection can be seen as an interstitial infiltrate, although a more advanced condition may cause diffuse alveolar disease with air bronchograms. This can progress to consolidation within several days. Occasionally, upper lobe air-filled cysts progress to pneumothorax or bronchopleural fistula. These latter findings mimic tuberculosis, but with PCP, adenopathy and pleural effusions are rare. A solitary pulmonary nodule can be due to unusual infections such as *Aspergillus*, *Nocardia*, and *Legionella*.

In patients with AIDS, there can be diffuse or nodular pulmonary involvement with lymphoma or Kaposi's sarcoma. Kaposi's sarcoma usually appears as indistinct focal pulmonary infiltrates rather than as well-defined discrete masses. A nuclear medicine gallium scan is not positive in patients with Kaposi's sarcoma but is positive in PCP, most other infections, and lymphoma. Isolated hilar adenopathy in AIDS patients is more likely due to lymphoma than to mycobacterial infections.

Aspiration

A common indication for ordering a chest radiograph is to exclude aspiration pneumonia. The question of aspirated gastric contents may occur as the result of a seizure, a cardiac resuscitation attempt, an alcoholic binge, a stroke, or a swallowing disorder. In the case of aspiration, the chest radiograph is often normal within the first hour or so. A normal chest x-ray interpretation after a recent suspected aspiration should be followed up with another chest radiograph in approximately 12 hours. It often takes several hours for the gastric contents to react with the lung to cause fluid exudate and an alveolar infiltrate (Fig. 3–28).

Foreign Bodies

Foreign bodies are usually the result of aspiration or swallowing an object that was in the mouth.

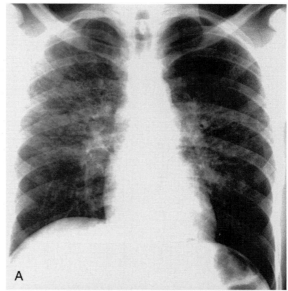

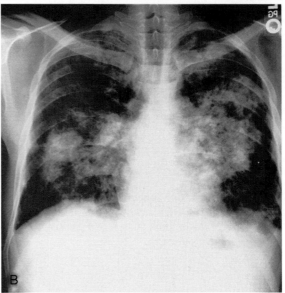

FIGURE 3–27. **AIDS complications.** A PA chest radiograph in an HIV-positive patient shows a diffuse bilateral perihilar infiltrate due to *Pneumocystis* pneumonia *(A)*. In many patients with AIDS, the chest radiograph may be negative when *Pneumocystis* is present. A chest radiograph in a different patient with AIDS *(B)* shows bilateral dense patchy alveolar infiltrates, in this case representing Kaposi's sarcoma.

In the case of aspiration, depending on the density of the offending object, it may or may not be seen on a chest radiograph. Metal objects are easily seen, whereas items such as plastic toys and peanuts do not differ in density from soft tissues. As mentioned earlier, in cases in which a nonmetallic obstructing foreign body is suspected, inspiration and expiration PA chest views are indicated. In uncooperative children, right and left decubitus chest views are sometimes used. The side that does not decrease in volume during expiration or when placed dependently is abnormal.

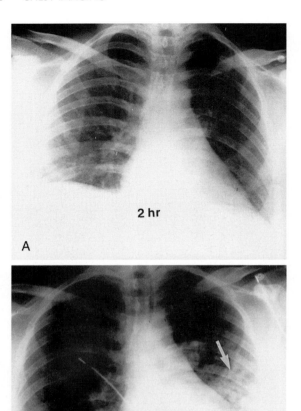

FIGURE 3–28. **Aspiration pneumonia.** A chest radiograph obtained immediately after aspiration may be quite normal *(A)*. The chemical pneumonia takes 6 or 12 hours *(B)* to cause an alveolar infiltrate *(arrow)*.

Tuberculosis

Routine screening chest radiographs to detect tuberculosis are not indicated. Screening is done by skin testing. Chest radiographs are often done on persons who have had a positive PPD skin test and 99% or more of the radiographs are normal. There are guidelines for the use of chest radiographs in tuberculosis detection in asymptomatic persons. One should ascertain the results of a recent chest radiograph on elderly persons being admitted to nursing homes (and who may not react to skin tests). A chest radiograph is also indicated in a person with a first-time positive PPD skin test or a converter to determine if there should be prophylaxis or multiple drug therapy.

It should be pointed out that a normal chest radiograph does not exclude active tuberculosis in other sites such as the kidneys or spine. When tuberculosis is visualized on a chest radiograph, the usual sequence of events is as follows. Primary tuberculosis is most commonly seen as a focal middle or lower lobe consolidation with lymphadenopathy and sometimes a pleural effusion. Cavitation is rare. Hilar adenopathy is present about 95% of the time and is more commonly seen in children than in adults. A pleural effusion is present about 10% of the time. Reactivation of a primary focus causes infiltrates in the posterior segments of the upper lobes and the superior segments of the lower lobes. Sequelae are miliary tuberculosis, cavitation (40%) (Fig. 3–29), and empyema. In reactivation tuberculosis, adenopathy is rare compared with primary infectious tuberculosis. Healed tuberculosis may present as fibrous changes in the apices or as areas of calcification, either within the lung parenchyma or in the region of the hilar or mediastinal lymph nodes. Most commonly, however, such focal calcifications are due to old histoplasmosis rather than tuberculosis.

Miliary tuberculosis is seen as a diffuse bilateral process with very small nodules scattered throughout both lungs. Numerous very small lung nodules can also be seen with histoplasmosis, varicella pneumonia, and metastatic thyroid cancer.

Fungal Lesions

A wide variety of fungal lesions can affect the lung. These may present as focal infiltrates or as discrete lesions. Occasionally, a fungus ball (mycetoma) can be seen within a pulmonary cavitary

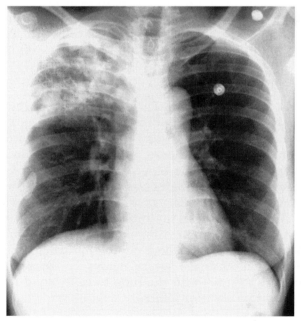

FIGURE 3–29. **Tuberculosis.** The classic appearance of reactivation tuberculosis is that of an upper lobe infiltrate with cavities. Over time, there will be healing and fibrosis, which will pull the hilum up on the affected side.

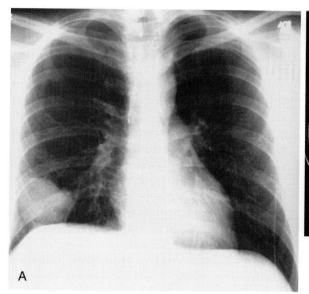

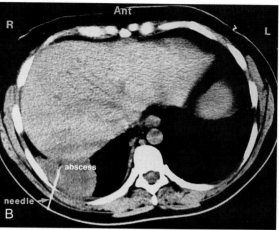

FIGURE 3–30. **Lung abscess.** On a chest radiograph, a lung abscess may look to be a solid rounded lesion *(A)*, or, if it has a connection with the bronchus, there may be an air-fluid level in a thick-walled cavitary lesion. CT scanning *(B)* can be used to localize the lesion and to place a needle for drainage and aspiration of contents for culture.

lesion. A cryptococcal lesion can be seen as a small cavitary lesion within the lung, and sometimes there are small satellite nodules nearby.

Lung Abscess

Inhaled particulate matter or necrotic pneumonias can result in a lung abscess. A typical appearance is that of a lesion several centimeters in diameter that either looks solid (Fig. 3–30) or has a lucent (dark) air-filled center and a shaggy, thick wall. The wall is typically about 5 mm in thickness. The major differential diagnosis of a thick-walled cavitary lesion in the lung is a lung abscess or a cavitating neoplasm (usually squamous cell carcinoma). Lung abscesses may have an air-fluid level in the central portion but so may infected cavitary neoplasms. Bronchoscopy or CT-directed needle biopsy is used to obtain cultures and cytology. CT is indicated to characterize the lesion in an otherwise healthy patient without a prior history of lung abscess and in immunocompromised patients. In a patient with a prior history of a lung abscess, a CT scan is not usually indicated unless there is a persistent fever after 1 week of antibiotic therapy or if there is no improvement in the chest radiograph after 2 weeks of antibiotic therapy. CT is routinely used for placement of drainage catheters.

Adult Respiratory Distress Syndrome

Adult respiratory distress syndrome (ARDS) results from the actions of multiple inflammatory cytokines on the integrity of the alveolar capillary walls with subsequent leakage of fluid from the alveolar capillary bed. It is typically seen in patients who have been in an intensive care unit for several days and in those who have been intubated. ARDS may occur in postoperative patients who have normal pulmonary function in the immediate postoperative period but who then develop tachypnea, anxiety, and breathing fatigue. Systemic nonpulmonary infections or other stressors can also result in damage to the pulmonary capillary bed and produce ARDS.

The usual pattern is that of diffuse or patchy alveolar infiltrates throughout both lungs (Fig. 3–31). The major difficulty in evaluating these patients is the exclusion of a concurrent bacterial pneumonia or CHF. The differential diagnosis is probably best made on clinical grounds, although if an alveolar infiltrate changes rapidly (within several hours or within 1 day), it most likely represents CHF or fluid overload. In patients with CHF, there are usually interstitial fluid (Kerley B lines), pleural effusions, increased heart size, and infiltrates that are perihilar or basilar. With ARDS, Kerley B lines should not be present, pleural effusions occur only late, heart size is often normal, and alveolar infiltrates often extend to the lung periphery.

Bacterial pneumonias often take a day or more to change, and patients with ARDS often have a relatively stable appearance for many days. The diagnosis of pneumonias is often made on the basis of bacterial cultures. Changes in the x-ray technique or in the amount of positive-pressure respira-

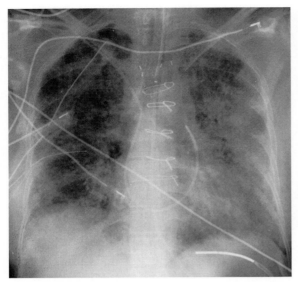

FIGURE 3–31. **Adult respiratory distress syndrome (ARDS).** The findings of ARDS in this patient who has had a coronary bypass graft are diffuse bilateral alveolar infiltrates. Similar findings may be due to diffuse pneumonia or even pulmonary edema, and the differential diagnosis is ranked on clinical findings.

tory therapy may cause significant changes in the appearance of the infiltrates in patients with ARDS.

Chronic Interstitial Lung Diseases

A wide variety of chronic lung abnormalities can occur. Bronchiectasis and COPD have been described earlier in this chapter. Given the non-specificity of the radiographic findings and the varied appearance of interstitial lung diseases, the diagnosis is best made by medical history and clinical findings. If the patient is not acutely ill, often no imaging need be done. If there are symptoms or decreased diffusing capacity, restrictive lung disease by pulmonary function tests and with interstitial prominence on chest radiograph, then a high-resolution CT scan can be done to look for early infiltrative lung disease (such as UIP [unusual interstitial pneumonitis]) while it may be treatable. If the patient is acutely ill, and atypical pneumonia or heart disease is suspected, a CT is not needed.

Diseases that preferentially affect the upper lobes are cystic fibrosis, ankylosing spondylitis, silicosis, sarcoid, eosinophilic granuloma, tuberculosis, and PCP. Silicosis may have "eggshell" calcifications in the hilar nodes in addition to uniformly distributed small (1 to 10 mm) nodules. These small nodules can coalesce to form upper lobe parenchymal masses (progressive massive fibrosis).

Sarcoid is a disease of unknown etiology that most commonly occurs in African Americans. The manifestations on a chest radiograph are hilar and mediastinal adenopathy and pulmonary parenchymal disease. About one third of patients demonstrate symmetric hilar lymph node enlargement and, occasionally, azygous adenopathy. About one third have pulmonary parenchymal disease manifested as either interstitial or alveolar infiltrates, and one third demonstrate both adenopathy and pulmonary parenchymal disease. In late stages, a linear interstitial fibrotic pattern develops.

Conditions that preferentially affect the lower lobes are bronchiectasis, collagen vascular diseases, drug toxicity, asbestosis, interstitial fibrosis, and unusual interstitial pneumonias. Diffuse chronic interstitial diseases include lymphangitic spread of tumor, inflammation (infection), fibrosis, and edema. For acute interstitial infiltrates, the mnemonic HEP refers to *h*ypersensitivity (allergic alveolitis), *e*dema, and *p*neumonia (viral).

Lymphangitic carcinoma and sarcoid can have extremely small nodules that are concentrated about the bronchi and blood vessels, although most of the other entities have nodules that extend to the periphery of the lung. Most collagen vascular diseases can cause interstitial (fine lines), reticular (mesh-like), or honeycombing (coarse mesh-like) pulmonary parenchymal abnormalities. These can be seen with rheumatoid arthritis, systemic lupus erythematosus, and a number of other entities.

Some chronic lung disease can cause diffuse interstitial changes, honeycombing, or focal patchy infiltrates. Sarcoid has already been mentioned. Other diseases that produce these varied findings include extrinsic allergic alveolitis (caused by a number of antigens such as mold or avian proteins), eosinophilic granuloma, bronchiolitis obliterans, and eosinophilic lung disease.

Hemoptysis

Bleeding from the gastrointestinal tract and nasopharynx are more common than true hemoptysis, and these sites should be excluded as a cause of the patients' complaints. The initial imaging study for hemoptysis is a standard PA and lateral chest radiograph. The most common cause is bronchitis, although an endobronchial neoplasm or pulmonary embolism should also be considered. If the chest radiograph is normal and the patient is at low risk for bronchogenic carcinoma, a CT scan with high-resolution cuts to exclude bronchiectasis is the most useful imaging study. If the chest radiograph is normal and the patient is at high risk for lung cancer (>10 pack-years of smoking) or has a malignancy elsewhere, bronchoscopy is usually performed, although CT can also be used. If an abnormality is seen on the chest radiograph, whether CT or bronchoscopy is used often depends on the nature of the abnormality. If it is peripheral in location, CT may be more helpful than bronchoscopy. If there is hemoptysis in a traumatized patient, a transected bronchus requiring surgery should be considered. In these cases the chest radiograph usually reveals an associated pneumomediastinum.

Solitary Pulmonary Nodule

In evaluating a patient with a solitary pulmonary nodule, it is useful to remember that any nodule that is less than 0.5 cm in diameter, easily seen, and quite dense is most likely a granuloma. Age is also a useful discriminating factor. In a person younger than 40 years, a lung cancer may occur, but it is extremely rare.

A solitary pulmonary nodule can be a granuloma or lung cancer, but other etiologies include a single metastatic lesion, septic embolus, arteriovenous malformation, hamartoma, or even a small area of rounded atelectasis (Table 3–5). There are several steps after having identified what appears to be a solitary pulmonary nodule on a plain chest radiograph. First, determine that the nodule is within the lung and not a nipple shadow or overlying skin lesion. Locate the nodule in a horizontal plane on the frontal chest radiograph (e.g., at the level of the aortic arch). Look at the lateral chest radiograph (again at the horizontal plane of the aortic arch) and see whether you can find the nodule at the same level projecting within the chest on both views. If there is any doubt, you can obtain shallow oblique views; if the nodule is truly within the thoracic cavity, it should rotate less than the anterior and posterior ribs.

The second step is to characterize the nodule. If it can be characterized as benign, the work-up ends. If the nodule is well defined and round, it is much more likely to be benign than if it is irregular or indistinct in its margins. Calcification that is dense (Fig. 3–32) or within a nodule suggests that it is most likely a granuloma. The calcification, however, should be centrally located in the nodule. If calcification is eccentrically located in a nodule, consider a neoplasm.

The third step of importance is to determine whether the nodule is new or old. A careful review of all available chest radiographs and phone calls to pertinent hospitals should be made before expensive or invasive studies are ordered. A nodule that has remained unchanged in size for 2 years can be considered benign. Stability for a period of 1 year is not enough, since slow-growing tumors may not change appreciably in a 12-month interval. For ex-

TABLE 3–5 Common Differential Diagnosis of Pulmonary Nodule(s)

Solitary
  Less than 3 cm
    Granuloma (especially if calcified)
    Lung cancer
    Single nipple shadow
    Wart on the skin
    Benign lung tumors
    Metastasis
    Rounded atelectasis
    Septic embolism
  Large
    Lung cancer
    Round pneumonia
    Large solitary metastases
    Lung abscess
Multiple
  Granulomas
  Metastases
  Septic emboli
Cavitary
  Septic emboli
  Tuberculosis
  Fungal
  Squamous cell cancer
Benign Characteristics
  Small (<3 cm)
  Round
  Well defined edges
  Slow growing (no appreciable change in 2 yr)
  Central calcification
  Solid (not cavitated)
Malignant Characteristics
  Large (>3 cm)
  Irregular shape
  Poorly defined edges
  Obvious growth in <2 yr
  Asymmetric or no calcification
  Cavitated

ample, even if a 1-cm nodule doubles the number of cells that it contains, its diameter grows only to 1.2 cm. A difference this minimal is difficult to appreciate on a chest radiograph.

Further evaluation of a nodule can be obtained by doing a chest CT scan consisting of thin cuts at the level of the nodule and regular scanning of the entire lungs. Since CT scanning is more sensitive than a chest radiograph, multiple nodules may be identified on the CT scan. If the nodule is less than 2 cm, is smooth, has central calcification, or contains fat, the nodule may be observed for stability over a 2-year period. If it does not meet these characteristics, biopsy is usually indicated.

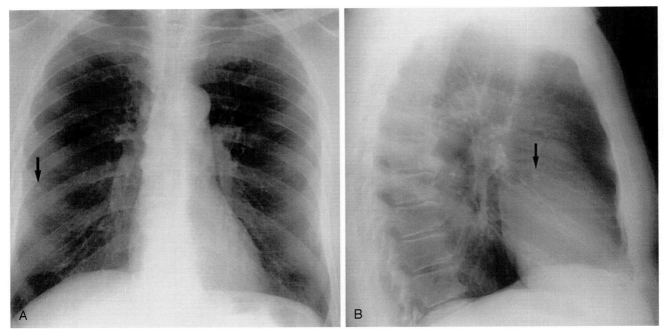

FIGURE 3–32. **Solitary calcified granuloma.** A very dense pulmonary nodule is seen on both PA (A) and lateral (B) chest radiographs. This can be confidently called a granuloma; it needs no further work-up, since it is much denser than even the surrounding ribs and therefore is clearly densely calcified.

Lung Cancer

Almost invariably, a chest radiograph is the imaging method by which lung tumors are initially detected. Screening chest radiographs in high risk persons (e.g., heavy smokers) have not been shown to be effective in reducing mortality. As a result, lung cancers are usually found on chest radiographs that are done for other reasons.

Primary lung cancers have a number of appearances. Adenocarcinoma occurs peripherally, whereas squamous cell types are central or peripheral. Squamous cell tumors of any origin tend to cavitate. Small cell carcinomas often present as an indistinct hilar or perihilar mass. A unilateral hilar mass or persistent infiltrate in an adult older than 40 years should always raise the suspicion of a lung cancer (Fig. 3–33). The diagnosis is usually made by sputum cytology or bronchoscopy. Dysplasia by sputum cytology should be evaluated by a chest radiography and bronchoscopy. If these are negative, a CT scan is indicated.

A CT scan is the most valuable imaging method for staging lung cancers (Fig. 3–34). Often, intravenous contrast is used with the CT scan so that the tumor, adenopathy, and pulmonary vessels can be differentiated. CT scanning is indicated when a mass on a chest radiograph is: (1) larger or new compared with findings of a previous radiograph, (2) greater than 3 cm, (3) less than 3 cm in a person

older than 35, or (4) has equivocal, eccentric, or no calcification.

Lung cancers commonly metastasize to the opposite lung, liver, bones, brain, and adrenal glands. The liver is the most common site, and the adrenal glands are involved in about 30% of patients. For

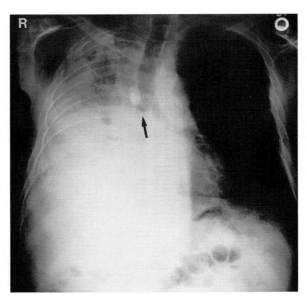

FIGURE 3–33. **Tumor obstructing right mainstem bronchus.** A sharp cutoff of the air column is clearly identified (arrow). The obstruction has caused a postobstructive infiltrate, with resorption of the air from the right lung, volume loss, and resultant shift of the mediastinum to the right.

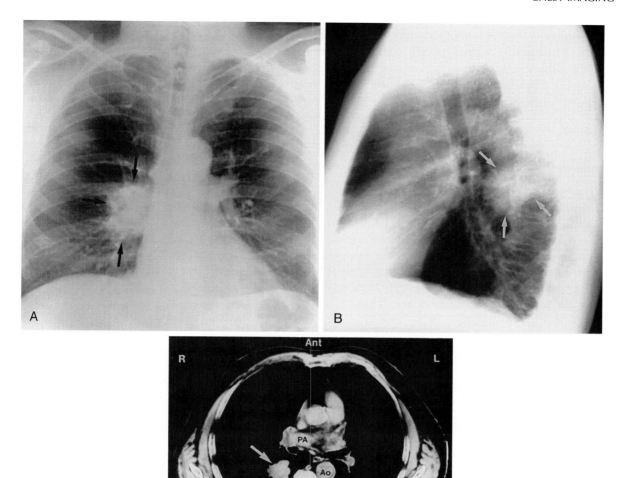

FIGURE 3–34. **Lung cancer.** An ill-defined mass is noted on the PA chest radiograph *(A)*. While this appears to be located near the right hilum, the lateral chest radiograph *(B)* clearly shows the mass to be posterior to the hilum. Its shaggy appearance is very suggestive of carcinoma. Further evaluation by CT scan *(C)* clearly shows the mass in relationship to the mediastinal structures, such as the pulmonary artery and aorta.

this reason, a chest CT scan done for a suspected lung cancer should be extended far enough down to visualize these organs.

In the absence of worsening symptoms or findings, follow-up of known lung tumors should be done by chest radiography. This is generally not necessary to be performed more frequently than every 2 cycles of chemotherapy and at the end of either chemotherapy or radiation therapy. For tumors that involve the mediastinum, CT scanning is necessary to evaluate any change in lymph node size.

Hilar Enlargement

This is another finding that may be seen on a chest radiograph. The three major etiologies are enlarged pulmonary arteries, lymphadenopathy, or a lung neoplasm. If the cause is unknown or there is a possibility of effective therapy, a contrast-enhanced CT scan is indicated for further evaluation.

Lymphoma

Lymphomas, particularly Hodgkin's disease, are most commonly visualized on the chest radiograph as either a large anterior mediastinal mass or a hilar adenopathy. If the lymphomatous mass is large and is up against the aorta, the mass can easily be mistaken for an aortic aneurysm. Hilar adenopathy is often difficult to distinguish from enlarged central pulmonary arteries. Extensive adenopathy can be recognized by multiple lumps or bumps rather than the single one from a prominent main pulmonary artery. Adenopathy may also fill in the normal concavity between the left main pulmonary artery and the aortic arch. If there is any question, a CT scan can easily sort out the differences (Fig. 3–35). Lymphoma and Hodgkin's disease can cause pulmonary infiltrates or nodules, although these are a relatively uncommon presentation.

Metastatic Lesions

The pulmonary parenchyma is a common site for metastatic deposits because the lungs act as a filter for large particles or cells. Most metastatic disease has two predominant patterns in the lung. One is the familiar nodular lesions. These are typically referred to as *hematogenous metastases*. This type

of metastatic lesion in the pulmonary parenchyma varies from being small nodules to extremely large (cannonball) masses. The pulmonary metastases of thyroid cancer typically create a snowstorm of very small nodular lesions. Other tumors, such as colon and renal cell carcinomas, typically produce metastatic lesions that range from approximately 1 cm to several centimeters in diameter. When there are extremely large multiple masses (about the size of a tennis ball), metastases from a sarcoma should be suspected (Fig. 3–36).

The second common appearance of metastases is streaky or linear infiltrates throughout the lungs. This lymphangitic pattern occurs quite commonly with stomach cancer (Fig. 3–37). Breast cancer can produce either the rounded hematogenous metastases or the lymphangitic pattern.

Clinicians commonly ask how often a periodic

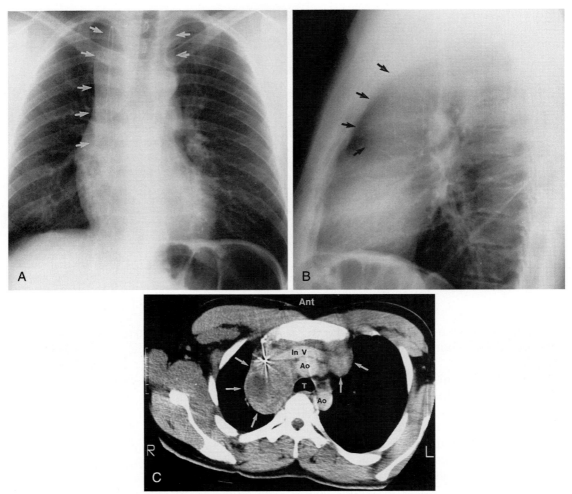

FIGURE 3–35. **Hodgkin's disease.** In this 20-year-old male with low-grade fevers, a PA chest radiograph *(A)* shows marked widening of the middle and superior mediastinum *(arrows)*. On the lateral chest radiograph *(B)*, there is filling in of the retrosternal space by an ill-defined anterior mediastinal mass *(arrows)*. The transverse contrast-enhanced CT scan *(C)* through the upper portion of the chest shows the innominate vein, ascending and descending aorta, and trachea. They are all enveloped by a mass of nodes *(arrows)*.

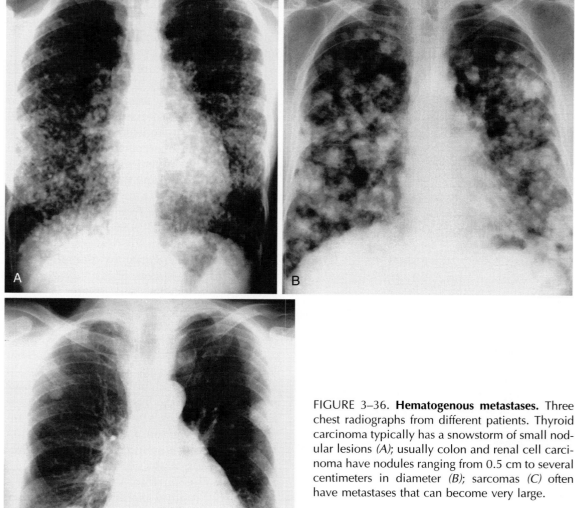

FIGURE 3–36. **Hematogenous metastases.** Three chest radiographs from different patients. Thyroid carcinoma typically has a snowstorm of small nodular lesions *(A)*; usually colon and renal cell carcinoma have nodules ranging from 0.5 cm to several centimeters in diameter *(B)*; sarcomas *(C)* often have metastases that can become very large.

chest radiograph should be obtained on a patient with a known cancer so as to exclude pulmonary metastases. It is rarely efficacious to get films monthly, and most oncologists order chest radiographs only on a 6-month or annual basis and only if the results may affect therapy. In a cancer patient, if there are worsening symptoms such as cough, shortness of breath, hoarseness, or wheezing, a chest radiograph should be obtained. If there is a new abnormality, a chest CT scan is indicated.

CT scanning can detect more and smaller pulmonary metastases than a chest radiograph. In spite of this, CT scanning is not indicated except when curative resection or treatment of the metastases is being considered. If there is a normal chest radiograph, CT scanning is usually done before therapy of germ cell or testicular tumor, renal cell carcinoma, sarcoma, and lymphoma or Hodgkin's disease.

Hypertension

Most hypertension is idiopathic in origin. A small percentage is due to renal artery stenosis. Plain chest radiographs are occasionally ordered on hypertensive patients. These are not indicated since the yield of positive findings is extremely low. Chest pain in a hypertensive patient should suggest either a thoracic aneurysm or coronary artery disease.

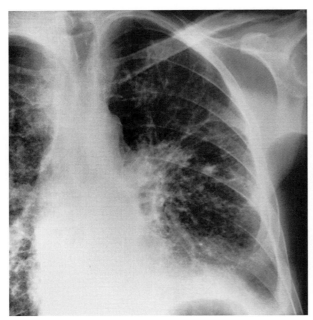

FIGURE 3–37. **Lymphangitic metastases.** The streaky appearance in the lung parenchyma is due to metastatic disease, in this case stomach carcinoma. The term "lymphangitic" is really a misnomer, since these actually do represent hematogenous metastases in the pulmonary interstitium.

These conditions in addition to an investigation of hypertension caused by renal artery stenosis are discussed in Chapter 5.

Chest Pain and Dyspnea

Both chest pain and dyspnea can be due to a wide variety of causes including traumatic, infectious, neoplastic, and circulatory. A plain chest radiograph is almost always indicated if the patient has an abnormal physical examination; has been traumatized; or has a fever, weight loss, or a cardiac condition. In a patient older than 40 years who has chest pain or dyspnea, a chest radiograph is usually done, even if the physical examination is normal. For patients younger than 40 years who have a normal physical examination, there is no consensus about whether a chest radiograph should be done. The next imaging study to order (if any) depends on whether the chest radiograph is positive or negative and what the radiographic and clinical findings suggest the diagnosis to be. Issues related to angina and cardiac conditions are discussed in Chapter 5.

Congestive Heart Failure and Pulmonary Edema

In the upright position, substantially more blood flows to the lung bases than to the apices. On a normal chest radiograph, the vessels should be distinct from the peripheral one third of the lung back centrally to the hila, and they should be much more apparent in the lower lung zones than in the upper lung zones.

In CHF, a spectrum and progression of findings are normally identified on an upright chest radiograph. In the early stages, there may be minimal cardiomegaly and redistribution of the pulmonary vascularity, with almost equal flow to upper and lower lung zones (correlating with mean pulmonary capillary wedge pressures of 15 to 25 mm Hg). Also, at this time the diameter of upper lobe vessels is equal to or greater than that of lower lobe vessels at the same distance from the hilum. Another way to detect early CHF is by noting the presence of pulmonary vessels in the first intercostal space that are greater than 3 mm in diameter. These signs are invalid on a supine chest radiograph, since the pulmonary blood flow will change in a normal person as a result of gravity. Do not be fooled into making the diagnosis of minimal CHF on a supine chest radiograph.

As CHF worsens and the mean pulmonary capillary wedge pressure is 25 to 30 mm Hg, fluid may be seen in the interlobular septa at the lateral basal aspects of the lung. These are referred to as *Kerley B lines*. They are always located just inside the ribs and are horizontal in orientation (Fig. 3–38). Remember, these cannot be blood vessels, because you should normally not see lung markings in the peripheral one fourth of the lungs.

As CHF becomes more pronounced, vessels near the hila become indistinct owing to fluid accumulating in the interstitium. Symmetric and bilateral hilar indistinctness should immediately suggest the possibility of CHF (Fig. 3–39). Pleural effusions may be present, as evidenced by blunting of the lateral or posterior costophrenic angles. With pronounced CHF, fluid accumulates in the alveolar spaces, and frank pulmonary edema becomes apparent. This is seen as bilateral, predominantly basilar and perihilar alveolar infiltrates (pulmonary capillary wedge pressure >30 mm Hg).

There are some common variations of CHF. In patients who have been lying down, on either their right or left side, relatively more accumulation of pulmonary edema is on the dependent side because the fluid pressure is greater. Patients who are in renal failure often have findings of CHF, particularly with a perihilar indistinctness and a bat-wing infiltrate centered about the hila. Typically, this is seen predialysis. In postdialysis, the infiltrate resolves almost immediately. Remember that pulmonary edema may occur from noncardiogenic causes. In the absence of cardiomegaly, drug overdose, head injury (with central nervous system de-

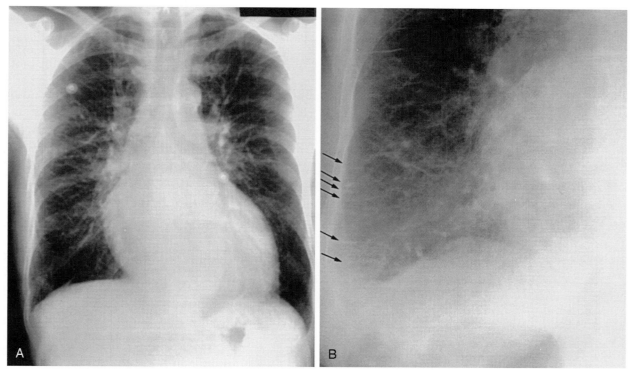

FIGURE 3–38. **Early findings of congestive heart failure.** The major signs on upright PA chest radiograph *(A)* are cardiomegaly and redistribution of the pulmonary vascularity. Normally, the vessels to the lower lobes are more prominent than those in the upper lobes; however, here they appear at least equally prominent. On a close-up view in another patient *(B)*, small horizontal lines can be seen at the very periphery of the lung *(arrows)*. These are known as Kerley B lines and represent fluid in the interlobular septa.

pression), and acute inhalations of noxious agents should be considered as possible etiologies.

■ PLEURAL PATHOLOGY

Pneumothorax

Pneumothorax refers to air in the pleural space. This is most often caused by trauma (e.g., stabbing or motor vehicle accidents). It also commonly results from attempted introduction of subclavian venous catheters or after liver biopsy (the pleural space extends down quite a way between the liver and the lateral and posterior abdominal wall). A pneumothorax may occur spontaneously (as a result of bleb rupture) or even as a result of some unusual tumors, such as histiocytosis X or metastatic osteogenic sarcoma.

Because the pleural space is continuous around each lung, if the patient is in an upright or semi-upright position, air in the pleural space typically goes toward the apex. Thus, the first place to look for a pneumothorax is in the right and left upper hemithorax (Fig. 3–40). The most common appearance is an area adjacent to the ribs where no lung vascularity is seen and where there is a thin white line, which represents the visceral pleura that has been separated from the parietal pleura by air. You will need to look very carefully for this line, because it is often difficult to distinguish from the bony cortex of nearby ribs. If the pneumothorax is small and the pleural line is behind the rib, it can be almost impossible to see. In such circumstances, it may be useful to obtain an expiration chest radiograph in addition to the usual inspiration chest radiograph. On an expiration view, the lung becomes somewhat denser and smaller as expiration occurs. The amount of air in the pleural space does not change in size or density, and thus the pneumothorax appears relatively larger during expiration (Fig. 3–41).

How much the lung collapses with a pneumothorax is a function of how much air can get into the pleural space. In patients who have adhesive pleural changes between the visceral and parietal pleura as a result of previous inflammatory disease or scarring, complete collapse of the lung is not possible, even if a large amount of air is available. The same is true of patients who have diffuse lung disease, because their relatively stiff lungs do not allow complete collapse.

Total lung collapse can occur in patients with

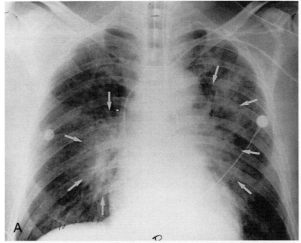

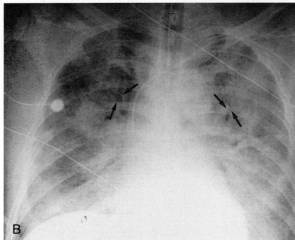

FIGURE 3–39. **Pulmonary edema.** Pulmonary edema, or fluid overload, can be manifested by indistinctness of the pulmonary vessels as they radiate from the hilum *(A).* This is sometimes termed a "bat wing" infiltrate. As pulmonary edema worsens *(B),* fluid fills the alveoli, and "air bronchograms" *(arrows)* become apparent.

normal lungs and without adhesions in the pleural space. This may or may not be accompanied by mediastinal shift. If mediastinal shift occurs or if there is depression of the hemidiaphragm with displacement of the heart and trachea away from the side with the pneumothorax, the patient has a potentially lethal condition known as a *tension pneumothorax* (Fig. 3–42).

Occasionally, a pneumothorax occurs when pleural fluid is present. This gives a rather characteristic, straight horizontal line as a result of the air-fluid level in the pleural space. This is termed a *hydropneumothorax.* A straight horizontal line, which extends to the chest wall with greater density below it, should raise consideration of a hydropneumothorax. Occasionally, you see a localized air-fluid level within a lung as a result of an abscess, but this is almost always surrounded by a thick wall

and should be easy to distinguish from a hydropneumothorax.

Quite commonly, a skinfold may cause an artifact that looks much like a pneumothorax. This artifact is caused by the patient's skin being folded over and pressed against the x-ray film cassette. The artifact is seen most often in patients who are either supine or semierect. It usually appears as an almost vertical line along the outer third of the upper lung zones. There are three ways to recognize this artifact. First, a skinfold line often extends above the lung apex into the supraclavicular soft tissues. Second, an increasing density or whiteness may become apparent as you look from the hilum toward the periphery of the lung, just before you reach the line that you think may be a pneumothorax. If there is increasing density (whiteness) as you proceed laterally, followed by sudden decrease in density, this probably represents a skinfold (Fig. 3–43). In the case of a small pneumothorax, both the lung and the pneumothorax are quite dark, and they are separated by a thin white line, which is the visceral pleura. Lastly, a skinfold line is often relatively straight, whereas a pleural line follows the curve of the inner aspect of the chest wall.

Because air tends to go to the highest position

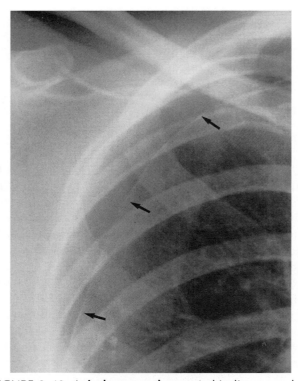

FIGURE 3–40. **Apical pneumothorax.** A thin line caused by the visceral pleura is seen separated from the lateral chest wall *(arrows).* Notice that no pulmonary vessels are seen beyond this line and that the line is curved. Notice also that the pleural line is white and that it is almost equally dark on the side of the pneumothorax and the side of the lung.

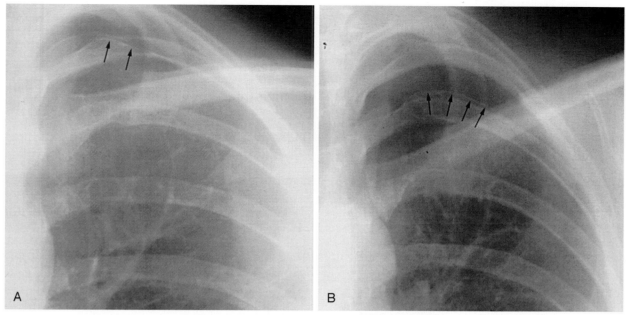

FIGURE 3–41. **Accentuation of the pneumothorax.** In this young male with chest pain, on a typical inspiration chest radiograph *(A)* a pneumothorax is barely visible. With expiration *(B)*, the lung becomes smaller, but the pneumothorax stays the same size; thus, relatively it appears bigger and is easier to see.

that it can find in the pleural space, it can be difficult to appreciate a small or even a moderate-sized pneumothorax on a frontal chest radiograph of a patient who is supine. With a supine AP chest projection, the x-ray beam is vertical, and the pneumothorax is layered horizontally along the anterior portion of the chest. In a supine adult, at least 500 cc of air needs to be in the pleural space for the pneumothorax to be visible. In supine infants and neonates, an anterior pneumothorax is common. Often the only way to see this pneumothorax is to obtain a supine lateral film and look for lucency (or a dark area) in the retrosternal region.

On the supine AP chest radiograph in the adult, one of the most reliable signs of a pneumothorax is what is known as the *deep sulcus sign* (Fig. 3–44). Normally, the lateral costophrenic angles are quite sharp or acute. The pleural space, however, goes much farther down along the edge of the lateral aspect of the liver and spleen than most people think. If air is in the pleural space, it can easily track down, making the costophrenic angle or sulcus much deeper and the angle much more acute than is normally seen. Thus, an extremely sharp or deep costophrenic angle or a costophrenic angle that becomes progressively deeper and sharper on sequential supine chest radiographs is an important sign to look for. If it is present, a pneumothorax has probably occurred.

Most of the findings that we have discussed describe the situation in which the air in the pleural space can move freely. In patients who have had prior inflammatory processes and adhesions in the pleural space, the air may not be able to move freely, and there may be a loculated pneumothorax. This can be difficult to appreciate, but if you see a dark area of lucency either around the edge of the lung or along the cardiac border, consider the possibility of a loculated pneumothorax.

A number of issues arise with regard to appropriate clinical management of a pneumothorax. Often, clinicians want to know how large the pneumothorax is. A few radiologists may give the volume in terms of percentage, although this is quite inaccurate. It may be simplest to refer to them as small, medium, large, and tension pneumothoraces. Experiments have been done on cadavers indicating that, on an upright film, if 50 cc of air has been placed in the pleural space, the apex of the lung has dropped approximately to the level between the second and third posterior ribs. One centimeter of space lateral to the lung constitutes about a 10% pneumothorax. One inch of space between the lateral chest wall and the lung margin signifies about a 30% pneumothorax.

After a chest tube has been placed, you should note not only the size of the residual pneumothorax and the position of the tip but also the location of the side port of the chest tube, if it has one. This is seen as a discontinuity of the opaque line in the catheter; it should be projecting inside the chest cavity and not out in the soft tissues. When a chest tube is properly placed—connected to a vacuum and unobstructed—if there is persistence of the pneu-

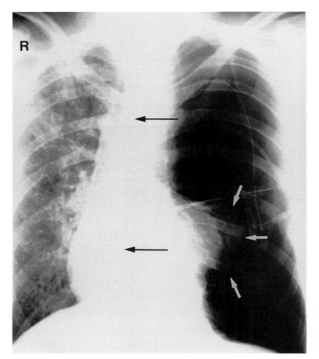

FIGURE 3–42. **Tension pneumothorax.** On this PA chest radiograph, the left hemithorax is very dark or lucent because the left lung has collapsed completely *(white arrows)*. The tension pneumothorax can be identified by the fact that the mediastinal contents, including the heart, are shifted toward the right, and the left hemidiaphragm is flattened and depressed.

mothorax, you should consider the possibility of a bronchopleural fistula. This is usually a result of blunt trauma with a tear in the region of a major bronchus. Other possibilities are a loculated pneumothorax or an anterior pneumothorax (with a posteriorly placed chest tube in a supine patient).

Pneumomediastinum

Air within the mediastinum is often (although not always) associated with a pneumothorax. With a pneumomediastinum, air collections within the upper portion of the mediastinum and lower neck are typically vertical. On the lateral view, you can sometimes see air in front of or behind the trachea (Fig. 3–45). A pneumomediastinum can be the result of a tracheobronchial tear. This entity carries up to a 50% mortality rate if not treated. A posttraumatic patient who has an abnormal air collection in the chest that does not resolve with placement of a chest tube should raise the suspicion of a pneumomediastinum or a bronchopleural fistula.

Sometimes people have difficulty distinguishing between a pneumomediastinum and a pneumopericardium. Pneumopericardium in an adult is very rare, typically resulting from a stab wound. The

pericardium envelops the heart and reaches only as high as the level of the hila. It does not extend around the hila or over the ascending aorta. Thus, in a pneumopericardium, air should be confined to the margins of the major chambers of the heart and not higher.

Subcutaneous Emphysema

Air in the soft tissues of the chest wall is often caused by blunt trauma with a pneumothorax and some broken ribs or by penetration, as with a stab wound or placement of a chest tube. Air in the soft tissues is seen as dark linear or ovoid ("bubbly") areas. Subcutaneous emphysema can extend into the supraclavicular and lower cervical regions. When this happens, however, it is important to distinguish subcutaneous emphysema from a pneumomediastinum that has extended up into the lower cervical area. When subcutaneous emphysema is extensive, it can dissect into the pectoral

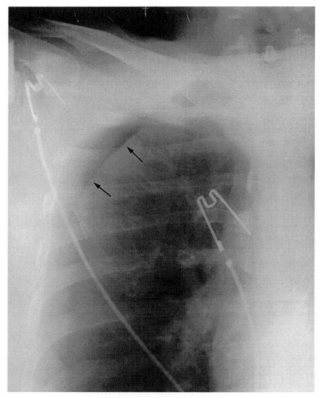

FIGURE 3–43. **Skinfold simulating a pneumothorax.** A near-vertical line is seen projecting over the right hemithorax *(arrows)*. This is a fold of skin caused by the patient pressing up against the film cassette. A skinfold can be differentiated by noting if it extends outside the normal lung area, by seeing pulmonary vessels beyond this line, or, as in this case, by noting that the lung is increasing in density or getting whiter from the hilum out to this line, then becoming darker. A pneumothorax will be seen as a white line that is dark on both sides.

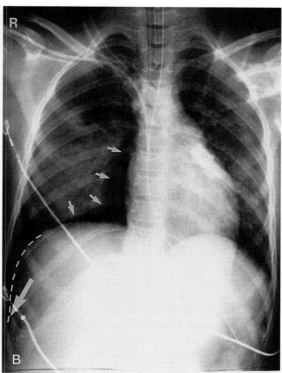

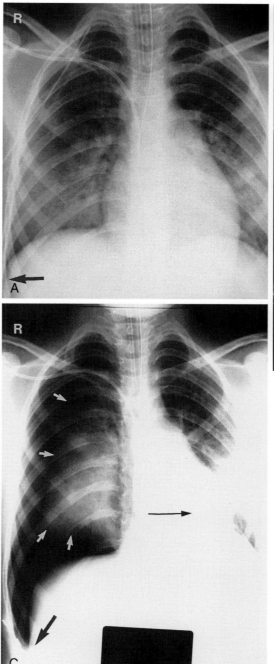

FIGURE 3–44. **Deep sulcus sign of pneumothorax.** On a PA chest radiograph *(A)*, the costophrenic angle is normally acute *(arrow)*. In a supine patient, a pneumothorax will often be anterior, medial, and basilar. On a subsequent supine film *(B)* the dark area along the right cardiac border and lung base got bigger *(small arrows)*, and the costophrenic angle became much deeper and more acute than normal *(large arrow)*. These findings were not recognized, and, as a result, the same patient developed a tension pneumothorax *(C)* with an extremely deep costophrenic angle *(large black arrow)* and almost completely collapsed right lung *(small white arrows)* and shift of the mediastinum to the left.

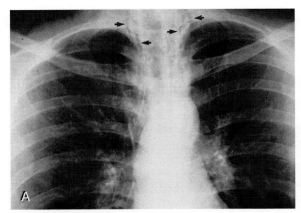

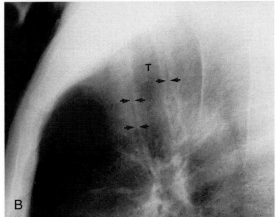

FIGURE 3-45. **Pneumomediastinum.** Vertical dark (lucent) lines representing air within the mediastinum are usually seen at or above the level of the aortic arch. On the PA view *(A)* these can be seen extending up into the lower cervical soft tissues. On the lateral view *(B)*, dark linear air collections can be seen in front of and behind the trachea (T).

muscles, producing a bizarre fan-shaped appearance of the air as it outlines the muscle fibers (Fig. 3-46).

Pleural Effusions

The appearance of pleural effusions or other fluid collections depends upon their size and location. Pleural effusions usually are at least 100 cc if they are seen on a routine upright chest radiograph. The most typical location of an effusion is in the dependent portions of the pleural space; therefore, they are seen best on upright chest radiographs. There will be blunting of the lateral costophrenic angles identified on the anterior or posterior chest radiograph and blunting of the posterior costophrenic angle seen on the lateral view. Somewhat larger effusions may extend into the inferior aspect of the major fissure (Fig. 3-47), and large effusions displace and compress lung tissue.

The appearances of larger effusions vary according to the position of the patient when the ra-

diograph was obtained. On the upright chest radiograph, increased basilar density (whiteness) and loss of the normal lung/hemidiaphragm interface are noted (Fig. 3-48). If the patient is supine when the radiograph is obtained, the effusion is typically layered out horizontally in the posterior pleural space. Because the x-ray beam is vertical for a supine chest radiograph, all that may be seen is a relatively increased density or whiteness of the affected hemithorax as compared with the normal side. In cases of doubt or to determine if a pleural fluid collection is free moving, you can obtain a decubitus chest radiograph. If you suspect that an effusion is on the right, you should order a right lateral decubitus view, that is, with the right side down when the radiograph is taken.

Pleural effusions have two other appearances sufficiently common to note. The first is a subpulmonic pleural effusion. This is more common on the right side. The tip-off to its existence is that the hemidiaphragm on the right is slightly higher than normal, with the highest portion of the dome more lateral than usual. The highest portion of the dome of the right hemidiaphragm is normally in the midclavicular line or slightly medial to this. If the high-

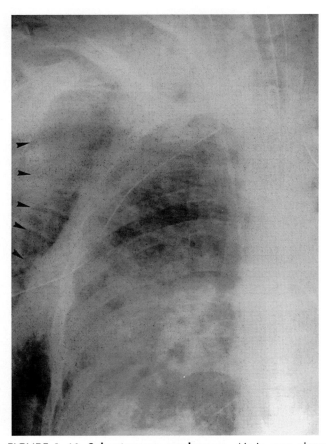

FIGURE 3-46. **Subcutaneous emphysema.** Air is seen along the lateral soft tissues of the chest outside the rib cage dissecting into the pectoral muscles creating fan-shaped dark lines over the upper chest *(arrowheads).*

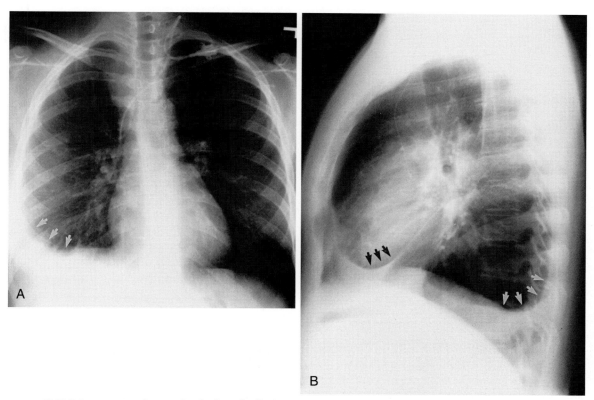

FIGURE 3–47. **Moderate-sized pleural effusion.** On this upright PA chest radiograph *(A)*, there is blunting of the right costophrenic angle due to pleural fluid. On the lateral view *(B)*, fluid can be seen tracking up into the major fissure *(black arrows)*, and there is blunting of the right posterior costophrenic angle *(white arrows)*.

est portion is lateral, suspect a subpulmonic effusion.

A loculated pleural effusion located within a fissure may be mistaken for an intrapulmonary lesion (a pseudotumor). On careful examination, loculated effusions in a fissure are typically lenticular or oval (not round) and are located in the expected position of the major or minor fissure.

Chest radiographs cannot be used to differentiate between a transudate and an exudate. The cause of an effusion, however, can sometimes be inferred. Massive effusions are usually malignant in origin. Pancreatitis is associated with left-sided effusions, whereas cirrhosis is associated with right-sided effusions. Most cardiogenic effusions are bilateral and are associated with cardiomegaly and other signs of CHF. About 40% of pneumonias are associated with a small effusion. When there is a moderate or large pleural fluid collection with a pneumonia, an empyema or malignancy should be suspected. If there is a pneumonia on chest radiograph and a decubitus film reveals fluid thicker than 11 mm from the chest wall, a thoracentesis should be obtained to exclude a complicated effusion. CT scanning is indicated to localize loculated effusions or empyemas before chest tube insertion or surgery.

Empyemas

An empyema is pus within the pleural space. It is the result of a primary infectious process 60% of the time, and is postsurgical (20%) or post-traumatic (20%) the rest of the time. On a chest radiograph, an empyema may look very much like a pleural effusion or pleural thickening, but an empyema does not move freely and will not layer on a decubitus chest radiograph (Fig. 3–49). It is often elliptic, with the long axis along the lateral chest wall, and the lung will be compressed or displaced. Empyemas are often loculated and have septa. A CT scan is the easiest way to visualize empyemas and locate them for potential drainage. Occasionally, an empyema may contain gas or air. If this is the case, the air-fluid level is often a different length on the frontal and lateral chest radiographs. The gas is most commonly the result of a bronchopleural fistula and much less frequently a result of gas-forming bacteria or a prior thoracentesis.

Pleural Calcification and Pleural Masses

Most pleural calcifications are the result of an old calcified empyema or asbestosis. Calcification

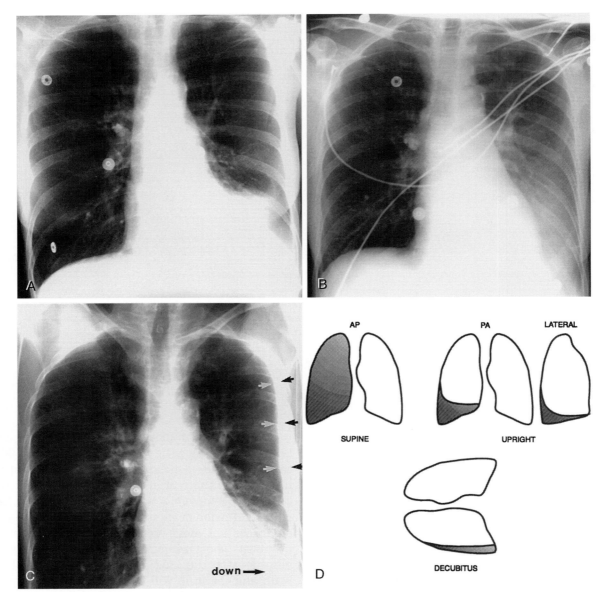

FIGURE 3–48. **The appearance of pleural effusions depending upon patient position.** On an upright PA chest radiograph *(A)*, a large left pleural effusion obscures the left hemidiaphragm, the left costophrenic angle, and the left cardiac border. On a supine AP view *(B)*, the fluid runs posteriorly, causing a diffuse opacity over the lower two thirds of the left lung; the left hemidiaphragm remains obscured. This can easily mimic left lower lobe infiltrate or left lower lobe atelectasis. With a left lateral decubitus view *(C)*, the left side of the patient is dependent, and the pleural effusion can be seen to be free-moving and layering *(arrows)* along the lateral chest wall. These findings are shown diagrammatically as well for a right pleural effusion *(D)*.

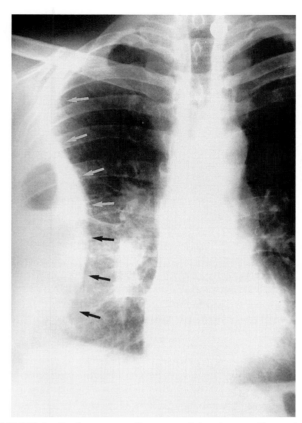

FIGURE 3–49. **Empyema.** On an upright chest radiograph, a lenticular density is seen along the lateral chest wall. An air-fluid level is also seen within this.

from an empyema is almost always unilateral and can be quite dense, whereas after asbestos exposure, calcification is often bilateral and not quite as dense (Fig. 3–50). Asbestosis can also produce an interstitial or reticulonodular pulmonary parenchymal pattern and occasionally a shaggy-looking heart. Mesotheliomas occur spontaneously or after asbestos exposure, and a focal pleural mass or thickening should raise suspicion of this tumor. However, the most common tumor after asbestos exposure is a lung cancer, not a mesothelioma and mesothelioma may occur in the absence of asbestos exposure.

■ MEDIASTINAL LESIONS

A large number of diseases present in the mediastinum are seen on the anterior chest radiograph as a widening or bulge in the central soft tissues of the chest. A contrast enhanced CT scan is almost always indicated for work-up of suspected mediastinal lesions. Perhaps the only exception to this is when the clinical suspicion is of a substernal thyroid or goiter. In that case a nuclear medicine thyroid scan should be obtained.

The differential diagnosis will change depending

on the location of the lesion in the mediastinum. The silhouette sign can be helpful in determining the site of a pathologic process. Normally the border of a soft tissue object (such as the aorta or heart) in the chest is seen because it is bounded by air. If there is a pathologic soft tissue mass in contiguity with a normal structure, the air interface will be lost. For example, if on a frontal chest radiograph a lesion is on the left upper mediastinum and if the descending aorta (in the posterior mediastinum) and the left pulmonary artery (in the middle medi-

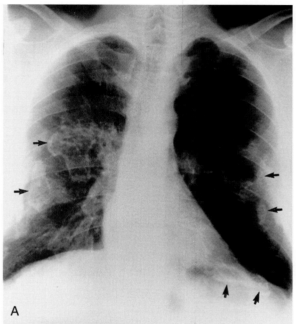

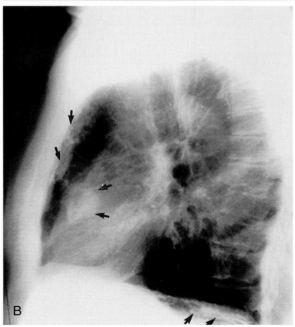

FIGURE 3–50. **Asbestosis.** Both the PA chest radiograph *(A)* and the lateral view *(B)* show areas of plaque-like calcification along the pleura and the hemidiaphragms *(arrows)*. Pleural lesions often appear to project within the lung parenchyma.

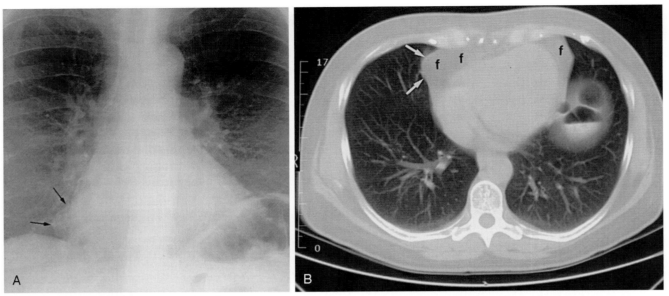

FIGURE 3–51. **Pericardial fat pad.** *A,* A soft tissue mass *(arrows)* is seen in the right cardiophrenic angle on the frontal chest radiograph. *B,* A CT scan shows the mass *(arrows)* to be bulging fat (f) around the heart.

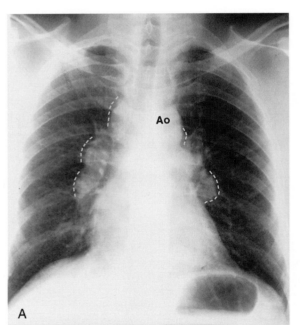

FIGURE 3–52. **Sarcoid.** Marked lymphadenopathy *(dotted lines)* is seen in the region of both hila in the right paratracheal region *(A).* The transverse contrast-enhanced CT scan of the upper chest *(B)* clearly shows the ascending and descending aorta (Ao) as well as the pulmonary artery (PA) and superior vena cava. The right and left mainstem bronchus area is also seen. The arrows indicate the extensive lymphadenopathy.

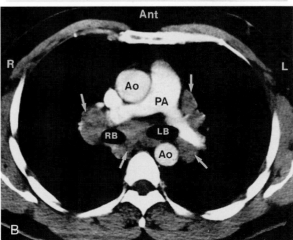

astinum) are seen well, an anterior mediastinal lesion is probably present.

The next and simplest way to localize the lesion is to look at the lateral chest radiograph. If there is filling-in of the space behind the top of the sternum and the ascending aorta, an anterior mediastinal lesion is probably present. The following four types of lesions tend to occur in the anterior mediastinum: substernal thyroid glands, thymic lesions, germ cell tumors (much more common in males), and lymphomas. Occasionally, retrosternal and internal mammary lymph nodes can become enlarged from metastases of breast cancer, or from leukemia. One can remember most of the anterior mediastinal lesions by using the four Ts. This stands for *t*hymoma, *t*hyroid lesions, *t*eratoma, and *T* cell lymphomas. A benign normal variant is the pericardial fat pad (Fig. 3–51). This almost always is found at the right cardiophrenic angle.

Lesions in the middle mediastinum include thoracic aortic aneurysms, hematomas, neoplasms, adenopathies (Fig. 3–52), esophageal lesions, diaphragmatic hernias (hiatal or Morgagni type), and duplication cysts. Morgagni's hernias tend to be on the right side. Any middle mediastinal lesion associated with the aorta should be considered an aneurysm until proved otherwise.

Posterior mediastinal lesions are seen on the lateral view projecting over the spine and are also paraspinous on the frontal chest radiograph. Most (90%) posterior mediastinal lesions are neurogenic. They may represent neuroblastomas in young children but in adults are more likely to be neurofibromas, schwannomas, or ganglioneuromas. Other posterior mediastinal lesions include hernias (hiatal or Bochdalek type), neoplasms, hematomas, or extramedullary hematopoiesis. Bochdalek's hernias are most often on the left side.

■ DIAPHRAGMATIC RUPTURE

Rupture of the diaphragm may occur after blunt trauma. The diaphragm is most frequently ruptured on the left side, perhaps because the liver

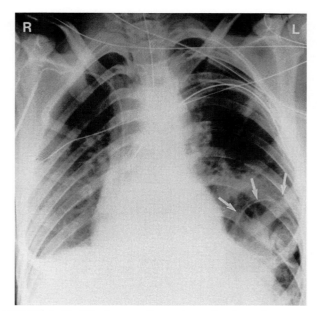

FIGURE 3–53. **Diaphragmatic rupture.** Six days after an auto accident, bowel loops can be seen in the left lower chest *(arrows)*. Diaphragmatic rupture is more common on the left than on the right.

may dissipate some of the force on the right caused by an abdominal blow, lessening the likelihood of rupture of the right hemidiaphragm. The most common appearance is loops of bowel protruding into the lower chest cavity without the normal dome-shaped structure of the hemidiaphragm (Fig. 3–53). The manifestations of a ruptured diaphragm can be delayed, and sometimes the bowel herniates through the diaphragm 1 or 2 weeks after the initial accident. The patient may remain asymptomatic for months or years.

GENERAL SUGGESTED READINGS

Juhl JH, Crummy AB, Kuhlman JE: The Chest, Section V. *In* Juhl JH, Crummy AB, Kuhlman JE (eds): Paul and Juhl's Essentials of Radiologic Imaging, 7th ed. Philadelphia, Lippincott-Raven, 1998.

Meholic A, Ketai L, Lofgren R: Fundamentals of Chest Radiology. Philadelphia, WB Saunders, 1996.

Potchen EJ, Grainger RG, Greene R: Pulmonary Radiology. Philadelphia, WB Saunders, 1993.

4

BREAST IMAGING

■ BREAST IMAGING MODALITIES

Breast imaging usually refers to mammography. Ultrasonography can be a useful adjunctive method but should not be relied on as a screening method for breast cancer. All breast imaging is complementary to physical examination. Tumors may be apparent by either physical examination or mammography. The primary purpose of mammography is to detect small breast cancers and, by so doing, to improve survival. In younger women, the breast is extremely dense; the density of the parenchymal tissue is the same as the density of a carcinoma. In this group, not only is the incidence of breast cancer low, but it is also extremely difficult to tell whether a cancer is present amid the normal dense tissue. As women age, there is fatty infiltration of the breast and atrophy of the parenchyma. Because the fat is lucent (dark) on a mammogram and a cancer is dense (white), tumors are more easily visualized as a woman ages (Fig. 4–1).

There is often great variation in the appearance of the breast tissue between women. Fortunately, most women have quite symmetric tissue when one breast is compared with the other breast. Any asymmetries in density should be examined carefully, because they may represent a cancer (Fig. 4–2). In addition to asymmetric masses, another sign of breast cancer is grouped, tiny calcifications. Often called *microcalcifications*, these are usually extremely fine (about 1 mm or less) and sand-like and sometimes can be seen to have a branching

structure. Most women, as they age, have calcifications within the breast that are benign. These are usually rounded calcifications greater than 2 mm in diameter (Fig. 4–3). In women older than 60 years, serpiginous calcifications can normally be seen within blood vessel walls.

Mammograms are usually obtained in what are referred to as the *craniocaudal* (top to bottom) and *axillary oblique* views. Appropriate indications for breast imaging are shown in Table 4–1. Once a suspicious lesion is identified on both craniocaudal and axillary oblique views, further investigation usually ensues, in the form of a magnified mammo-

TABLE 4–1 Appropriate Breast Imaging and Screening

Screening	
Physical examination	Yearly by healthcare provider and monthly self-examination
Mammography	
Younger than age 35	Mammography only if high risk
Age 35–49	Baseline and individual informed decision (see text)
Older than age 50	Annual mammography
Palpable Mass	
Younger than age 30	Ultrasonography if cystic, possibly aspirate if solid, biopsy
Older than age 30	Mammography and ultrasonography if solid, biopsy

FIGURE 4–1. **Normal mammogram and the process of aging.** On the axillary oblique view of the right breast (A), the normal breast parenchyma is seen as an ill-defined white density, predominantly located behind the nipple. In young women, the breast tissue can be extremely dense with only a small amount of interspersed fat, making tumors difficult to see. Another mammogram (B) on the same patient several years later shows fatty replacement of most of the breast tissue. The breast tissue can become dense again if the woman is placed on estrogen therapy.

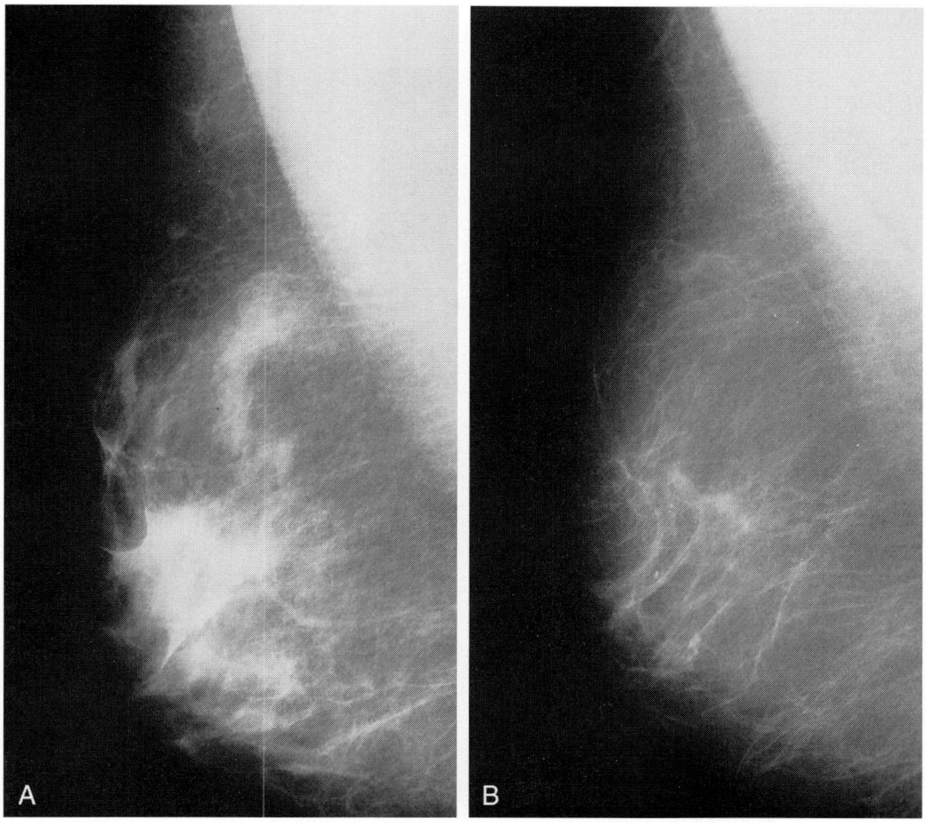

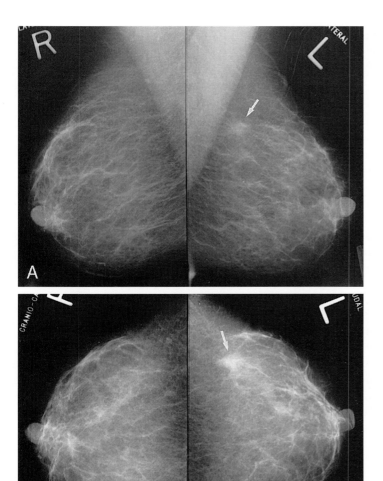

FIGURE 4–2. **Breast cancer.** Axillary oblique (A) and craniocaudal (B) views of the right and left breast show an asymmetric density (arrows) in the upper outer aspect of the left breast. Any asymmetric density should be suggestive of a neoplasm.

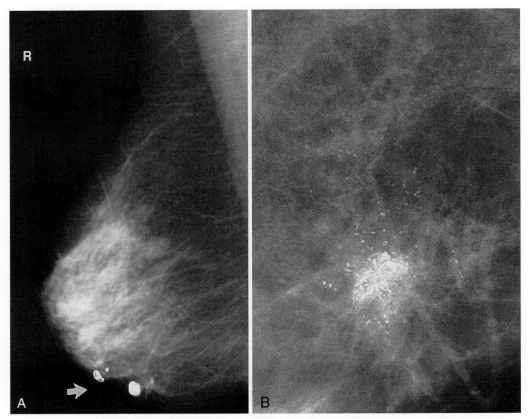

FIGURE 4–3. **Breast calcifications.** A lateral view of the right breast *(A)* shows several well-defined rounded or lobular calcifications. These are almost always benign. Malignant calcifications *(B)* tend to be quite small, sand-like, and clustered, as seen in this enlarged view from a mammogram in a different patient with breast cancer.

gram, an ultrasound examination, or a biopsy. Ultrasound examination of the breast is improving, but it cannot reliably differentiate carcinomas from fibroadenomas or other benign solid lesions. It is very useful for differentiating solid lesions from a cyst. If a lesion is solid on an ultrasound study or if on a mammogram there is asymmetric or stellate density or if there are grouped microcalcifications, an intensive search should be undertaken for prior mammograms to be used for comparison. However, if the lesion is new or if old films are not available and the lesion is thought to be suspect, a biopsy is recommended. The biopsy may be in the form of a needle aspiration, core biopsy, or needle localization followed by a surgical biopsy. A surgical biopsy results in scar tissue, and scar tissue may leave an asymmetric radial density that can look like a neoplasm. Magnetic resonance imaging and nuclear medicine techniques have been used to evaluate potential breast cancers but the accuracy of these tests remains limited.

▪ SCREENING FOR BREAST CANCER

Only mammography is effective for screening asymptomatic patients. In spite of this, only half of

older women have ever had a mammogram. Many managed care programs are not implementing preventive care requirements that include mammography. There has been great discussion during the past decade as to the indications for screening mammography. Most screening guidelines currently utilized for non–high risk women call for annual screening for women older than 49 years and a baseline mammogram at age 35 to 40. There is controversy about the utility of screening between the ages of 40 and 50 years. At present a number of guidelines produced by different groups suggest a baseline examination and biannual screening during this period. However, the National Institute of Health consensus statement concluded that there should not be a universal recommendation and that each woman should decide for herself based on educational material, objective analysis of scientific evidence, individual medical history, and personal perception of value and risk. Women classified as high risk for breast cancer include those with a prior breast cancer, abnormal biopsy results, or breast cancer family history in a first-order relative. It should be noted, however, that 75% of patients with breast cancer have none of these risk factors. As mentioned previously, ultrasound examination by itself is not a reliable tool for detecting occult breast cancer. When a small breast cancer is detected (stage 1) in an asymptomatic patient and blood chemistries are normal, imaging studies are not indicated to rule out metastases.

■ MANAGEMENT OF A PALPABLE BREAST MASS

The management of a palpable breast mass differs depending on the age of the patient. In women younger than 30 years, cancer is unlikely, and an ultrasound is indicated to determine if the lesion is cystic. If the lesion is solid, needle aspiration or biopsy is often done. If the woman is older than 30 years, mammography is usually performed first followed by an ultrasound examination. The mammogram may show signs that are highly suggestive of malignancy or indicate other nonpalpable areas that are suspect and need to be evaluated by ultra-sonography or biopsy. A normal mammogram should never deter biopsy of a clinically suspicious palpable lesion.

■ PROSTHESIS EVALUATION

Mammography can be used in the evaluation of a breast prosthesis. Normally, the prosthesis can be seen as an oval rim of fibrous density in the breast. A complication that can arise is calcification, which can occur around the prosthesis, and this is sometimes visualized on chest radiographs. Leakage of a prosthesis can be identified if the leakage has been enough to cause deflation of the prosthesis. Leaking saline cannot be visualized directly on a mammogram.

GENERAL SUGGESTED READING

Kopans DB: Breast Imaging. Philadelphia, Lippincott Williams & Wilkins, 1997.

5

CARDIOVASCULAR SYSTEM

■ IMAGING TECHNIQUES

The normal anatomy and configuration of the heart on a chest radiograph is discussed in Chapter 3. Perhaps the next most common noninvasive imaging modalities are ultrasound imaging (echocardiography) of the heart and duplex ultrasonography of large vessels. Nuclear medicine techniques are also widely used. Computed tomography (CT) and magnetic resonance imaging (MRI) are used occasionally for specialized applications, and these should not be considered primary or secondary cardiac imaging techniques. Angiograms are indicated when cardiac or vascular surgery or interventional procedures are being considered. Appropriate imaging for cardiovascular problems is shown in Table 5–1.

■ COMMON CARDIOVASCULAR PROBLEMS

Generalized Cardiomegaly

The appearance of the pulmonary vessels and lungs on a chest radiograph is discussed in Chapter 3. The width of the heart should not exceed half the width of the chest at its widest point. This measurement is only reliable on an upright posteroanterior (PA) chest film; on an anteroposterior chest radiograph, the heart often exceeds this mea-

surement owing to magnification. On a supine film, there is even more magnification and high position of the hemidiaphragms. This high position pushes the heart upward and outward, making it appear wide. In patients with chronic obstructive pulmonary disease (COPD), the diaphragms are low. The heart elongates and may appear normal in width when it is actually enlarged.

Cardiomegaly or an enlarged cardiac silhouette can be due to valvular disease, cardiomyopathy, congenital heart disease, pericardial effusion, and mass lesions. Both cardiomyopathies and pericardial effusions generally lead to symmetric enlargement, whereas valvular disease and congenital heart disease often have specific chamber enlargement. The dilated cardiomyopathies most commonly result from ischemia, infections, and metabolic disorders. Other causes include collagen vascular disease and toxic agents such as alcohol and chemotherapeutic drugs (Fig. 5–1).

If there is acute marked enlargement of the cardiac silhouette (within several days or weeks), the most likely diagnosis is a pericardial effusion. Under these circumstances, the heart has quite a pendulous appearance and is much wider at the base. This is often referred to as a *water bag appearance* (Fig. 5–2). Pericardial effusions must be greater than 250 mL to be detectable radiographically. If a pericardial effusion is suspected, the imaging procedure of choice is echocardiography.

TABLE 5–1 Appropriate Imaging and Other Studies for Cardiovascular Problems

Clinical Problem	Imaging Study
Most cardiac problems	Initial posteroanterior and lateral chest radiography
Congestive heart failure (new or worse)	Chest radiography and ejection fraction; wall motion evaluation by nuclear medicine or echocardiography
Congestive heart failure (chronic)	Chest radiography
Hypertension (suspected essential)	No imaging indicated
Hypertension (suspected renal artery stenosis)	Nuclear medicine captopril renogram
Left ventricular ejection fraction	Gated nuclear medicine blood pool study or echocardiography
Chest pain or shortness of breath (suspected pulmonary embolism)	Chest radiography and nuclear medicine ventilation/perfusion scan
Shortness of breath (suspected cardiac origin)	Chest radiography and echocardiography or nuclear medicine myocardial perfusion study
Acute chest pain (suspected myocardial infarction [<6 hours])	Electrocardiography, chest radiography, and coronary angiography
Chronic chest pain (suspected cardiac origin)	Electrocardiography, chest radiography, nuclear medicine myocardial perfusion or coronary angiogram
Coronary ischemia	Electrocardiography; if negative then stress electrocardiogram, nuclear medicine myocardial perfusion study or stress echocardiogram; if positive then coronary angiogram
Congenital heart disease	Chest radiography, echocardiography, or cardiac catheterization
Endocarditis	Echocardiography
Valvular disease	Echocardiography
Pericardial effusion	Echocardiography
Constrictive pericarditis	Echocardiography, if equivocal then computed tomography
Aortic trauma	Angiography or computed tomography with contrast
Thoracic aortic dissection	Computed tomography with contrast or transesophageal ultrasonography
Abdominal aortic aneurysm	Computed tomography with contrast if symptomatic; ultrasonography for follow-up
Deep venous thrombosis	Duplex ultrasonography
Carotid bruit	Duplex ultrasonography; if high-grade stenosis then contrast angiography
Claudication	Doppler ultrasonography of lower extremity

Congestive Heart Failure

Discussion of the pulmonary x-ray findings of congestive heart failure (CHF) have been discussed in Chapter 3. The diagnosis of CHF is made on the basis of the patient's medical history and physical examination; chest radiography is confirmatory. Because assessment of cardiac function by chest film is rather crude and insensitive, quantitative evaluations of cardiac ejection fraction are usually made by nuclear medicine gated blood pool or multiple gated acquisition (MUGA) studies and echocardiography. Both are quite accurate. Computer analysis of the MUGA allows calculation of an ejection fraction. The normal left ventricular ejection fraction (LVEF) is between 55 and 75%. In older persons, the lower limit of LVEF is probably about 50%. If exercise treadmill, nuclear medicine, or echocardiography results are positive or if the LVEF is less than 35%, an angiogram may be indicated.

Specific Chamber Enlargement

It is difficult to differentiate right atrial from right ventricular enlargement on a chest radiograph. In most adults, when one of the right chambers is enlarged, so is the other. On the frontal chest radiograph, right atrial enlargement is suggested by an increased convexity of the right cardiac border. Isolated right ventricular enlargement is very difficult to appreciate. On the lateral view, both right ventricular and right atrial enlargement will cause a filling-in of the anterior clear space behind the sternum. Normally on the lateral view, the anterior portion of the heart fills in only approximately one third or less of the anterior clear space, unless there is enlargement of the right atrium or right ventricle.

Isolated left atrial enlargement most commonly occurs as a result of mitral stenosis. Enlargement is noted as prominence of the left atrial appendage

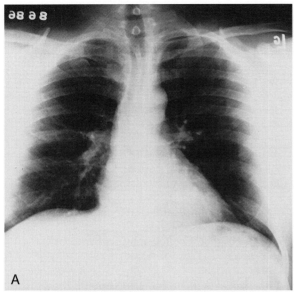

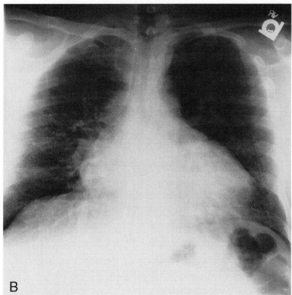

FIGURE 5–1. **Cardiomyopathy.** In this case, cardiomyopathy is due to cancer chemotherapy with doxorubicin. An initial chest x-ray examination (A) demonstrates a normal-sized heart. After several therapeutic courses of doxorubicin (B), there has been marked enlargement in the cardiac silhouette due to multichamber dilatation.

on the PA view and splaying or widening of the inferior carinal angle. The normal inferior carinal angle should not exceed 75 degrees. An extremely enlarged left atrium can be seen on the PA radiograph as a double density behind the heart and below the carina (Fig. 5–3).

The classic appearance of a mitral (rheumatic) heart on a PA chest radiograph is easily recognized by four bumps along the left cardiac border. This is also sometimes called the *ski mogul heart.* Going from superior to inferior, the bumps represent the aortic arch, pulmonary artery, left atrium, and left

ventricle. Left atrial enlargement is also seen in patients with congenital cardiac lesions that have intracardiac shunts and in those who have left ventricular failure. Prosthetic valves are often identified in postsurgical rheumatic patients (Fig. 5–4).

On a frontal chest radiograph, left ventricular enlargement produces a round left cardiac border and a downward displacement of the apex. On the lateral view, the posterior aspect of the heart, where it intersects the hemidiaphragm, is usually posteriorly displaced behind the inferior vena cava. The Hoffman-Rigler sign can also be used. To use this sign, find the intersection of the inferior vena cava

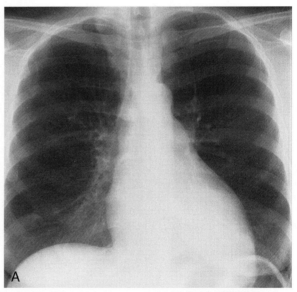

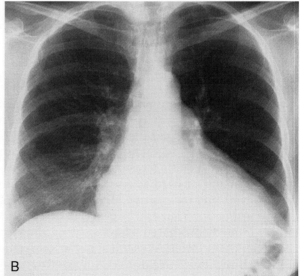

FIGURE 5–2. **Pericardial effusion.** In a patient with a viral syndrome, a posteroanterior chest radiograph (A) shows mild cardiomegaly with prominence of the left cardiac border. One week later (B), a marked and sudden increase in the transverse diameter of the heart is caused by a pericardial effusion. A definitive diagnosis is best made by using cardiac ultrasound imaging.

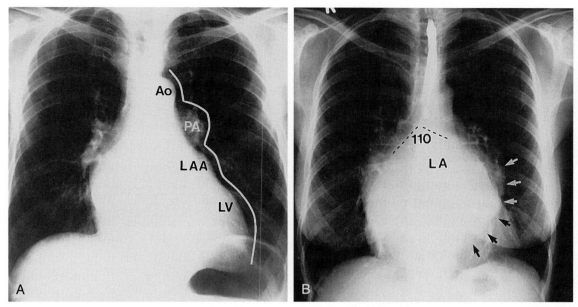

FIGURE 5–3. **Mitral stenosis.** On a posteroanterior chest radiograph *(A)*, there is a four-bump or ski mogul heart. The four bumps are created by the aorta (Ao), pulmonary artery (PA), left atrial appendage (LAA), and left ventricle (LV). The LAA normally does not bulge out. Late findings of left atrial enlargement on the posteroanterior chest radiograph *(B)* are a double density behind the heart *(arrows)* and a splaying of the subcarinal angle (110 degrees in this case), which normally does not measure more than 75 degrees.

with the hemidiaphragm on the lateral film and then measure 2 cm up and 2 cm back. If the heart projects posterior to this point, there is probably left ventricular enlargement. Because an enlarged right side of the heart can sometimes push the left ventricle back, look at the space behind the sternum. Only the lower one third should be filled by soft tissue. If more space is filled, there is at least right heart enlargement and possibly left heart enlargement.

Left ventricular dilatation can be due to a number of causes, including coronary artery disease (CAD), aortic stenosis, aortic regurgitation, and left ventricular aneurysm. Ventricular aneurysms most commonly occur near the apex, anteriorly, and are associated with a high rate of mortality. Left ventricular hypertrophy is difficult to detect radiographically. It may be present in patients who have a normal cardiac configuration on chest radiograph. If this is suspected, an echocardiogram (ultrasound) is the test of choice.

Endocarditis

Endocarditis usually occurs in patients with pre-existing valvular heart disease and most commonly involves the left side of the heart. As a result, septic emboli are found in the spleen, kidneys, and brain. Drug addicts may develop endocarditis in the right side of the heart and then shower septic emboli to the lungs. Imaging studies in patients with suspected endocarditis are usually limited to an initial chest radiograph and are followed by an echocardiogram to visualize vegetative growths on the valves and bicuspid valves, atrial septal defect (ASD), ruptured chordae tendineae, and dilatation of the heart or valve ring. If there are suspected emboli in the spleen, brain, or kidneys, additional imaging studies such as CT or MRI of these organs may be helpful.

Pericardial Disease

Pericardial effusions are often clinically unsuspected. As mentioned earlier, a rapidly enlarging heart or one with a water bag appearance should suggest a pericardial effusion, and echocardiography is the procedure of choice. It is also the procedure of choice with penetrating trauma when a cardiac tamponade is suspected. Constrictive pericarditis is usually manifested by right cardiac failure (hepatomegaly, distended neck veins, ascites, and peripheral edema). An echocardiogram is again the procedure of choice. If this is nondiagnostic, a CT may be helpful.

Aortic Stenosis and Insufficiency

Aortic stenosis may be difficult to detect on a plain film of the chest, and sometimes the only

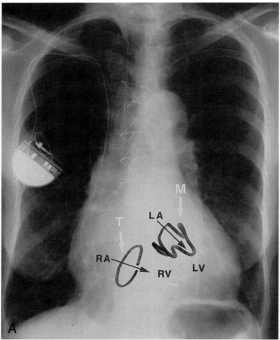

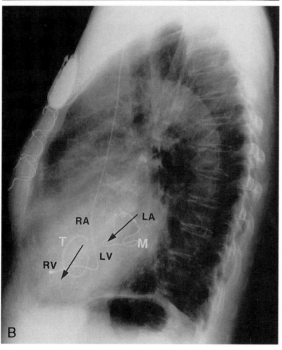

FIGURE 5–4. **Prosthetic mitral and tricuspid valves.** The mitral (M) and tricuspid (T) valves are difficult to appreciate on the posteroanterior view of the chest *(A)* and are therefore drawn in. They are easily seen on the lateral view *(B)* in the expected regions between the left atrium (LA) and left ventricle (LV) and between the right atrium (RA) and right ventricle (RV). Also, note the cardiac pacer that comes down the superior vena cava through the RA and into the RV. These two valves are normally relatively large owing to relatively low pressure gradients across these valves.

finding is a calcified aortic valve. Initially, with aortic stenosis, there is left ventricular hypertrophy. The heart is normal in size and may show slight rounding of the cardiac apex. When left ventricular dilatation occurs, the left cardiac border elongates, and the apex of the heart moves downward toward the left hemidiaphragm. The aortic knob is normal in size, although the ascending aortic arch is enlarged, causing a convexity of the right upper cardiac margin. The enlargement of the ascending aorta is due to poststenotic dilatation.

With aortic insufficiency, the left ventricle be-

comes much larger. On a PA chest radiograph, the apex of the heart may project below the most superior portion of the left hemidiaphragm. The ascending aorta still shows some enlargement.

Pulmonary Artery Enlargement

Enlargement of the pulmonary artery is fairly easy to recognize on the PA chest radiograph by a bulging along the left cardiac border just below the aortic arch (Fig. 5–5). Pulmonary artery enlarge-

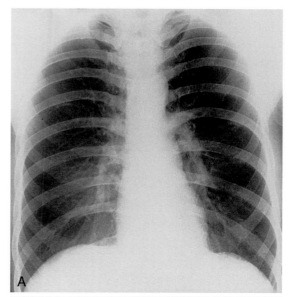

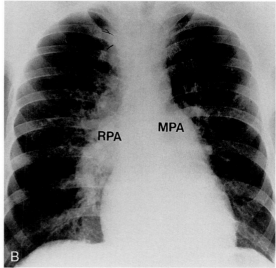

FIGURE 5–5. **Progressive pulmonary arterial hypertension.** This patient initially presented with a relatively normal chest radiograph *(A)*. However, several years later *(B)*, there is increasing heart size as well as marked dilatation of the main pulmonary artery (MPA) and right pulmonary artery (RPA). Rapid tapering of the arteries as they proceed peripherally is suggestive of pulmonary hypertension and is sometimes referred to as *pruning*.

ment can be due to a number of causes, but probably the three most common are pulmonic stenosis (with poststenotic dilatation), pulmonary artery hypertension, and abnormalities in which there is increased flow through the pulmonary artery, such as a patent ductus arteriosus or an ASD.

If enlargement of both the left and the right main pulmonary arteries is present, consider the diagnosis of pulmonary arterial hypertension. In this condition, in addition to the large central pulmonary arteries, there is rapid pruning of the vessels as they proceed peripherally in the lung. Even

though the central vessels are quite large, it is unusual to be able to see vessels at the very edge of the lung. Pulmonary hypertension may be idiopathic or due to a number of causes, including ASD and ventricular septal defect (VSD), patent ductus arteriosus, arteriovenous shunt, left ventricular failure, mitral valve disease, pulmonary embolism (PE), parenchymal lung disease, chronic obstructive lung disease, drug abuse, and other less common conditions.

Congenital Cardiac Disease

Rather than including every entity, a few examples are presented to provide an approach to interpretation. There are several important factors to assess in the evaluation of congenital cardiac disease. These include the age of the individual; the clinical findings, such as murmurs; whether the patient is cyanotic or acyanotic; specific chamber enlargement; and pulmonary vascularity (increased, decreased, or normal).

Probably the easiest place to begin is in the determination of whether the individual is cyanotic or not. A cyanotic infant who has normal or decreased pulmonary vascularity and a normal heart size probably has a tetralogy of Fallot. Tetralogy of Fallot includes pulmonic stenosis, VSD, an overriding aorta, and right ventricular hypertrophy. On x-ray examination, there is usually decreased pulmonary vascularity and a boot-shaped heart with an uplifted apex and a concavity along the left cardiac border. If there is cardiomegaly with an enlarged right atrium, the differential diagnosis includes Ebstein's malformation, tricuspid atresia, and pulmonic atresia. In Ebstein's anomaly, there is a giant right atrium, with a shoulder along the right side of the heart, and a small pulmonary artery. In this entity, there is downward displacement of the tricuspid valve, with the right ventricle being partially atrialized.

Causes of cyanotic heart disease with increased pulmonary vascularity include transposition of the great vessels (which is most common), truncus arteriosus, total anomalous pulmonary venous return, tricuspid atresia, and a single ventricle. Radiographic features of transposition of the great vessels include a heart that is said to have an *egg-on-side shape* and a narrow superior mediastinum secondary to a hypoplastic thymus.

Similarly, acyanotic congenital heart disease should initially be evaluated by determination of pulmonary vascularity. In those with normal vascularity, aortic stenosis, pulmonic stenosis, coarctation, and interruption of the aortic arch should be considered. Acyanotic heart disease with increased pulmonary vascularity should be investigated next by looking for left atrial enlargement. This is not present in ASD, and an endocardial cushion defect may be considered.

An ASD is the most common congenital cardiac anomaly in adults, yet it is rarely symptomatic in infancy or childhood. The common radiologic finding in an ASD, in addition to enlargement of the pulmonary artery, is an increase in the size of the right atrium and right ventricle. This is often best seen as filling-in of the retrosternal clear space on the lateral view (Fig. 5–6). The imaging modality of choice, if an ASD is suspected, is echocardiography.

If there is acyanotic heart disease with increased pulmonary vascularity and left atrial enlargement, look at the aorta. If the aorta is enlarged, a patent ductus arteriosus should be suspected, because there is excess blood flow through the aortic arch that is shunted to the pulmonary arteries. If the aorta is not enlarged, consider a VSD.

Pulmonary Embolism

PE is a potentially fatal entity. Typical symptoms include sudden onset of dyspnea (80% of patients), tachypnea (>16 resp/min, 80%) pleuritic chest pain (70%), rales (60%), fever (45%), tachycardia (>100 beats/min, 40%), and hemoptysis (20%). A low-grade fever may occur with PE, but a high-grade fever and leukocytosis suggest a pneumonia. About 35% of patients with PE also have clinically evident phlebitis. However, the converse is more important; that is, about two thirds of patients with PE do not show evidence of phlebitis.

The chest x-ray findings in a patient with pulmonary emboli are relatively nonspecific, and the major reason for ordering a chest radiograph is to exclude other causes of the patient's symptoms. Occasionally, a small pleural effusion, atelectasis, or an elevated hemidiaphragm may be present. If there has been infarction of a portion of the lung as a result of the embolism, there may be a wedge-shaped infiltrate present (Fig. 5–7).

After a chest radiograph, the next essential study to be performed is a nuclear medicine ventilation/perfusion (V/Q) lung scan. Ventilation is assessed by having the patient inhale and then exhale a radioactive gas or an aerosol containing radioactive particles (Fig. 5–8). Perfusion is assessed by intravenously injecting a number of biodegradable radioactive particles that are unable to pass through the pulmonary capillary bed. Because these are trapped in the capillary bed and give off radiation, images of the lungs can be obtained in various projections (Fig. 5–9). The ventilation and perfusion lung images are then compared. Interpretation of the per-

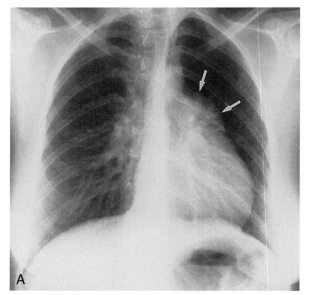

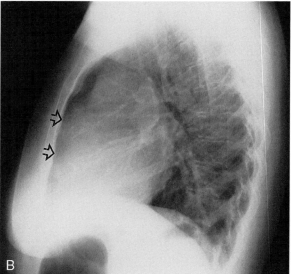

FIGURE 5–6. **Atrial septal defect.** *A,* Extra blood flow from the left side of the heart back to the right side *(arrows)* increases the size of the main pulmonary artery (best seen here on the posteroanterior chest radiograph). *B,* There is also an increase in the size of the right ventricle (best seen here on the lateral view) as soft tissue filling-in the lower and middle retrosternal space *(arrows).*

fusion scans first entails the identification and classification of any defects according to their appearance. Defects corresponding to anatomic divisions should be classified as lobar, segmental, or subsegmental. Those that are not anatomic or do not respect segmental boundaries may be considered nonsegmental and unlikely to represent pulmonary emboli. A PE causes a defect on the perfusion scan that is not seen on the ventilation scan (a mismatched defect). The reason for this is that a PE generally does not interfere much with ventilation. Abnormalities such as tumors, pneumonia, and bul-

and it is unlikely that these defects are the cause of the patient's symptoms.

Occasionally, mismatched (large but not completely segmental) defects are seen, or the patient has a large amount of COPD, making the scan difficult to interpret. These scans are interpreted as intermediate probability for pulmonary embolus. If a patient has a positive ultrasound test for deep venous thrombosis (DVT), and clinical suspicion is high, the individual is usually treated. If tests for DVT are negative, yet clinical suspicion remains high, CT angiography or pulmonary angiography is usually performed.

The accuracy of any test is dependent on the number of patients in the test population who actually have the disease (pretest probability). In general, when a V/Q scan is interpreted as high probability or high likelihood, there is an excellent chance that pulmonary emboli are present regardless of the pretest probability in the patient population. The same is true of low probability interpretations; that is, there is a relatively low chance of pulmonary emboli. In contrast, when the intermediate category is determined, there is a significant impact of the pretest probability. Thus, when an intermediate interpretation is rendered, careful attention should be paid to the type of patient, the medical history, and the clinician's suspicion level in arriving at a conclusion regarding patient therapy.

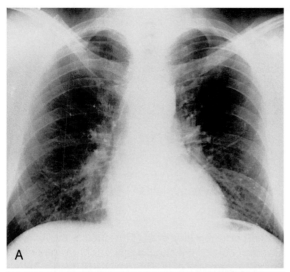

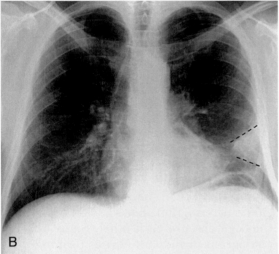

FIGURE 5–7. **Pulmonary embolism and infarction.** *A,* Immediately after an acute episode of shortness of breath because of a pulmonary embolism, the posteroanterior chest radiograph is essentially normal. *B,* If the pulmonary embolism actually leads to infarction, a peripheral wedge-shaped infiltrate (dotted lines) develops.

lae would cause both a ventilation and perfusion abnormality (a matched defect).

If a significant number of segmental defects are seen on the perfusion scan and are not identified on the ventilation scan, the images are interpreted as high probability for PE (Fig. 5–10). Under these circumstances, there is an 80% or greater chance that the patient has PE. There is rarely any need to perform pulmonary angiography on a patient with a high probability scan, unless there is a significant contraindication to anticoagulation.

If the perfusion scan is normal or shows only small subsegmental defects, the examination is interpreted as either low probability or normal. Under these circumstances, there is less than a 20% chance that the individual has pulmonary emboli,

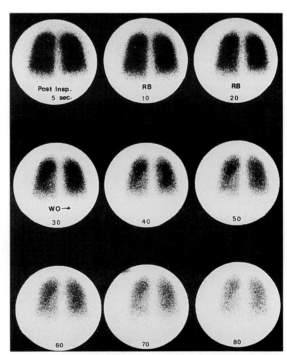

FIGURE 5–8. **Normal ventilation lung scan.** These are images of the lungs made from the patient's back. The patient inhales radioactive gas and rebreathes (RB) it for several seconds; additional images are made as the radioactive gas is allowed to wash out (WO) of the lungs, during 30 to 80 seconds.

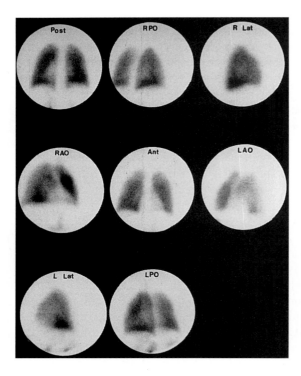

FIGURE 5–9. **Normal perfusion lung scan.** This nuclear medicine study is performed by intravenously injecting numerous, tiny particles that lodge in the pulmonary capillary bed. This allows perfusion images of the lungs to be obtained in a number of projections. The defect, or lack of activity between the lungs, is due to the spine and the heart. Post = posterior; RPO = right posterior oblique; R Lat = right lateral; RAO = right anterior oblique; Ant = anterior; LAO = left anterior oblique; L Lat = left lateral; LPO = left posterior oblique.

Some clinicians believe that in a patient with severe COPD, a lung scan should not be performed. Their reasoning is that the V/Q scan is most likely interpreted as intermediate probability. In fact, if the V/Q scan is done and multiple segmental defects are seen, there can be an interpretation of high probability even in the presence of COPD, obviating the need for pulmonary angiography. In addition, there is a high complication rate of pulmonary arteriography in patients with COPD and elevated pulmonary artery pressures. Additionally, the V/Q lung scan may identify a particular lung segment of interest, enabling the radiologist to perform a selective arteriogram on that segment. Performance of the V/Q scan also allows the radiologist to choose the optimal projection, because a single view of a pulmonary arteriogram shows a lot of overlying vessels that can obscure each other. Signs of a PE on an arteriogram include an abrupt termination of a vessel or an intraluminal filling defect (Fig. 5–11).

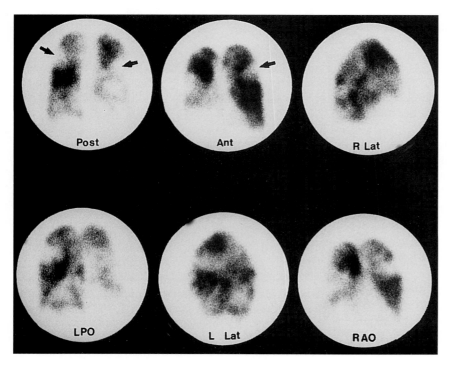

FIGURE 5–10. **Multiple pulmonary emboli.** This young lady with shortness of breath had a normal chest radiograph and a normal ventilation lung scan. The images here are from the perfusion portion of the nuclear medicine lung scan. Note that there are multiple segmental and subsegmental areas without perfusion *(arrows)* throughout both lungs. This is indicative of a high probability of pulmonary emboli. Post = posterior; Ant = anterior; R Lat = right lateral; LPO = left posterior oblique; L Lat = left lateral; RAO = right anterior oblique.

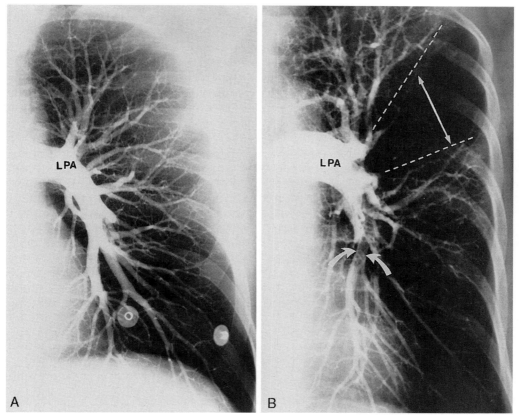

FIGURE 5–11. **Pulmonary emboli.** The gold standard for evaluation of pulmonary emboli is pulmonary angiography. In this technique, contrast agent is injected directly into the left main pulmonary artery (LPA). A normal angiogram *(A)* shows the typical branching structures of the pulmonary artery. The pulmonary arteriogram in a patient with pulmonary emboli *(B)* shows a large area of nonperfusion *(double-ended arrows).* This is suggestive of, but not specific for, pulmonary emboli. What is much more specific is the filling defect seen within the lumen of the left lower lobe pulmonary artery *(curved arrows).*

An area where no perfusion was identified on angiography does not necessarily mean that there is a pulmonary embolus, because there can be a bulla in this area.

A radiologist sometimes makes a correlation between the likelihood of PE, based on the size of an infiltrate seen on the chest radiograph and the size of a perfusion defect seen on a nuclear medicine lung scan. An embolus typically has a larger area of nonperfusion than the size of the resultant infiltrate. In the presence of PE, infiltrate on the chest radiograph most often represents infarcted lung. With a pneumonia, there is usually a large area of infiltrate on chest radiograph, but on the perfusion lung scan, the area of decreased perfusion is often relatively smaller. If the perfusion defect and the infiltrate are almost the same size, the probability of pulmonary embolus is intermediate.

Spiral CT scanning can also be used to evaluate pulmonary emboli, but the scans are somewhat more difficult to interpret, and they are less sensitive for small peripheral emboli than are V/Q scans. The gold standard for detection of pulmonary emboli is a selective pulmonary angiogram. Usually this is not done unless there is an intermediate probability V/Q scan or a significant discrepancy between the clinical suspicion and the V/Q scan interpretation.

Septic pulmonary emboli are common in intravenous drug users. They are usually seen as ill-defined pulmonary nodules, but they can cavitate (Fig. 5–12). Differentiation from metastatic disease is made mostly on the basis of patient history, and, in the case of septic emboli, positive blood cultures and presence of fever. V/Q lung scans are of little value in either suspected septic or fat embolism.

Coronary Artery Disease and Angina

CAD can be asymptomatic, be associated with stable or unstable angina, or be evident as the result of a myocardial ischemic event. Angina is considered stable if it occurs with a predictable level of exertion and has not changed in pattern for more than 60 days. It usually lasts 0.5 to 10 minutes and

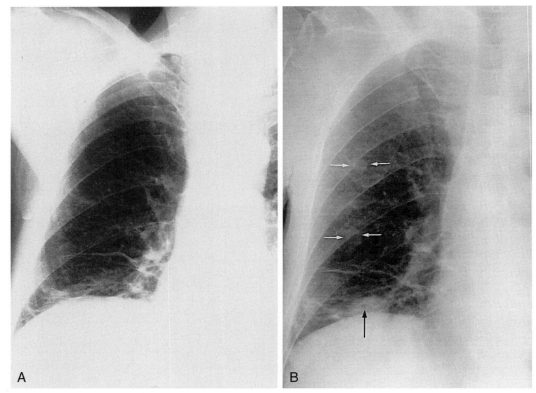

A   B

FIGURE 5–12. **Septic emboli.** In this patient, who is a drug abuser with a fever, the initial chest radiograph *(A)* shows some linear interstitial infiltrates just above the right hemidiaphragm. Several days later, a repeated chest radiograph *(B)* shows that several nodules had developed *(white arrows)* as well as an ill-defined lesion at the right lung base with a central area of cavitation *(black arrow).*

quickly subsides with rest or nitroglycerin. Unstable angina is pain at rest or with minimal exertion, typically lasting 20 to 30 minutes or increasing in frequency, duration, or severity. It is caused by insufficient oxygenation of the myocardium. Laboratory abnormalities (e.g., elevated CK-MB levels) of a myocardial infarction (MI) are not present.

Most patients with CAD have relatively normal chest radiographs. As CAD progresses, however, there may be cardiac decompensation with enlargement of the cardiac silhouette and signs within the pulmonary parenchyma of CHF. Although it is quite rare, occasionally, one can identify tram-tracking or parallel calcifications in the coronary arteries on a plain film (Fig. 5–13). Although calcification is a reliable marker for atherosclerosis, it does not indicate a hemodynamically significant coronary artery stenosis. With conventional CT, about 90% of patients who had coronary artery calcification had some stenosis, although not necessarily of significant size (more than 50% reduction in diameter). The major lesson is that if a chest CT does not show any coronary calcification, the risk of CAD is low but that presence of calcification does not imply a significant stenosis.

Evaluation of CAD usually involves a determina-

tion of whether the patient with chest pain has a hemodynamically significant stenosis, unstable plaque with ischemia, or an MI. The normal initial work-up includes tests of cardiac enzymes and electrocardiography (ECG) to exclude an MI. The indications for an initial noninvasive stress test are shown in Table 5–2. The utility of exercise ECG for diagnosing CAD is limited by both sensitivity (70%) and specificity (80% at best). As a result, both nuclear medicine and echocardiography techniques may be indicated in patients with normal exercise ECG results.

The least invasive imaging methods for evaluation of CAD are nuclear medicine myocardial perfusion studies and echocardiography. Nuclear medicine studies show the actual perfusion and therefore may be preferred.

A nuclear medicine study can use a number of radioactive myocardial agents (such as thallium-201 chloride or technetium-99m sestamibi) to image the musculature of the left ventricle. Images are typically obtained in slices or tomographic cuts. Patients are imaged both with and without the heart having been stressed either by exercise or by chemical agents (dipyridamole, adenosine, or dobutamine). If a defect is seen on both exercise and rest

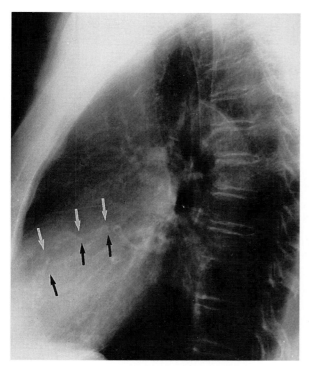

FIGURE 5–13. **Coronary artery calcification.** On this lateral view of the chest, calcification of the coronary arteries can be easily seen *(arrows)*.

images, there is a high probability of scar; if a defect is seen only on stress images, this implies ischemia (Fig. 5–14).

Echocardiography is based on stressing the patient and then looking for a regional wall motion abnormality, caused either by induced ischemia or by a previous infarction. Echocardiography provides indirect evidence of ischemia and tells little about loss of myocardial viability vs. abnormal motion caused by chronic ischemia.

TABLE 5–2 Indications for an Initial
Noninvasive Cardiac Stress Test*,†

Patients with a known history of coronary artery disease.
A male older than 60 years or a female older than 70 years with definite angina.
Patients experiencing hemodynamic changes or electrocardiographic changes during an episode of pain.
Patients who describe a change in angina pattern.
Patients with an electrocardiogram that reveals ST-segment elevation or depression of 1 mm or more.
Patients with an electrocardiogram that reveals marked symmetric T-wave inversion in multiple precordial leads.

*In patients with chest pain in whom a myocardial infarction has been excluded.

†Exercise stress test, pharmacologic stress test, nuclear medicine myocardial stress test, or echocardiographic stress test.

Patients with two or more episodes of chest pain and one risk factor should have a cardiac stress test. Stress tests are usually performed on patients 6 weeks after hospital discharge for an MI. They are also indicated in patients with a prior positive stress test, as well as for periodic assessment of those patients with a CAD event or as a result of progression of angina.

Visualization of the individual coronary arteries and the location, extent, and severity of stenosis is best done by coronary angiography. Because this is an invasive, expensive procedure and the radiation dose is high, it is not used as a screening test. Obviously, angiography must be done if bypass surgery or percutaneous catheter therapy is contemplated. Catheter techniques include dilating of a particular area of coronary stenosis (angioplasty), placement of a rigid device in the lumen (stent), or infusion of a clot-lysing agent.

Myocardial Infarction

An acute MI is usually diagnosed by history, ECG changes, and laboratory abnormalities (e.g., elevated CK-MB levels). If the patient is within 6 hours of the onset of chest pain, a coronary angiogram is indicated in a facility where balloon angioplasty, stent placement, or thrombolytic therapy is performed. Coronary angiography is also indicated if there is cardiogenic shock, papillary muscle rupture, LVEF less than 35%, or an ischemic VSD, or the patient has an arrhythmia and is a cardiac arrest survivor. If the patient presents later than 6 hours with evidence of an MI, initial evaluation is done either by rest or stress ECG, nuclear medicine myocardial scan, or echocardiogram.

▓ AORTA

Anatomy and Imaging Techniques

A number of anomalies of the aortic arch may occur, the most common of which is a right-sided aortic arch (Fig. 5–15). Right-sided aortic arches are associated with congenital heart disease in 5% of cases.

Calcification of the aortic arch is common in persons older than 60 years and is easily seen on a chest radiograph. It is fairly unusual before the age of 50 years, and calcification suggests a higher than average incidence of atherosclerotic disease in such patients (Fig. 5–16).

Injection of contrast material directly into the aorta (contrast angiography) yields the most definitive evaluation of normal and anomalous anatomy. Effective imaging can also be done with CT or MRI

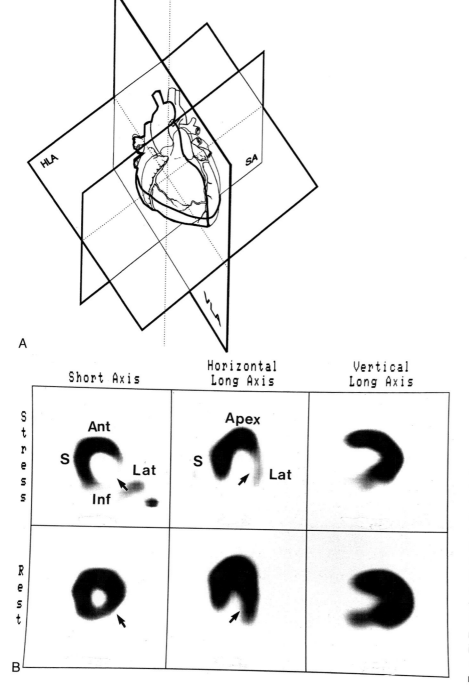

A

	Short Axis	Horizontal Long Axis	Vertical Long Axis

S
t
r
e
s
s

R
e
s
t

B

FIGURE 5–14. **Assessment of myocardial perfusion.** There are a number of nuclear medicine agents that can label the myocardium. *A,* Utilizing computer techniques, images of the left ventricular wall can be obtained in the short axis (SA), horizontal long axis (HLA), and vertical long axis (VLA). By imaging during stress and rest, it is possible to tell whether there is an area of reversibility (ischemia), or whether there is a fixed defect (scar or infarction). *B,* In this case, the *arrows* demonstrate the defect during stress that reverses or fills-in during rest images, indicating ischemia of the inferolateral wall of the left ventricle. S = septum; Ant = anterior; Inf = inferior; Lat = lateral.

scanning and to a lesser extent with transesophageal ultrasound imaging.

Coarctation of the Aorta

Coarctation is a congenital narrowing of the proximal descending thoracic aorta, which usually occurs in the vicinity of the ductus arteriosus. Symptoms are rarely, if ever, present during childhood. The diagnosis is usually discovered during a physical examination by noting diminished or absent

femoral pulses or by finding that the patient has hypertension of the upper extremities.

On the chest radiograph, the heart may be normal or may have slight left ventricular enlargement. There is prominence of the ascending aorta. Occasionally, the actual site of the coarctation can be visualized as narrowing in the proximal portion of the descending aorta. In addition, there is often prominence along the left paratracheal region in continuity with the outline of the aortic knob caused by dilatation of the left subclavian artery. A rather characteristic finding is notching of the inferior as-

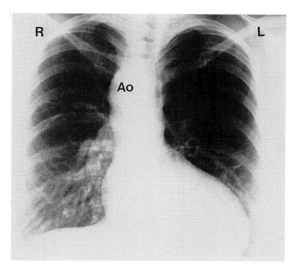

FIGURE 5–15. **Right-sided aortic arch.** While the heart is in its normal left-sided configuration, the ascending, transverse, and descending thoracic aorta (Ao) are on the right side.

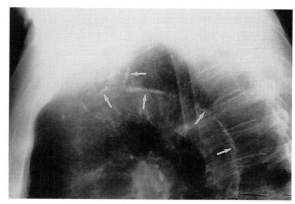

FIGURE 5–16. **Calcification of the aortic arch and great vessels.** The lateral view of the upper chest clearly shows areas of increased density in the walls of the aortic arch *(arrows)* and in the great vessels.

pect of the ribs due to erosion by tortuous and dilated intercostal arteries (Fig. 5–17). The actual site of stenosis is best visualized by either contrast angiography or MRI. Treatment is surgical, consisting of resection of the coarctated segment.

Aortic Tears

Traumatic disruption of the aorta usually occurs as a result of an automobile accident. In fact, rupture of the aorta causes 15 to 40% of the fatalities resulting from motor vehicle accidents. Rapid deceleration can cause the aorta to tear, usually in the proximal portion of the descending aorta at the level

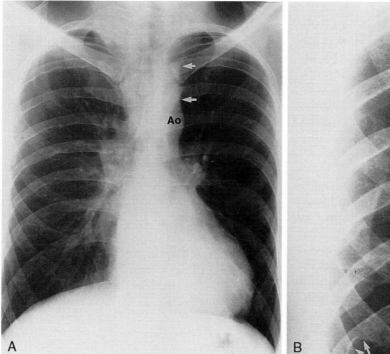

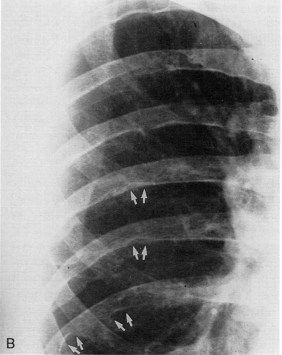

FIGURE 5–17. **Coarctation of the aorta.** A chest radiograph *(A)* was obtained in this patient who had high blood pressure in both upper extremities. It demonstrates prominence of the left cardiac border (due to left ventricular hypertrophy). There is also a dilated left subclavian artery *(arrows)* due to increased flow, because blood has difficulty getting down the descending aorta (Ao). A close-up view *(B)* of the chest shows notching along the inferior aspects of the ribs *(arrows)* as a result of dilated intercostal arteries.

of the attachment of the ligamentum arteriosum. Ninety-five percent occur at this level, and approximately 5% occur at the level of the aortic root. Signs of a tear on an anteroposterior chest radiograph include a mediastinal width of more than 8 to 10 cm at or above the level of the aortic arch, apical pleural density (capping) caused by blood above the left apical portion of the lung, deviation of the trachea or nasogastric tube to the right, and depression of the left mainstem bronchus. Usually, there is also poor definition of the aortic arch and opacification of the aortopulmonary window (Fig. 5–18). CT scanning is the initial test of choice to exclude aortic injury and to evaluate the rest of the chest and abdomen for other associated traumatic injuries. About 10% of patients have equivocal findings and require an aortogram.

Thoracic Aortic Aneurysms

Aneurysms of the aortic arch and descending thoracic aorta may be the result of atherosclerosis; inflammatory, mechanical, traumatic, or congenital causes; fibromuscular dysplasia; and cystic medial necrosis. An aneurysm of the ascending aorta historically was most likely caused by syphilis. This is quite rare at the present time, and Marfan's syndrome is a more likely cause.

Aneurysms may be discovered incidentally, or the patient may present with pain, rupture, new pulse deficit, unexplained hypotension, or thromboembolic complications. Aneurysms of the thoracic aorta are fairly easy to identify on chest radiographs as widening of the ascending aorta (>5 cm) or aortic arch (>3.5 cm) (Fig. 5–19). Sudden onset of chest pain in a patient with hypertension or atherosclerosis should suggest aortic rupture or ongoing dissection.

Detailed evaluation of an aneurysm can be easily performed using CT scanning with a bolus of intravenous contrast material. This allows the lumen to be visualized as well as clot along the inner wall of the aneurysm. Many patients have portions of the clot that come loose and lead to distal thromboembolic events. An arteriogram is not the best initial method for evaluation of aneurysms, because usually all that is visualized is the patent lumen and not the outer wall or the thickness of intraluminal clot. In addition, a catheter in the aorta raises the possibility of knocking portions of clot loose. MRI can be used, but imaging times are longer than on CT scanning. Further, if the patient is unstable, it is difficult to manage life support owing to the high magnetic field strength and the inability to bring ferromagnetic materials into the MRI room.

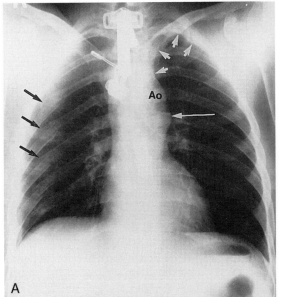

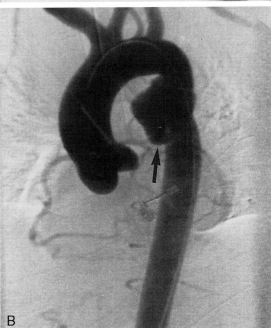

FIGURE 5–18. **Aortic tear.** A chest radiograph *(A)* obtained in an individual who was in a motor vehicle accident shows multiple rib fractures *(black arrows)*, filling-in of the normal concavity of the anteroposterior window *(long white arrow)*, and fluid over the apex of the left lung *(short white arrows)*. These latter two findings are suggestive of mediastinal hemorrhage. A digital subtraction contrast aortogram *(B)* shows a bulge of contrast material *(arrow)* caused by a tear in a typical location.

Aortic Dissection

Aortic dissection is the result of an intimal tear causing separation of the layers of the wall of the aorta. It is more common in men than in women and usually occurs between the ages of 45 and 70 years. The incidence is higher in patients with Mar-

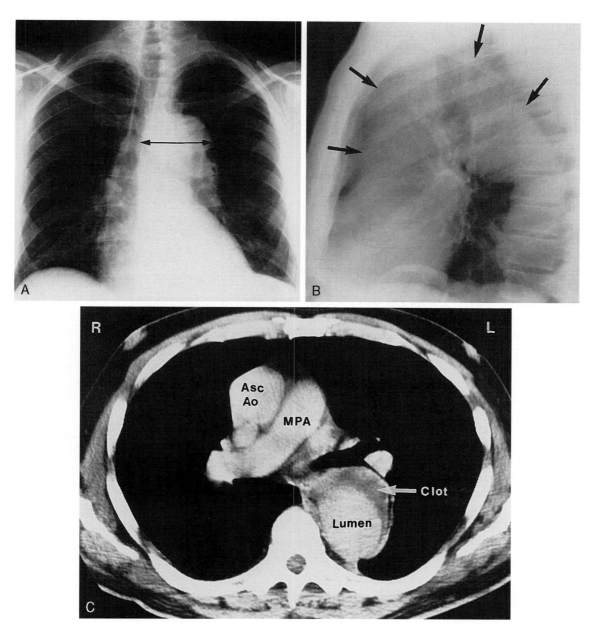

FIGURE 5–19. **Aortic aneurysm.** A posteroanterior chest radiograph *(A)* demonstrates a markedly widened aortic arch *(double-ended arrow)*. The lateral view *(B)* shows marked dilatation of the entire aortic arch *(arrows)*. A contrast-enhanced transverse computed tomography scan *(C)* shows the ascending aorta (Asc Ao), the main pulmonary artery (MPA), and marked dilatation of the proximal portion of the descending thoracic aorta. The contrast-enhanced lumen and mural clot are seen as well.

fan's syndrome, coarctation of the aorta, and bicuspid aortic valve disease. Aortic dissection also commonly occurs in patients with aortic atherosclerosis, particularly those who are hypertensive. Dissection carries a high mortality if undiagnosed and untreated. Dissection of the thoracic aorta proximal to the left subclavian artery is a surgical emergency, whereas dissections of the descending thoracic aorta are usually managed by medical treatment of the patient's hypertension.

The dissection can allow blood to flow in between the layers of the aortic wall, causing a false lumen.

Sometimes, this false lumen re-enters the true lumen farther down the aorta. Generally, aortic dissection begins either in the ascending aorta or in the descending aorta just distal to the left subclavian artery. About one third of patients have extremity pain, and another one third have a central nervous system abnormality if the dissection involves the ascending aorta and great vessels.

Aortic dissection should be suspected in a hypertensive patient with known atherosclerosis and chest pain, particularly if there is a new central nervous system event, pulse deficit, or 10 mm Hg or greater systolic blood pressure difference between the arms. Dissection should also be suspected if on a chest radiograph there is a double contour of the aortic arch, if there is progressive serial enlargement, or if there is displacement of intimal calcification more than 6 mm from the outer aortic margin. This last sign has to be interpreted with caution, because a minor degree of rotation of the chest may cause anterior arch calcification to project eccentrically over the posterior arch. On chest radiograph, most patients with a dissection have a dilated aorta with a widened mediastinum and cardiomegaly.

Enlargement of the aortic arch on a single film is not specific for a dissection, inasmuch as the aortic arch can frequently be enlarged in patients with hypertension or atherosclerosis. Lack of enlargement of the aortic arch should not be taken as evidence that a dissection is not present, because the arch is of normal size in 25% of dissection cases.

An angiogram can sometimes show the true and false lumens (Fig. 5–20). The diagnosis of dissection can also be made by a contrasted CT or an MRI study. CT scanning is somewhat quicker, and it is easier to manage a patient who may suddenly decompensate. Demonstration of an intimal flap on CT is conclusive evidence of a dissection. An intimal flap and the false lumen can be seen in 70% of patients. Transesophageal ultrasound imaging can be used to evaluate dissections or aneurysms of the descending thoracic aorta, because the esophagus is in such close proximity. Generally, however, surgeons want a more complete evaluation, such as that provided by CT, before they operate on a patient.

Abdominal Aortic Aneurysm

In patients with extensive atherosclerosis, striking calcification of the abdominal aorta and iliac arteries (Fig. 5–21) is often seen on plain radiographs, particularly the lateral view of the lumbar spine. The abdominal aorta should not exceed 2.5 cm in diameter. As with the thoracic aorta, once the diameter exceeds 5 cm, there is an increased likelihood of rupture (Fig. 5–22).

An easy noninvasive examination of the abdominal aorta can be done using abdominal ultrasonography. Not only can the aorta be visualized but also other vessels, such as the superior mesenteric artery and vein, can be seen (Fig. 5–23). Abdominal ultrasonography is indicated for suspected abdominal aortic aneurysm in an asymptomatic patient or for follow-up. Ultrasonography follow-up is indicated in persons who have had a prior examination demonstrating abdominal aortic diameter of 4 to 4.9

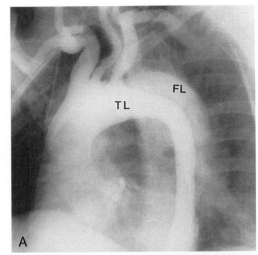

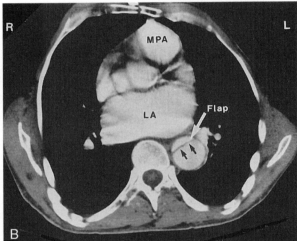

FIGURE 5–20. **Aortic dissection.** A standard contrast aortogram in the left anterior oblique projection *(A)* shows contrast material in the true lumen (TL) and the great vessels. Contrast material is also seen in the false lumen (FL), which is a channel within the wall of the aorta. A contrast-enhanced transverse computed tomography scan *(B)* easily shows the intimal flap between the TL and the FL. MPA = main pulmonary artery; LA = left atrium.

cm. This is done at 6 months and annually thereafter. If there is an interval change of 0.5 cm or more or the diameter exceeds 5.0 cm, a surgical consultation is indicated. In a symptomatic patient whose condition raises concern of clot within the aorta, dissection, or rupture, a CT scan with an intravenous bolus of contrast material is the initial test of choice.

■ PERIPHERAL VESSELS

Imaging Modalities

The gold standard for evaluation of peripheral arteries is done by using contrast angiography. This typically involves percutaneous access to the femo-

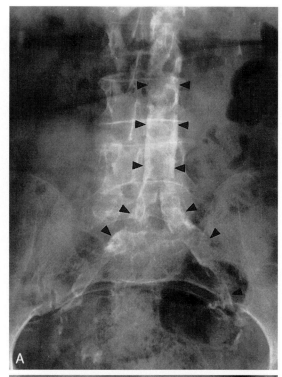

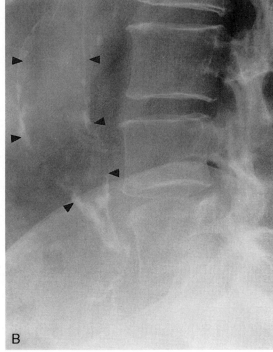

FIGURE 5–21. **Calcification of the abdominal aorta.** *A,* A plain radiograph of the abdomen shows extensive calcification of the abdominal aorta and iliac vessels. *B,* Calcification of the abdominal aorta is usually much easier to see on the lateral view. If the distance from the anterior calcified wall back to a vertebral body exceeds 5 cm, an abdominal aortic aneurysm is present.

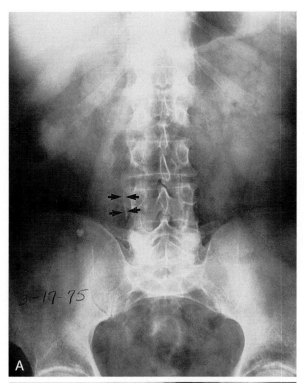

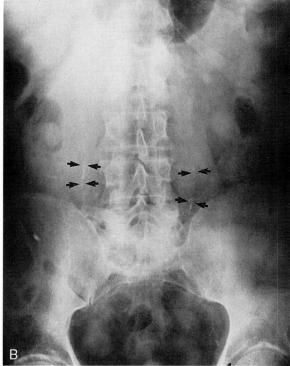

FIGURE 5–22. **Progressive development of an abdominal aortic aneurysm.** A plain radiograph *(A)* of the abdomen of a patient done in 1975 showed a small area of linear calcification overlying the right side of L5 *(arrows)*. This represents calcification within the wall of the aorta. A repeated radiograph 10 years later *(B)* showed bilateral linear areas of calcification *(arrows)*. The distance between these two linear calcifications represents the width of the aneurysm.

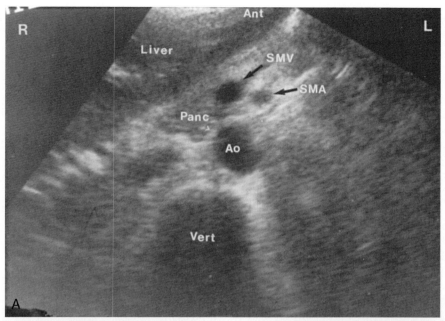

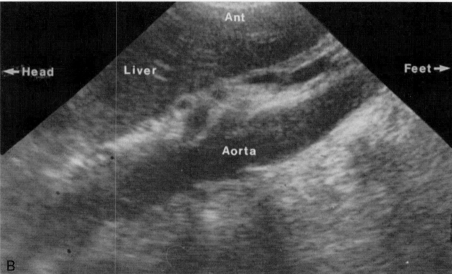

FIGURE 5–23. **Ultrasound demonstration of normal vascular anatomy in the upper abdomen.** A transverse sonogram *(A)* shows the liver, pancreas (Panc), vertebral body (vert), the superior mesenteric artery (SMA), superior mesenteric vein (SMV), and abdominal aorta (Ao). A longitudinal view just to the left of midline (B) shows the liver and abdominal aorta as well as the origin of the celiac axis and superior mesenteric artery.

ral artery and placement of the catheter up the aorta with selective catheterization of the individual vessels. The contrast angiogram shows exquisite detail and can easily demonstrate areas of stenosis or aneurysm.

All contrast angiography of the vessels of the head and neck carries a small risk of stroke, due to injection of air bubbles, and of vascular spasm or clotting, due to the catheter. Recently, advances in CT and MRI have allowed noninvasive visualization of blood vessels. Whereas, both methods are useful, neither of these has the detail of an angiogram.

Many peripheral vessels are routinely evaluated by using duplex ultrasonography. *Duplex* refers to the machine's ability to obtain images as well as to use Doppler ultrasound to evaluate magnitude and direction of flow. Typically, images and evaluations

are done for limited sections of relatively large vessels such as the femoral or carotid artery.

Carotid Bruit

A carotid bruit may be identified as part of a stroke or transient ischemic attack work-up or as an incidental result of a physical examination done for other reasons. Carotid bruits are not sufficiently predictive of high-grade symptomatic carotid stenoses to identify those that are amenable to surgery. As a result, both asymptomatic and symptomatic patients with a bruit should be evaluated with duplex ultrasonography to determine the degree and extent of stenosis. Interpretation is based on the image of the vessel walls and the flow across the area in question. Patients with a high-grade (>60 to 80%) stenosis may benefit from a carotid endarterectomy. The role of surgery in low-grade stenoses or in asymptomatic patients remains debatable. Surgery is considered in those patients with recurring transient ischemic attacks while receiving medical therapy and those with severe carotid ulceration. Although CT and MRI can demonstrate evidence of CAD, they are not considered capable of providing precise estimates of stenosis; therefore, conventional arteriography is indicated before surgery.

Carotid ultrasound imaging is also indicated in patients with other vascular disease and before cardiac surgery or aortic aneurysm repair. It is also widely done in patients with other peripheral vascu-lar disease, for example, those with foot pain at rest, nonhealing foot ulcers, gangrenous changes of the feet, and a resting ankle-brachial index at or below 0.5.

Stenosis of Peripheral Vessels

Evaluation of abdominal and pelvic vessels other than the aorta is best done by contrast angiography. Not only can the major vessels, such as hepatic artery and renal arteries, be identified, but also all their branches can be seen in great detail. Even small lumbar arteries can be visualized. Atherosclerotic changes and areas of stenosis are also easily identified.

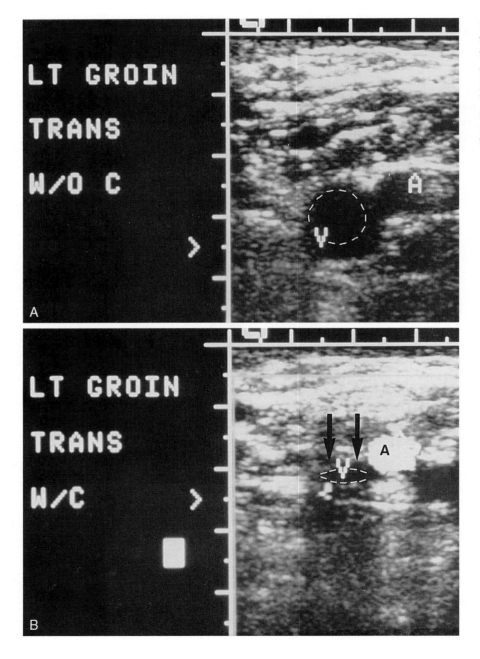

FIGURE 5–24. **Normal ultrasound of the femoral vein.** A transverse view of the left inner thigh is obtained without compression *(A)* and then with compression *(B)*. Without compression, the vein is seen to be round, but with compression the vein is easily flattened *(arrows)*. The artery is seen just lateral to the vein. V = vein; A = artery.

After identification of areas of stenosis, it is possible to insert a catheter that has a balloon on the end and to dilate the areas of stenosis. This is called *percutaneous transluminal angioplasty.* The method involves fracturing the vascular intima and media and stretching the adventitia, thus expanding the diameter of the vessel. Atherosclerotic plaques themselves are quite hard and are rarely fractured by dilatation. The success rate depends on the vessel, and the success of angioplasty is greatest in the larger vessels such as the iliac arteries.

Renal Artery Stenosis and Hypertension

Only 1 to 2% of hypertension is due to renal vascular disease. The clinical features that help distinguish this from other forms of hypertension are occurrence at an unusual age (<30 years or >50 years) or poor response to medical therapy. Physical examination may reveal a bruit in the flank or upper abdomen. Laboratory evaluation may rarely yield evidence of hyperaldosteronism, including hypokalemia and metabolic acidosis. The appropriate initial imaging test is not an intravenous urogram but rather a nuclear medicine captopril renogram. The captopril causes the affected kidney to temporarily have poor function. If this occurs, the study is repeated without captopril and if this is normal (because the kidney compensates for the renal artery stenosis), an angiogram and possible angioplasty are indicated.

Deep Venous Thrombosis

Deep venous thrombosis (DVT) fails to produce clinical signs in half the patients who have it. Thrombosis in calf veins is usually insignificant in that it rarely leads to PE; however, in the femoral veins and pelvic veins, thrombi are significant and require immediate anticoagulation. Risk factors for

FIGURE 5–25. **Ultrasound demonstration of femoral vein thrombosis.** Images of the left thigh are obtained without compression *(A)* and *(B)* with compression in the direction of the dark *arrows.* The vein could be seen in both instances, and it is not compressible because it contains clot. Additionally, there are echoes within the vein as a result of clot. V = vein; A = artery; C = clot.

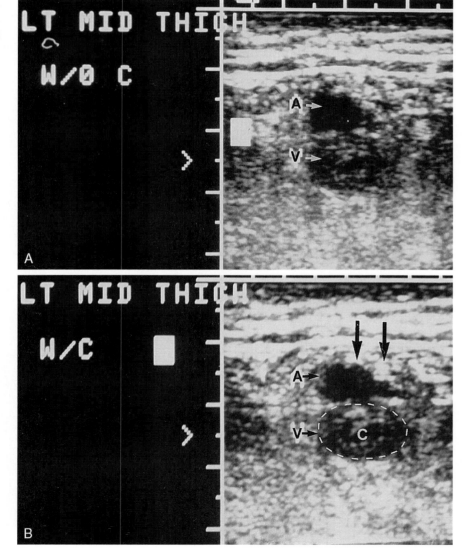

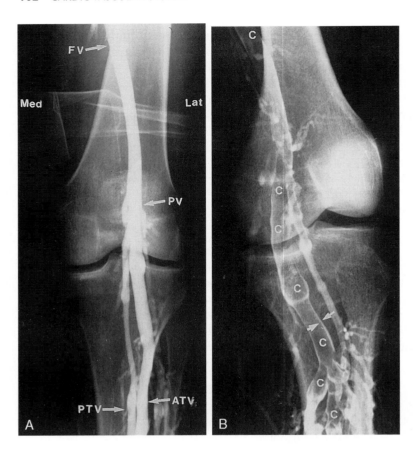

FIGURE 5–26. **Venous thrombosis about the knee.** A normal contrast venogram *(A)* near the knee shows the contrast material coming up the anterior (ATV) and posterior (PTV) tibial veins into the popliteal vein (PV) and then into the femoral vein (FV). A venogram *(B)* in a different patient with leg swelling demonstrates that the veins are filled with clot (C). A small amount of contrast agent is able to pass by and outline the clot in some veins *(arrows)*.

FIGURE 5–27. **Inferior vena caval filter.** An expandable wire mesh basket *(arrows)* has been placed in the inferior vena cava. This can be done by pushing the device out of a catheter and allowing it to expand in place. This keeps the large clots from traveling from the lower extremities and pelvis, up the inferior vena cava, and into the lung.

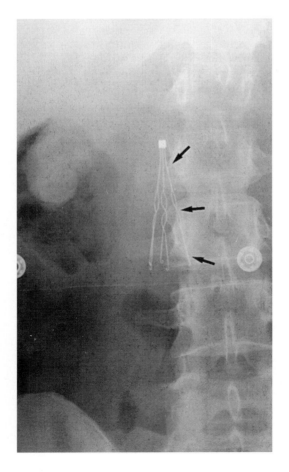

DVT include prolonged bed rest, immobilization of an extremity, pregnancy, oral contraceptives, malignancy, and postoperative and traumatic circumstances.

The initial imaging test of choice for a patient with suspected DVT is duplex ultrasonography of the thigh and inguinal region. Ultrasound imaging has a sensitivity and specificity of approximately 95%. For proximal DVT, the femoral artery and vein can both easily be visualized using ultrasonography. With pressure, the femoral vein normally compresses (Fig. 5–24). If there is a clot within the vein, echoes are seen within the lumen, and no compression is identified (Fig. 5–25). Color Doppler ultrasonography can be used to classify flow in the vein into none or partial flow. Thrombolytic therapy can often be instituted on the basis of ultrasound results.

The most accurate method for imaging veins is contrast venography. With this approach, contrast material is injected into the veins on the dorsum of the foot and the contrast material is visualized as it proceeds up the veins of the leg and into the pelvis. Contrast venography allows visualization of the deep venous system but not of the superficial venous system. Clots can be seen as intraluminal defects with contrast material surrounding them (Fig. 5–26). Total obstruction with visualization of collateral veins can also be seen with DVT. One of the problems with contrast venography is that it involves the use of intravenously administered iodinated contrast material. Sometimes venous access is difficult in patients who have a grossly swollen leg. It is possible that the contrast material itself may cause some inflammation of the vein and may carry a low but real complication rate of thrombophlebitis.

Recurrent DVT or DVT that is not successfully treated with heparin can result in multiple episodes of PE. Owing to the life-threatening nature of this problem, methods have been developed to keep the thrombi from migrating into the lung. Probably the most frequently employed method is placement of a filter in the inferior vena cava (Fig. 5–27). Access is gained through the femoral vein, and contrast material is injected to make sure that no clot is in the iliac vein or inferior vena cava itself. After this, a catheter is advanced to the level just below the renal veins, and an expandable wire net or basket is pushed out the end of the catheter. At this time the most commonly used device is a Greenfield filter.

Work-Up of Claudication

Claudication is most commonly caused by chronic arterial ischemia from atherosclerosis. The atherosclerosis can involve any site from the aortoiliac region distally. The simplest method to document lower extremity arterial occlusive disease is with ultrasonography. This is most often done in a vascular laboratory; Doppler ultrasonography is used to derive an ankle-brachial index. A normal ankle-brachial index is 1.0 or greater. Before any type of surgical intervention, an arteriogram that includes visualization of the aortoiliac, femoral, popliteal, and tibial arteries is required. There are few imaging tests that are useful in evaluating extremity pain caused by venous or small vessel insufficiency, or for neurologic or muscular pain.

GENERAL SUGGESTED READINGS

Crummy AB, McDermott JC, Baron MG: The Cardiovascular System. *In* Juhl JH, Crummy AB, Kuhlman JE (eds): Paul and Juhl's Essentials of Radiologic Imaging, 7th ed. Philadelphia, Lippincott-Raven, 1998, pp 1197–1268.

Gedgaudas E, Moller JH, Castaneda-Zuniga WR, Amplatz K: Cardiovascular Radiology. Philadelphia, WB Saunders, 1984.

Juhl JH, Kuhlman JE: Circulatory Disturbances. *In* Juhl JH, Crummy AB, Kuhlman JE (eds): Paul and Juhl's Essentials of Radiologic Imaging, 7th ed. Philadelphia, Lippincott-Raven, 1998, pp 987–1010.

Shelton DK: Cardiovascular Radiology, Section V. *In* Brant WE, Helms CA (eds): Fundamentals of Diagnostic Radiology, 2nd ed. Philadelphia, Lippincott Williams & Wilkins, 1999, pp 525–650.

6

ABDOMINAL IMAGING

■ ANATOMY AND IMAGING TECHNIQUES

The most common imaging study of the abdomen is referred to as *kidneys, ureter, bladder (KUB)* or supine plain film (Fig. 6–1). When examining this film, look at the bony structures, the lung bases, and the soft tissue and gas patterns (Table 6–1). The soft tissue pattern should include evaluation of the lateral psoas margins. Whether or not you see them bilaterally, only faintly, or throughout their length depends on the shape of the psoas and the amount of retroperitoneal fat in that particular individual. It can be normal not to see the psoas margin on either side. If the psoas margin is visible on one side but not on the other, most commonly this is due to normal anatomic variation. In about 25% of cases, however, pathology is evident on the side of the obscured psoas margin.

The liver is seen as a homogeneous soft tissue density in the right upper quadrant. The spleen can sometimes be seen as a smaller homogeneous density in the left upper quadrant. Except if it is a massive enlargement, minimal to moderate enlargement of either one of these organs is difficult to ascertain. Clinical palpation and percussion are at least as accurate.

Evaluation of the gas pattern is also important (Table 6–2). Because people routinely swallow air and often drink carbonated beverages, the stomach

---

TABLE 6–1 Items to Look for on a Plain Abdominal Film (KUB)

Gas Patterns Stomach, small bowel, and rectosigmoid Abnormal or ectopic collections
Organ Shapes and Sizes Liver Spleen Kidneys Soft tissue pelvic masses
Calcification
Asymmetric Psoas Margins
Skeleton
Basilar Lung Abnormalities

KUB = kidneys, ureter, bladder.

TABLE 6–2 Evaluation of Gas Patterns on a Plain Film of the Abdomen

Collections Normally Present Look for dilatation of structure and assessment of wall or mucosal thickness in stomach, small bowel, colon, and rectosigmoid
Collections Not Normally Present Free air under the diaphragm (upright film) Free air on supine films (double bowel wall sign) Right upper quadrant: Portal vein (peripheral in liver), biliary system (central in liver) Small bubbles in an abscess Emphysematous cholecystitis, pyelonephritis, or cystitis

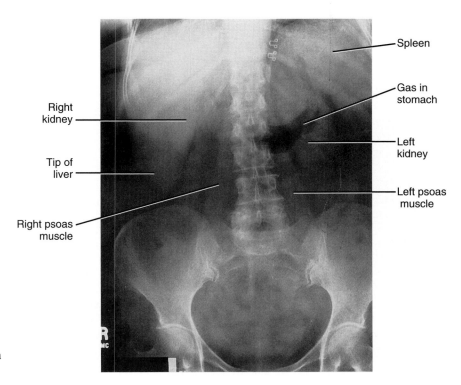

Spleen

Gas in stomach

Left kidney

Left psoas muscle

Right kidney

Tip of liver

Right psoas muscle

FIGURE 6–1. **Normal anatomy seen on a supine radiograph of the abdomen.**

almost always has some gas within it. When a person is lying on his or her back, the air goes to the most anterior portion of the stomach, which is the body and antrum; this is seen as a curvilinear air collection, just along the left side of the upper lumbar spine (Fig. 6–2). If the person has swallowed a lot of air, there are gas bubbles within the entire gastrointestinal (GI) tract extending from the stomach to the rectum. Gas in the small bowel can usually be identified, because small bowel mucosa has extremely fine lines that cross all the way across the lumen. Most small bowel gas is located in the left midabdomen and the lower central abdomen. The colon can often be traced from the cecum in the right lower quadrant to both the hepatic and the splenic flexures and down to the sigmoid. The colon often has a bubbly appearance representing a mixture of gas and fecal material. Colonic air often has a somewhat cloverleaf-shaped appearance caused by the haustra of the colon. Normal small bowel should not exceed 3 cm in diameter, and the colon should not exceed 6 cm. The cecum can normally be somewhat larger than the rest of the colon and may be up to 8 cm in diameter.

In addition to a supine abdominal film, a three-way view of the abdomen is often obtained. The additional two views are an upright posteroanterior (PA) chest radiograph and a view of the abdomen taken with the patient standing upright. The reason for taking the PA view of the chest is to look for chest pathology that may be mimicking or causing abdominal symptoms, as well as to look for free air underneath the hemidiaphragms. The reason for the standing view of the abdomen is to look at the air-fluid levels within the bowel to differentiate between an obstruction and the ileus.

Computed tomography (CT) scanning is the most common procedure used to image nonintestinal abdominal pathology. CT anatomy is presented in Figure 6–3. With new scanners, the entire abdomen and pelvis can be imaged in several minutes. The patients are commonly prepared by having them drink oral contrast agent for an hour or so before the examination. This is important because it allows differentiation of bowel from other soft tissues. If there is suspected pelvic pathology, rectal contrast agent should also be given at the time of the examination. For most examinations, if renal function is normal, intravenous contrast agent is also given. This clearly outlines the vascular structures and provides excellent visualization of the kidneys, ureter, and bladder.

Ultrasonography is used primarily to image the liver, kidneys, gallbladder, common bile duct, and, to a lesser extent, the pancreas and appendix. Ultrasound imaging is often limited by the inability of the sound to penetrate air and by loops of bowel that may obscure underlying pathology. Ascites is easily detected and localized for paracentesis.

Nuclear medicine scans provide physiologic information that is often not available using other imaging techniques. It is often used to quantitate gas-

Text continued on page 111

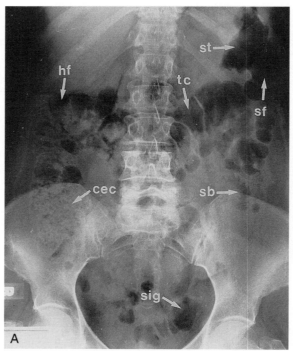

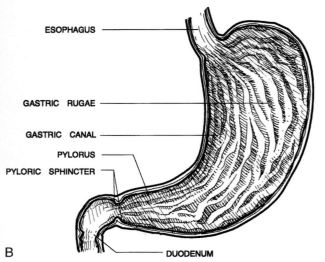

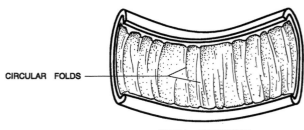

CIRCULAR FOLDS

SMALL INTESTINE

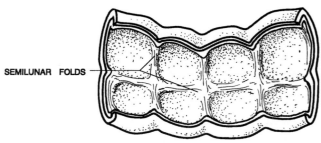

SEMILUNAR FOLDS

C

LARGE INTESTINE

FIGURE 6–2. *A to C,* **Normal bowel gas pattern.** Gas is normally swallowed and can be seen in the stomach (st). Small amounts of air normally can be seen in the small bowel (sb), and this is usually in the left midabdomen or central portion of the abdomen. In this patient, gas can be seen throughout the entire colon, including the cecum (cec). In the area where the air is mixed with feces, there is a mottled pattern. Cloverleaf-shaped collections of air are seen in the hepatic flexure (hf), transverse colon (tc), splenic flexure (sf), and sigmoid (sig).

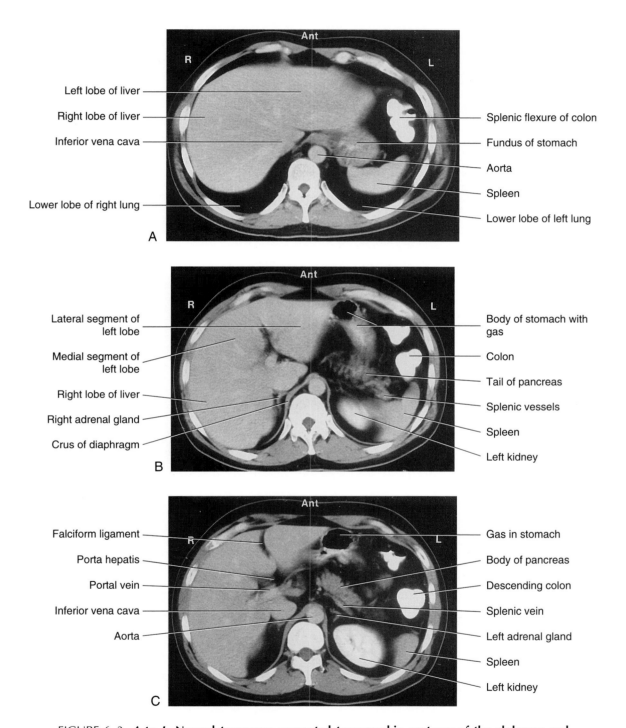

FIGURE 6–3. *A to L,* **Normal transverse computed tomographic anatomy of the abdomen and pelvis.** The patient has been given oral, rectal, and intravenous contrast media.

Illustration continued on following page

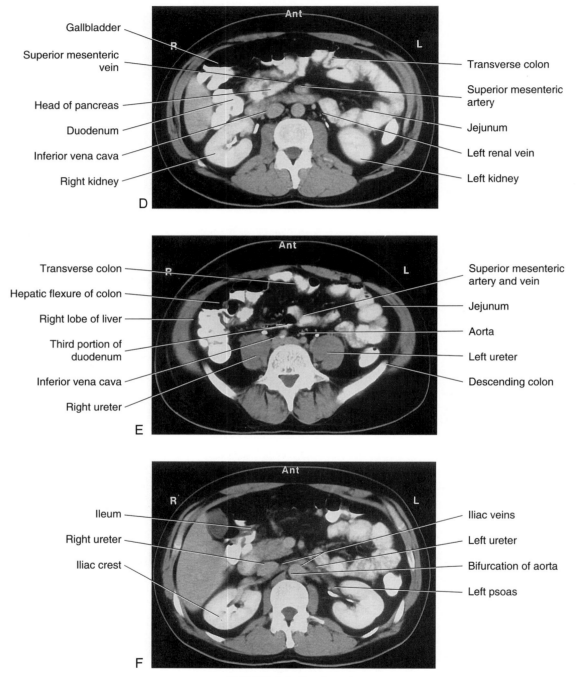

Gallbladder
Superior mesenteric vein
Head of pancreas
Duodenum
Inferior vena cava
Right kidney

Transverse colon
Superior mesenteric artery
Jejunum
Left renal vein
Left kidney

D

Transverse colon
Hepatic flexure of colon
Right lobe of liver
Third portion of duodenum
Inferior vena cava
Right ureter

Superior mesenteric artery and vein
Jejunum
Aorta
Left ureter
Descending colon

E

Ileum
Right ureter
Iliac crest

Iliac veins
Left ureter
Bifurcation of aorta
Left psoas

F

FIGURE 6–3 *Continued*

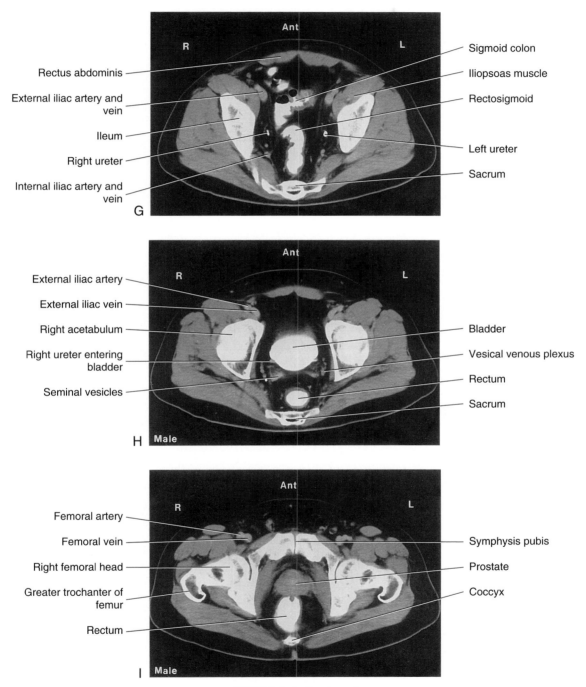

FIGURE 6–3 *Continued*

Illustration continued on following page

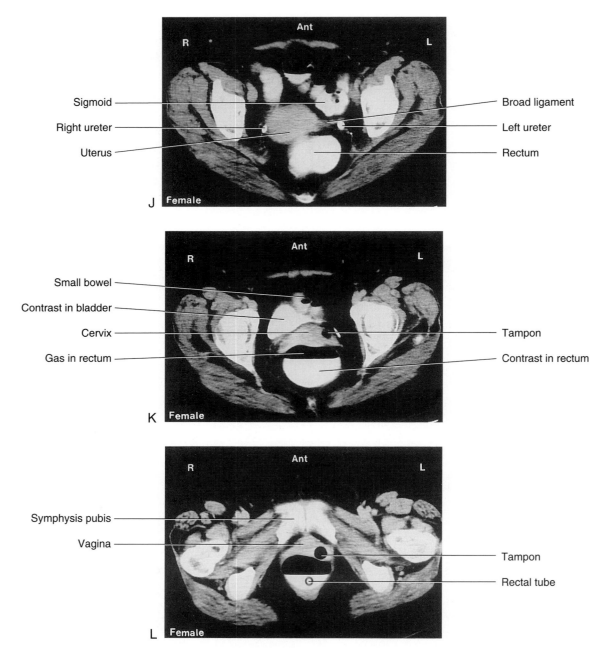

FIGURE 6–3 *Continued*

tric esophageal reflux and gastric emptying, diagnose acute cholecystitis and biliary leaks, and determine the site of GI bleeding.

Both contrast x-ray studies and endoscopy can be used to evaluate most of the tubular GI tract with the exception of the small bowel. The latter can only be effectively imaged with contrast material. Primary care providers often wonder which type of procedure to order. Both have advantages and disadvantages. Contrast x-ray studies are much cheaper and do not require sedation. In addition to anatomic detail, they can provide information about motility. Endoscopy has the advantage of providing direct visualization and allowing for biopsies and for occasional therapeutic interventions such as cauterization or injection. Endoscopy is the only technique consistently available for evaluation of the pancreatic duct. For most clinical problems, no randomized studies are available indicating clear superiority of one technique over the other. As a result, in this chapter we have chosen to present what we believe is the current status of practice. For some presenting symptoms (such as positive fecal occult blood test [FOBT]), the choice of procedure is affected by patient age. Bleeding from upper GI lesions is more common in patients younger than 40 years, and bleeding from lower GI lesions is more common in older individuals.

Pneumoperitoneum

It is easiest to identify small amounts of free air in the peritoneal cavity by doing an upright chest radiograph. In this manner, as little as 3 or 4 mL of air may be visualized (Fig. 6–4). An upright abdominal film is usually not useful to look for free air, because the domes of the diaphragms are often off the upper edge of the film. It is quite difficult to appreciate even relatively large amounts of free air within the peritoneal cavity by looking at a supine (KUB) view of the abdomen. If there is a lot of free air, the bowel wall may be outlined by air. If the patient is too sick to stand up, a left lateral decubitus view of the abdomen can suffice. In this manner, with the patient lying on the left side (for 10 to 15 minutes), small amounts of air can be seen tracking up over the lateral aspect of the right lobe of the liver.

Intra-abdominal Abscesses and Fever of Unknown Origin

Air can be seen within some, but by no means all, abscesses. Although a large abscess may be appreciated on a plain film, it is often difficult to tell whether the air is within the bowel or in some other structure. For this reason, when an abdominal or pelvic abscess is suspected, the imaging test of choice is a CT scan (Fig. 6–5). Under these circumstances, it is important that the CT scan be done with GI contrast so that the entire bowel is opacified. If this is not done, it may be difficult, even on a CT scan, to differentiate a collection of bowel that has air and fluid within it from an abscess. If CT is not available, ultrasonography is good for evaluating the liver, pelvis, and, to a lesser extent, the pancreas and appendix. Ultrasound imaging is poor for the detection of abscesses in the lower retroperitoneum or in between bowel loops.

The imaging work-up of a patient with a fever of unknown origin usually begins with a chest radiograph. Most infectious processes in the chest are quite obvious. Once intrathoracic pathology has been excluded, the next place to look is in the abdomen and pelvis. Assuming that the physical examination of the abdomen and pelvis is negative, the choice is between a contrasted CT scan of the abdomen and pelvis or a nuclear medicine gallium or labeled white blood cell scan. Usually the CT scan is ordered because the price is about the same and the results are available sooner.

Feeding Tubes

As mentioned in Chapter 3, feeding tubes or nasogastric tubes are particularly recalcitrant medical devices. Not only can they inadvertently be passed into the trachea and major bronchus, but they also coil within the stomach. On the plain film, a well-placed enteric feeding tube can be seen coming down the esophagus, passing in an arc through the stomach toward the right of midline, progressing downward in a reverse arc through the duodenum, back to the left, and across the vertebral column. It is best to have the tip of these feeding tubes in the distal duodenal loop, ideally near the junction of the duodenum and jejunum (ligament of Treitz) (Fig. 6–6). An unacceptable position of a feeding tube tip is in the esophagus or at the gastroesophageal junction (Fig. 6–7) because there can be esophageal reflux with aspiration.

Abdominal Calcification

Abdominal calcifications are quite common and most of them have some characteristics that help determine their importance. Single or multiple calcifications in the right upper quadrant are usually gallstones or kidney stones. If the calcifications are multiple, are quite close together, and lie outside the normal expected area of the kidney, they most likely are gallstones. A simple way to tell the differ-

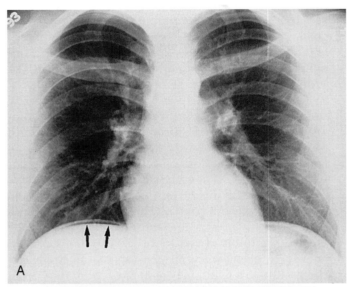

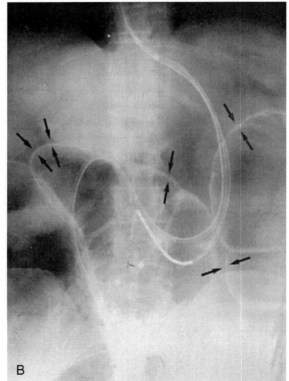

FIGURE 6–4. **Pneumoperitoneum.** *A*, A few milliliters of free air *(arrows)* can be identified under the right hemidiaphragm on this upright posteroanterior chest radiograph. *B*, A supine abdominal film obtained on a different patient with massive pneumoperitoneum shows the bowel wall *(arrows)* outlined by air.

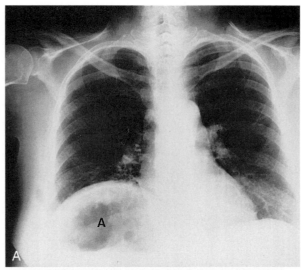

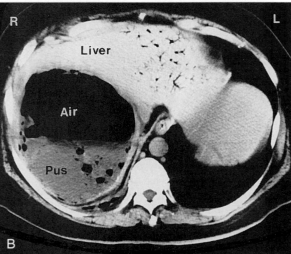

FIGURE 6–5. **Hepatic abscess.** This drug abuser presented with right upper quadrant pain and fever. *A,* On the upright chest film, a collection of air (A) is seen in the right upper quadrant. Notice that there is a thick and irregular margin between the air and the hemidiaphragm, indicating that this is not free air. *B,* A transverse computed tomography scan shows an air and pus collection as a result of a large abscess in the right lobe of the liver.

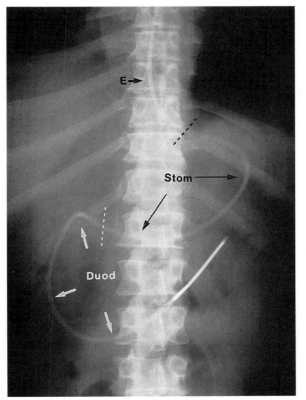

FIGURE 6–6. **Optimal positioning for an enteric feeding tube.** On an anteroposterior film of the upper abdomen, the feeding tube should be seen extending down the esophagus (E) slightly to the left of midline, taking a gentle curve to the right through the stomach, and then reversing its curve through the duodenum and going back to the left across the spine to the junction of the fourth portion of the duodenum and the jejunum (ligament of Treitz).

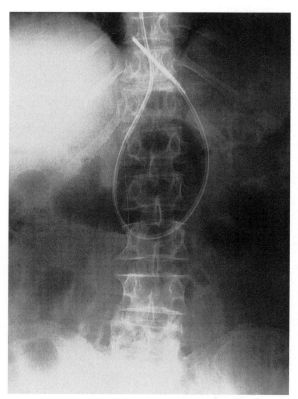

FIGURE 6–7. **Unacceptable position of feeding tube.** In this case, the tip of the feeding tube is in the distal esophagus with the remainder coiled within the body of the stomach. Feeding with the tube in this position is likely to cause aspiration.

ence between a renal calculus and a gallstone is to take a right posterior oblique view. A gallstone rotates anteriorly and does not move with the outline of the kidney. Another way to tell the difference is to order a right upper quadrant ultrasound study, on which gallstones are very easily identified (Fig. 6–8).

Left upper quadrant calcifications are nearly always related to the spleen. Multiple small punctate calcifications are the result of histoplasmosis. Serpiginous or rounded calcification in the left upper quadrant is usually related to splenic artery calcification or to a splenic artery aneurysm, respectively.

With chronic pancreatitis, there is often calcification of the pancreas. This can be seen as spotted or mottled calcification, usually lying in a somewhat horizontal distribution over the vertebral bodies of L1 and L2 and extending to the left. Remember, however, that on a plain abdominal radiograph most people with chronic pancreatitis do not have visible calcification. CT scanning is much more sensitive for pancreatic calcifications than a standard radiograph (Fig. 6–9), but clinical and laboratory history, not a CT scan, should be used to make the diagnosis of chronic pancreatitis.

Calcification of mesenteric lymph nodes can occur

as a result of previous infections. These are usually seen as somewhat rounded or popcorn-shaped calcifications in the right midabdomen. A tip-off is the significant downward movement of these calcifications on the upright views, because the mesentery is extremely mobile (Fig. 6–10).

In a patient who has right lower quadrant pain, one must look carefully in this area for calcification. A stone within the appendix (appendicolith) often projects over the right side of the sacrum (Fig. 6–11) and can be difficult to see. An appendicolith is present in approximately 10% of patients with appendicitis, and if there is an appendicolith in a patient with pain, appendicitis is a very high probability.

In adults, it is quite common to see rounded calcifications in the lower half of the pelvis. These are almost always 1 cm or less in diameter and represent phleboliths (calcification within pelvic venous structures). They are easy to identify, because they often have a lucent or dark center (Fig. 6–12). They can occasionally be confused with stones in the distal ureter. If a patient has symptoms of renal colic or obstruction and of red blood cells in the urine, an intravenous pyelogram or a noncontrasted CT scan may be indicated.

Uterine fibroids (leiomyomas) can be calcified. This type of calcification is quite similar to the popcorn type seen in the mesenteric lymph nodes. The difference is that fibroids are located in a suprapubic position and centrally in the pelvis. On occasion, these can be large and spectacular (Fig. 6–13).

Two special types of calcification can be seen in the male pelvis. The first, found immediately behind the symphysis pubis, is quite common and is the result of benign prostatic inflammatory disease (Fig. 6–14). The second, and more rare, type of calcification looks like a little set of antlers in the middle of the pelvis, projecting slightly above the symphysis pubis. This represents calcification of the vas deferens and almost always indicates that the patient has diabetes.

Acute Abdominal Pain

Acute atraumatic abdominal pain requires urgent evaluation. Evaluation of the location, onset, progression, and character of abdominal pain is necessary to begin a development of a reasonable differential diagnosis. A thorough medical history and physical examination is necessary because abdominal pain may be associated with GI, genitourinary, cardiovascular, or respiratory disorders. An electrocardiogram may be necessary to exclude myocardial causes of abdominal pain. In addition to physical examination of the chest and abdomen, pelvic and

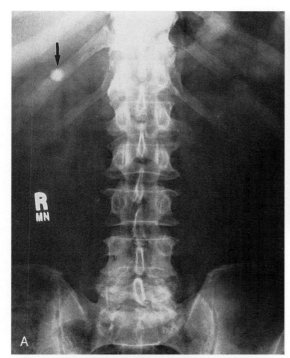

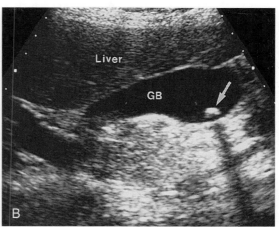

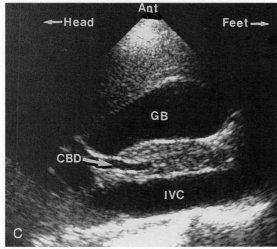

FIGURE 6–8. **Single gallstone.** *A,* On the plain film of the abdomen, a single calcification *(arrow)* is seen in the right upper quadrant. It is not possible to tell from this one picture whether this is a gallstone, kidney stone, or calcification in some other structure. *B,* A longitudinal ultrasound image in this patient clearly shows the liver, gallbladder (GB), and an echogenic focus *(arrow)* within the gallbladder lumen, representing the single gallstone. Also note that there is a dark shadow behind the gallstone. *C,* Another longitudinal ultrasound image slightly more medial also shows the inferior vena cava (IVC) and the common bile duct (CBD), which can be measured. Here it is of normal diameter.

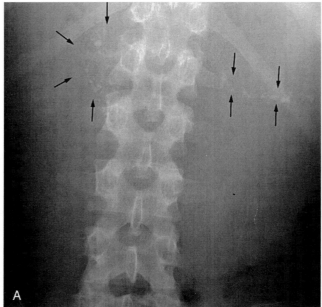

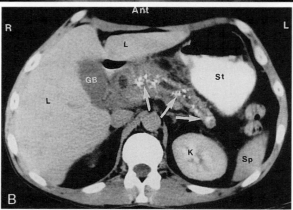

FIGURE 6–9. **Calcification in chronic pancreatitis.** Rarely, on a plain film of the abdomen *(A)*, a horizontal band of calcification can be seen extending across the upper midabdomen *(arrows)*. Calcification within the pancreas is much easier to see on a transverse computed tomography scan of the upper abdomen *(B)*. Calcification is seen as white speckled areas within the pancreas *(arrows)*. The darker areas within the pancreas represent dilated common and pancreatic ducts. L = liver; GB = gallbladder; St = stomach; K = kidney; sp = spleen.

rectal examinations may also yield useful information. Sudden onset of pain is often associated with bowel perforation, ruptured ectopic pregnancy or ovarian cyst, aneurysm, or ischemic bowel. Gradually increasing and localizing pain is more common in appendicitis, cholecystitis, and bowel obstruction.

After the primary care provider has assessed the patient clinically, a reasonable approach to imaging can be formulated. Initial examinations or procedures for various symptoms and suspected disorders is presented in Table 6–3. In most cases of acute abdominal pain, the best initial imaging study is a PA chest radiograph and a supine and

upright view of the abdomen. Ultrasonography is the best initial examination if gallbladder, obstetric, or gynecologic etiologies are suspected.

Acute Gastroenteritis

A diagnosis of acute gastroenteritis is made on the basis of clinical history and the presence of diarrhea. The patients may also have vomiting,

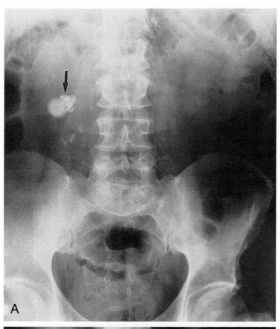

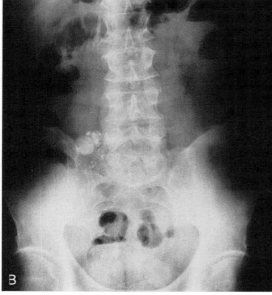

FIGURE 6–10. **Calcification in the mesenteric lymph nodes.** This is a benign finding. The calcification is typically located in the midabdomen to the right of midline, is somewhat popcorn shaped *(arrow)*, and is relatively easy to see on a supine film *(A)*. On an upright view of the abdomen *(B)*, these calcifications drop substantially owing to the mobility of the mesentery.

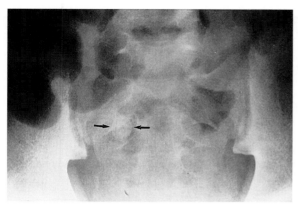

FIGURE 6–11. **Appendicolith.** This calcification within the appendix can be seen almost anywhere in the right lower quadrant but is especially difficult to see when it overlies the sacrum *(arrows).* A right lower quadrant calcification in a patient with pain in this area should carry an extremely high clinical suspicion of acute appendicitis.

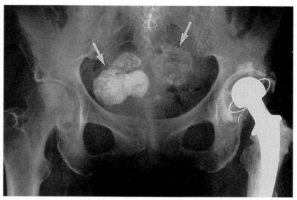

FIGURE 6–13. **Calcified fibroids.** Central pelvic calcification, which are somewhat amorphous, most commonly represent fibroids *(arrows).*

nausea, and abdominal pain. Dehydration is a common complication. The only procedure usually recommended is flexible sigmoidoscopy if blood is present in the stool.

Abdominal Masses

Abdominal masses can arise from any organ or structure in the peritoneal space, retroperitoneum,

aorta, and pelvis. As a general rule, most primary abdominal masses do not grow down into the pelvis, but pelvic masses often grow up into the abdomen. The initial imaging study should be a three-way view of the abdomen to look for associated thoracic pathology (such as metastases or effusions), abnormal gas collections, displacement of the bowel, renal outlines, or associated calcification. Although ultrasound imaging can be used to characterize an ab-

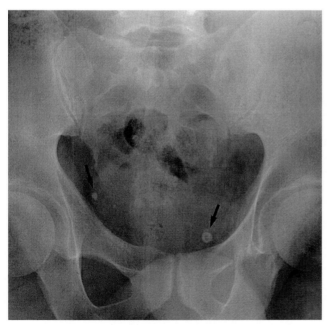

FIGURE 6–12. **Phlebolith.** These rounded vascular calcifications *(arrows)* within the pelvis are quite common and are of no clinical significance. They are usually round and less than 1 cm in diameter. They often have a lucent or dark center. They are typically seen in the lower half of the pelvic brim and can occasionally be difficult to differentiate from a ureteral calculus without an intravenous pyelogram.

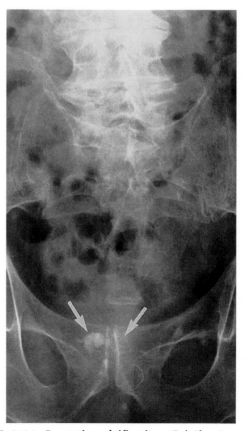

FIGURE 6–14. **Prostatic calcification.** Calcification situated immediately behind the pubis *(arrows)* in a male usually represents the sequelae of previous prostatitis.

TABLE 6–3 Initial Study to Order for Various Clinical Problems

Suspected Clinical Problem	Imaging Study
Gastroesophageal reflux	
Mild or transient symptoms	Medical therapy
Severe or persistent symptoms	Endoscopy with biopsy
Esophageal obstruction	Barium swallow
Esophageal tear	Gastrografin swallow
Bowel perforation or free air	Upright chest and supine abdominal plain film; supine and left lateral decubitus, if patient is unable to stand
Hematemesis	Endoscopy (less preferred, contrast UGI series)
Gastric or duodenal ulcer	Test for *Helicobacter pylori*; if medical therapy fails, endoscopy or double contrast upper GI series
Trauma, blunt or penetrating	Supine/upright abdomen and CT
Abdominal aortic aneurysm	Supine and lateral abdomen
	Ultrasound or CT
Pancreatic mass or inflammation	CT (intravenous and GI contrast)
Pancreatic pseudocyst follow-up	CT or ultrasound
Abscess	CT (intravenous and GI contrast)
Acute cholecystitis	Ultrasound or nuclear medicine hepatobiliary scan
Chronic cholelithiasis	Right upper quadrant ultrasound
Common duct obstruction	Right upper quadrant ultrasound
Jaundice	
Painful	Ultrasound and ERCP
Painless, suspect biliary obstruction	CT or ERCP
Painless, suspect liver	Ultrasound
Suspected bile leak	Nuclear medicine hepatobiliary study
Small bowel stricture or polyp	Enteroclysis with barium
Intestinal obstruction	Supine and upright film of abdomen as an initial study, followed by those listed below
Esophagus or stomach obstruction	UGI and small bowel series or endoscopy
Small bowel obstruction	CT
Distal small bowel or colon obstruction	Barium enema
Right upper quadrant pain (+ Murphy's sign, fever)	Nuclear medicine hepatobiliary scan or ultrasound
Right lower quadrant pain	Supine and upright film of abdomen; ultrasound, if female < 45 years old; CT, if suspect inflammatory process
Appendicitis	
Adults	CT
Children	Ultrasound
Abdominal abscess	Supine and upright plain film of abdomen, then CT with GI and intravenous contrast
Suspected pelvic abscess	CT or ultrasound
Ulcerative colitis	Colonoscopy (see text for screening); if incomplete or unavailable, barium enema
Ischemic colitis (without signs of peritonitis)	Plain radiograph, three-way view of abdomen then colonoscopy or contrast enema (see text)
Suspected ureteral stone	IVP or noncontrast CT
Pelvic pain (female)	Ultrasound
Bladder pathology	Cystoscopy; if not available, CT cystogram
Uterine or ovarian pathology	Ultrasound
Abdominal tumor	CT
Colon cancer	Colonoscopy (see text for screening); if incomplete or not available, barium enema
Abdominal trauma	CT
Acute diverticulitis	Plain film, CT
Rectal bleeding (obvious)	
Dark red	Esophagogastroduodenoscopy; if not available, UGI series
Bright red	Colonoscopy
Unknown source or colonoscopy nondiagnostic	Nuclear medicine bleeding study
Positive fecal occult blood test	
>age 40	Colonoscopy or barium enema
<age 40 with GI symptoms	*Helicobacter pylori* test, therapeutic trial; if fails, endoscopy or UGI series

GI = gastrointestinal; CT = computed tomography; ERCP = endoscopic retrograde cholangiopancreatography; IVP = intravenous pyelography; UGI = upper gastrointestinal.

dominal mass, CT scanning of the abdomen and pelvis with intravenous and GI contrast is the next procedure of choice and the most efficient. This allows complete evaluation of not only the mass itself but also of all other structures. CT scanning can also be used to direct a needle biopsy of the mass if indicated.

Immunosuppressed Patients

These patients may have a wide variety of pathology involving the GI tract and abdominal organs. Dysphagia may be the result of esophageal overgrowth with candida, cytomegalovirus, or herpes. Splenic lesions may occur as a result of a number of infections including *Pneumocystis carinii, Mycobacterium avium intracellulare,* and tuberculosis. Kaposi's sarcoma can occur anywhere in the GI tract but most commonly in the stomach. It is found in about 50% of patients who have skin lesions. If no skin lesions are present, Kaposi's sarcoma in the GI tract is unlikely. Immunosuppressed patients are also prone to lymphoma, typhlitis, cytomegalovirus in the terminal ileum, and pseudomembranous or cytomegalovirus colitis. The choice of imaging mode depends on the organ or structure involved or the presenting symptoms. These are discussed in the appropriate sections later in this chapter.

▪ ESOPHAGUS

Anatomy and Imaging Techniques

As mentioned earlier, the appropriate initial imaging study for a number of suspected clinical problems is shown in Table 6–3. Evaluation of the esophagus for many problems is best done by direct visualization (endoscopy). Because this is a major procedure requiring sedation, many physicians begin by ordering an upper GI examination or a contrast-enhanced esophagram. In addition to barium, other water-soluble contrast materials can be used. If a tear or perforation of the esophagus is suspected, it is best to initially use water-soluble contrast material rather than barium. If aspiration is suspected, barium is used because water-soluble contrast material can irritate the lung if aspirated.

The normal esophagus has a rather smooth lining. Two indentations, caused by an impression by the aortic arch and the left mainstem bronchus, can be seen along the left side (Fig. 6–15). Normally, a peristaltic wave, initiated by swallowing, propels food down the esophagus.

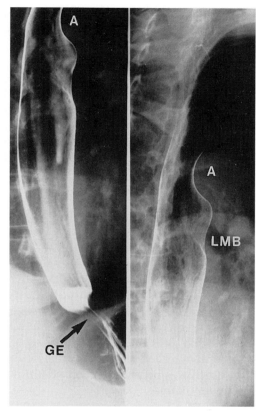

FIGURE 6–15. **Normal anatomy of the esophagus.** The upper portion of the esophagus is seen on the image on the right and the lower portion in the image on the left. An indentation along the left side of the esophagus occurs from the aorta (A) and another less significant one from the left mainstem bronchus (LMB). As the distal aspect of the esophagus goes through the diaphragm, the gastroesophageal junction (GE) can also be identified.

Dysphagia and Odynophagia

Initially, it is important to differentiate dysphagia (difficulty swallowing or sticking of food) from odynophagia (pain with swallowing). The most common cause of dysphagia is hiatal hernia with gastroesophageal reflux disease (GERD). Patients with mild dysphagia do not need imaging or endoscopy, but they should have a trial of GERD medical therapy. Patients with severe symptoms should be investigated with either a barium swallow or endoscopy.

Of patients in the 60 to 80 years-of-age range, many have dysmotility and do not pass food properly. They generally have vague symptoms. A contrast study is indicated to exclude other pathology. Patients who complain of food getting stuck often have a benign or malignant stricture. Such patients usually require endoscopy with biopsy.

Difficulty swallowing can also be the result of central nervous system pathology. There can be pharyngeal paresis with ineffective constriction of muscles due to abnormalities involving cranial nerves 9 and 10, stroke, or degenerative changes. In these patients, failure to close the glottis often results in aspiration.

Odynophagia is usually due to an infection or a medication that produces esophagitis. In these patients, a barium swallow can visualize ulcerations or other characteristic mucosal patterns (such as herpes). Endoscopy is more expensive but has the advantage of allowing biopsy of visualized abnormalities.

Esophageal Diverticula

In the lower cervical region, there is sometimes a pharyngeal diverticulum (known as Zenker's diverticulum) that projects posteriorly. The diverticulum pouch can distend with food, producing dysphagia. In the middle of the esophagus (near the carina), a traction diverticulum caused by scarring from mediastinal granulomatous disease may be present. Just above the stomach, a pulsion diverticulum can sometimes be found. The two latter types are rarely symptomatic.

Presbyesophagus

As a function of aging, tertiary deep contractions within the esophagus may develop. These are usually disordered and can interfere with normal peristaltic process and swallowing. These tertiary contractions are easily visualized as multiple transverse or ring-like contractions of the esophagus. Such a condition is quite common in persons older than 60 years, and no specific therapy is indicated.

Gastroesophageal Reflux Disease

A large number of adults suffer from "heartburn" or dysphagia, as a result of reflux of gastric contents into the esophagus. This may occur because of esophageal motility problems, incompetence of the lower esophageal sphincter, hiatal hernia, delayed gastric emptying, or increased intragastric or intra-abdominal pressure. In adults, the most common cause appears to be transient relaxation of the lower esophageal sphincter with reflux esophagitis.

With mild or transient symptoms, a trial of medical therapy is usually instituted without any imaging procedures being performed. If the symptoms are persistent or severe, endoscopy with biopsy is usually performed. In patients with swallowing difficulties, a barium study may be performed that can demonstrate a mass or stricture that requires endoscopic biopsy. A biopsy is also indicated in immunocompromised patients and those with known Barrett's esophagus. GERD can be documented by use of an intraesophageal pH probe, and nuclear medicine techniques are available to assess the volume of reflux. Neither of these are considered primary diagnostic techniques.

The most common type of hiatal hernia is the sliding type, in which the gastroesophageal junction and a portion of the fundus of the stomach slide upward into the thorax (Fig. 6–16). Large hiatal hernias can be seen on the chest radiograph, even without the use of barium. The typical finding is an air-fluid level or soft tissue mass located behind the heart but in front of the spine. GERD can sometimes be seen on an upper GI examination, but this test is insensitive, and the patient may still be refluxing at other times and under other conditions. A more sensitive imaging method uses nuclear medicine. A small amount of radioactive material is mixed with orange juice, which the patient drinks. A computer region of interest is set up over the chest, abdominal compression is applied, and the patient is imaged for about 1 hour. A positive study documents the presence of reflux. A negative study does not exclude reflux at other times. A more invasive but more accurate method used by gastroenterologists is to put a pH probe on the end of a tube and station this for some time above the gastroesophageal junction.

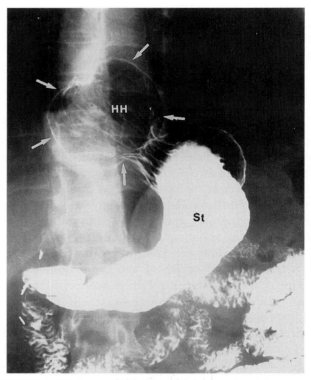

FIGURE 6–16. **Large sliding-type hiatal hernia.** A large portion of the fundus of the stomach has slipped up through the hemidiaphragm into the retrocardiac region *(arrows)* and can easily be identified on an upper gastrointestinal examination. HH = hiatal hernia; St = Stomach.

Foreign Bodies of the Esophagus

Most commonly, the foreign bodies lodged in the esophagus of children are coins. They often stick just above the level of the aortic arch. A number of other foreign bodies lodge at the gastroesophageal junction (Fig. 6–17). In adults, the most common object is a piece of inadequately chewed meat. Meat

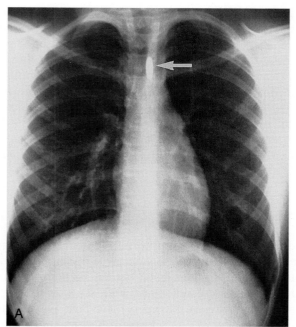

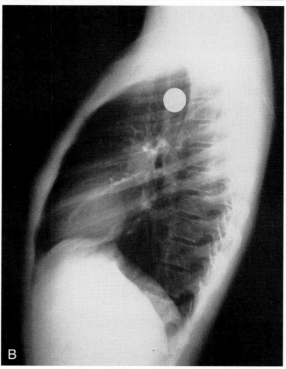

FIGURE 6–17. **Coin in the esophagus.** The coin *(arrow)* can easily be seen in both the posteroanterior chest radiograph *(A)* and the lateral view *(B)*. Objects often stick at this level because the esophagus is somewhat narrowed here by the impression of the aortic arch.

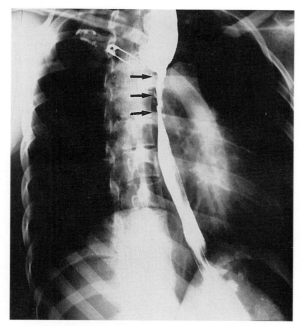

FIGURE 6–18. **Benign esophageal stricture.** This upper esophageal stricture *(arrows)* was due to attempted suicide by lye ingestion. Notice that the stricture does not have any overhanging edges and is relatively smooth and tapered. Essentially all patients with esophageal strictures should have esophagoscopy and biopsy to rule out malignancy.

is not visualized on a plain radiograph but can easily be seen during a contrast-enhanced esophagram. Endoscopy is used in most instances to remove foreign bodies and to biopsy any stricture that might be present.

Strictures and Dilatation

Strictures in the esophagus are a common cause of food lodging at a specific level. High esophageal strictures can occur as a result of scarring caused by (either deliberate or inadvertent) swallowing lye or corrosive alkaline material (Fig. 6–18). Middle and distal esophageal strictures may develop from scarring resulting from GERD or a tumor. Most benign strictures have a smooth appearance on esophagram. The diameter of a stricture can be assessed during a barium swallow by giving the patient a radiopaque pill of known diameter. These pills quickly dissolve (Fig. 6–19). Strictures caused by carcinomas most commonly are irregular and have overhanging edges. Usually, a biopsy is performed on even benign-appearing strictures to exclude malignancy.

There are two entities that can cause marked dilatation of the esophagus. These are achalasia and scleroderma. The esophagus may be so dilated that it can be visualized on chest radiograph as a tortuous structure in the post-tracheal and retrocardiac regions, and often a horizontal air-fluid level

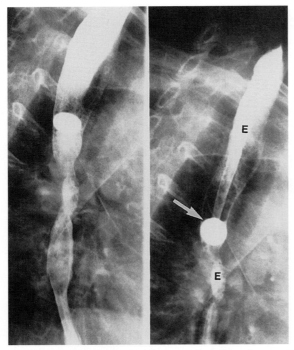

FIGURE 6–19. **Measurement of an esophageal stricture.** During a barium swallow, a radiopaque pill of known diameter *(arrow)* can be given. This will lodge above a stricture, but it will quickly dissolve. Knowing the size of the pill allows measurement of a stricture. E = esophagus.

can be seen in the upper esophagus. Air-fluid levels within the esophagus are definitely abnormal.

In achalasia (Fig. 6–20), the gastroesophageal sphincter fails to relax. The esophagus becomes massively dilated and tapers distally to a beak-like shape. There is usually no evidence of GERD. A massively dilated esophagus that looks like achalasia can also be seen in Chagas' disease, which is caused by an infection with *Trypanosoma cruzi.* This parasite releases a neurotoxin that destroys ganglion cells in the myenteric plexus. Scleroderma is a collagen vascular disease involving smooth muscle. The esophagus is usually only mildly dilated and has no primary contractions. Gastroesophageal reflux can occur with this condition, causing stricture and ultimately proximal dilatation.

Esophagitis and Tears

Ulceration and irregularity of the esophageal mucosa can be the result of reflux esophagitis. In these circumstances, the irregularities are extremely fine. In patients who are immunocompromised, *Candida albicans (Monilia)* infection of the esophagus can create a coarse irregular mucosal pattern (Fig. 6–21).

Tears of the esophagus occur in Boerhaave's syndrome and Mallory-Weiss syndrome. In Boerhaave's syndrome, spontaneous perforation of the esophagus because of a sudden increase in intraluminal esophageal pressure occurs. Clinically, the patient has severe epigastric pain, and dyspnea is common. Overall mortality in this syndrome is approximately 25%, but it approaches 100% if diagnosis is delayed 24 hours. An erect chest film is useful because it may demonstrate a left pleural fluid collection, left pneumothorax, or mediastinal air.

Mallory-Weiss tear is usually a longitudinal nontransmural tear in the lesser curvature of the stomach, often extending across the gastroesophageal junction. These tears are produced by prolonged vomiting, often in alcoholics, usually self-limited, and not painful, although there is hematemesis. There should be no evidence of a pneumomediastinum. In most cases, endoscopy is used because the diagnosis can be made and treated. In cases in which endoscopy is nondiagnostic, a barium swallow is indicated.

Varices

Long, tortuous, longitudinal, or vertical worm-like filling defects in the distal esophagus can be the result of varices because the large vascular channels in the esophageal wall are large enough to displace barium. However, the best way to appreciate varices is by endoscopy, because only when the varices are large and extensive are they seen on a barium swallow. In addition, endoscopy also offers therapeutic options.

Tumors

Mass malignant tumors of the esophagus are squamous cell carcinoma (95%) or adenocarcinoma (5%). Adenocarcinomas usually arise in the region of the gastroesophageal junction or have grown out of the stomach to involve the lower esophagus. Adenocarcinomas may also occur somewhat higher up in the esophagus in patients with chronic gastroesophageal reflux who develop islands of columnar mucosa (Barrett's esophagus).

■ STOMACH AND DUODENUM

Anatomy and Imaging Techniques

Lesions of the stomach and duodenum are most appropriately visualized using an upper GI examination or endoscopy. If a perforated viscus is suspected, Gastrografin (meglumine diatrizoate) or another water-soluble material should be used as a

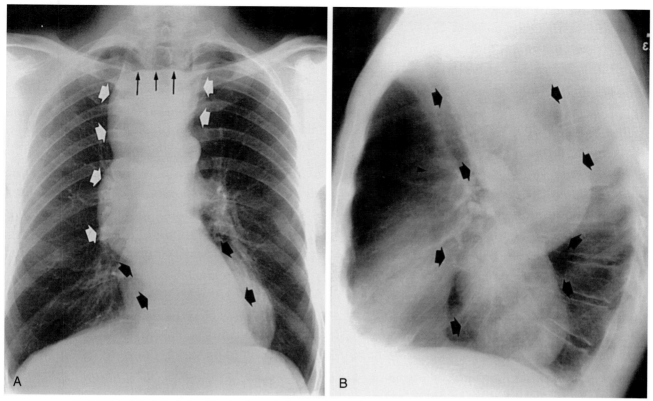

FIGURE 6–20. **Achalasia.** On the frontal chest radiograph *(A)*, a tortuous structure is seen extending from the cervical region down into the retrocardiac region *(thick arrows)*. An air-fluid level is also seen near the top *(thin arrows)*. This represents a massively dilated esophagus due to achalasia. The dilated esophagus *(arrows)* is also seen on the lateral chest radiograph *(B)*, because it is dilated and filled with fluid.

contrast agent rather than barium. CT is usually not an appropriate initial imaging mode for most stomach or intestinal pathology.

The appearance of the stomach on an upper GI study can be variable depending on whether the patient is prone or supine. With the patient supine, barium collects in the gastric fundus (the most dependent position of the stomach), and the normal mucosal patterns of the body and antrum are easily visualized (Fig. 6–22). The duodenal bulb projects upward to the right and posteriorly relative to the gastric antrum. It is important to obtain images with the bulb distended. Radiologists almost always take several pictures of the bulb in different stages of peristalsis.

Gastritis and Gastroduodenal Ulcer Disease

Helicobacter pylori is a bacteria responsible for about 80% of gastritis and gastric or duodenal ulcers. The presence of *H. pylori* is detected noninvasively by immunoglobulin G antibody serology or a urea breath test. Appropriate antibiotic therapy (such as bismuth, metronidazole, and tetracycline)

usually cures 95% of patients. Symptomatic patients should also be treated and discouraged from using alcohol, aspirin, or nonsteroidal anti-inflammatory drugs, and to refrain from smoking. If symptoms persist or an FOBT is positive, an endoscopy or an upper GI barium study is indicated.

The detection rate of gastric ulcers by upper GI examination is only approximately 70%. The nondetectable ulcers are often too superficial or too small to see. Occasionally, the ulcers are so large that the crater is overlooked.

Ulcers that are identified on upper GI examination should be characterized as benign, indeterminate, or malignant. In general, benign ulcers decrease to half their original size with several weeks of therapy and should show almost complete healing within 6 weeks. Unless an ulcer has all benign features, endoscopy with biopsy is usually recommended. There are four radiographic signs of a benign ulcer. If the mucosal folds are thin, regular, and extend up to the margin of the ulcer crater, the lesion is probably benign. Benign ulcers typically extend beyond the projected margin of the stomach (Fig. 6–23). A 1- to 2-mm lucent line may be around the mouth of the ulcer on a tangential view. Finally, normal peristalsis in the region and invagination of

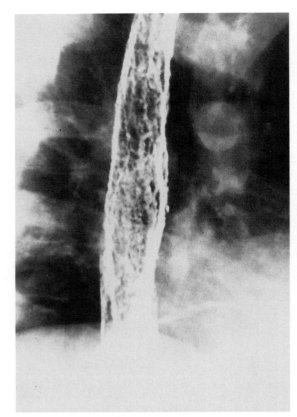

FIGURE 6–21. **Candida esophagitis.** In this immunocompromised patient with acquired immunodeficiency syndrome, the normal smooth esophageal mucosa has been replaced by a rough and irregular ulcerated mucosa extending the length of the esophagus. Tiny ulcerations can be seen tangent along the edge of the esophagus.

the wall opposite the ulcer are helpful signs to indicate benignity. At the present time, most benign ulcers are treated with antibiotics for *H. pylori* and proton pump inhibitors.

In fact, 95% of all gastric ulcers are benign, and only 5% are malignant. Of the malignant ulcers, 90% are due to carcinoma, and the rest are a result of lymphoma and other rare malignancies or metastases. With a cancer, there is usually a thickened and markedly irregular wall. Peristalsis is limited or decreased. The stomach may have decreased distensibility, and the mass or ulcer tends to lie within the projected outline of the stomach, rather than projecting beyond it. If the tumor becomes large enough to infiltrate most of the gastric wall, the stomach becomes rigid and nondistensible, and this is referred to as *linitis plastica* (leather bottle stomach).

Ulcers that arise within the first portion of the duodenum are benign at least 90% of the time. Ulcers that occur distal to the duodenal bulb should be considered malignant until proved otherwise. Duodenal ulcers are 2 to 3 times more common than gastric ulcers. Their location is bulbar in 95% of

cases and postbulbar in 5%. In the duodenal bulb, the anterior wall is the most common site of ulceration; these anterior ulcers can lead to perforation, peritonitis, and pneumoperitoneum. Ulcers in the posterior wall of the duodenal bulb may penetrate into the pancreas.

If the patient has sudden onset of severe abdominal pain and a perforated ulcer is suspected, a three-way view of the abdomen should be immedi-

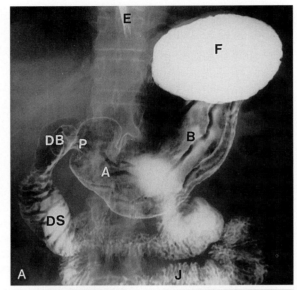

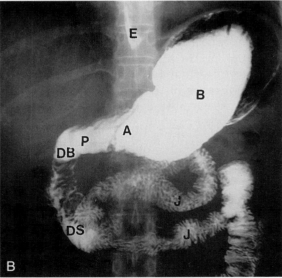

FIGURE 6–22. **Normal upper gastrointestinal contrast examination.** On the supine view *(A)*, note the barium layers in the most dependent portions. The esophagus (E), fundus (F), body (B), antrum (A), and pylorus (P) of the stomach are all easily identified. The normal longitudinal gastric mucosa is also seen. The duodenal bulb (DB), duodenal sweep (DS), and jejunum (J) are also identified with their predominantly transverse mucosal pattern. On a prone view *(B)*, the barium collects in the body (B) and antrum (A) of the stomach, because these are more dependent in that particular projection.

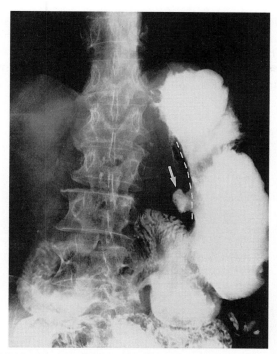

FIGURE 6–23. **Benign gastric ulcer.** A large ulcer *(arrow)* is seen along the lesser curvature of the stomach. Notice that the ulcer projects out beyond the normal expected lesser curvature *(dotted lines)*; this is one sign that the lesion is benign.

ately obtained to look for free air. Other than this, the timing of imaging studies for evaluation of a suspected ulcer is a matter of debate. Some physicians delay imaging procedures until after a trial of testing and treating for *H. pylori*. If the pain is severe and there is a long history of dyspeptic pain, weight loss, vomiting, dehydration, or radiating pain, imaging studies or endoscopy should be performed. Esophagogastroduodenoscopy is the preferred method because a diagnostic biopsy or therapeutic cauterization can be performed if necessary. The sensitivity of this procedure is more than 90%. This is similar to a double-contrast (barium and air) upper GI series, although single-contrast barium studies have a much lower sensitivity (about 60%).

Gastric Emptying

Patients with abnormal gastric motility may have either accelerated emptying of gastric contents (dumping) or delayed gastric emptying. The latter is quite common in diabetics. Because barium is not physiologic, nuclear medicine studies that tag food or liquid with a small amount of radioactive material are used to quantitate gastric emptying. Computer regions of interest are drawn over the stomach, and the emptying rate is calculated. For solid

foods, half the material should leave the stomach in less than 90 minutes.

Gastric Dilatation or Outlet Obstruction

Gastric distension can be due to a number of causes that can be divided into physiologic and metabolic or obstructive. An enlarged stomach may be seen on a plain radiograph of the abdomen in a patient with vomiting or loss of appetite. If causes of gastric dilatation and poor motility such as diabetes, narcotic drugs, and others are not evident, obstructive causes such as neoplasms need to be excluded. Either a barium upper GI series or an endoscopy is indicated. If an abdominal mass other than the stomach can be palpated, a CT scan should be performed.

■ LIVER

The most common method of imaging the liver and spleen is with a CT scan. In many institutions, CT scans are done both with and without intravenous contrast material. For most situations, however, a single CT scan using intravenous contrast material is often adequate and cheaper. The liver or spleen can also be imaged using ultrasonography or nuclear medicine, but there is less anatomic resolution and less complete imaging of other nearby structures.

Cirrhosis and Alcoholic Liver Disease

Probably the most common imaging manifestation of alcoholic liver disease is fatty infiltration. On a noncontrasted CT scan, the liver and spleen should be of the same density. If the liver is darker than the spleen or muscle, fatty infiltration should be suspected. Often the fatty infiltration is focal and not uniform (Fig. 6–24). The low density in an area of fatty infiltration can usually be differentiated from low density caused by malignancy or another abnormality, because fatty infiltration is usually geographic or with straight borders in its distribution. There is also lack of a mass effect, with normal vessels and architecture being preserved in the areas of the fat. The periportal region or medial segment of the left lobe is often spared.

Ascites is another common manifestation of alcoholic liver disease. If ascites is massive, gas in the small bowel is seen floating centrally or concentrated in the middle and anterior abdomen on a supine plain film, and a generalized gray haziness may overlie the whole abdomen (Fig. 6–25). Small amounts of ascites can easily be visualized on a CT

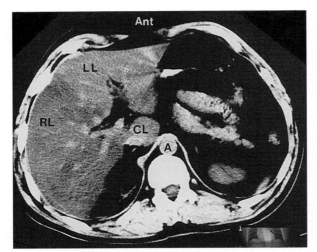

FIGURE 6–24. **Focal fatty infiltration of the liver.** On this transverse computed tomography scan (done without intravenous contrast material), the right lobe (RL) of the liver is darker than the left lobe (LL). This is due to fatty infiltration of the RL. Notice also that there has been sparing of the caudate lobe (CL). Normal vascular structures are seen in the RL, even without contrast enhancement, because they are surrounded by fat. A = aorta.

scan along the edge of the liver and in the pericolic gutters. If imaging is needed only to determine whether the patient has ascites or in locating a suitable area to tap the ascites, ultrasonography is an effective and much cheaper mode. The liver is sometimes imaged by using a nuclear medicine colloid liver-spleen scan. This test is ordered on patients in whom there is liver disease of uncertain etiology or in whom evaluation for the presence of portal hypertension is required.

Trauma

In penetrating abdominal injuries, the liver is the most commonly injured intra-abdominal organ, and it is the second most commonly injured organ in blunt abdominal trauma. Blunt abdominal trauma can cause hepatic lacerations, subcapsular hematomas, and intraparenchymal hemorrhage. Usually, in cases of blunt abdominal trauma, a CT scan is ordered to assess not only the liver but also the spleen, kidneys, and other organs. Hepatic laceration and hemorrhage usually manifest as areas of low density compared with the liver, although acute hemorrhage can be denser (whiter) than the liver (Fig. 6–26). Hepatic lacerations are often treated conservatively, if possible, because removal of a large portion of liver carries a high risk of mortality. Intraparenchymal liver hemorrhages may ultimately resorb.

Hepatic Tumors

The most common benign hepatic tumor is a cavernous hemangioma. This is often discovered incidentally on ultrasound examination, where it ap-

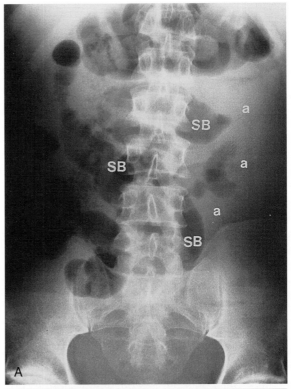

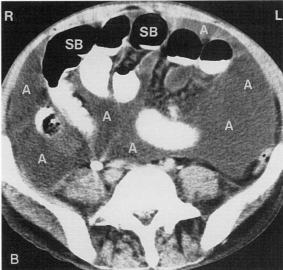

FIGURE 6–25. **Ascites.** On a plain film of the abdomen (A), only gross amounts of ascites (a) can be identified. This is usually seen because the ascites have caused a rather gray appearance of the abdomen and pushed the gas-containing loops of small bowel (SB) toward the most nondependent and central portion of the abdomen. A transverse computed tomography scan (B) shows a cross-sectional view of the same appearance with the air- and contrast-filled small bowel (SB) floating in the ascitic fluid (A).

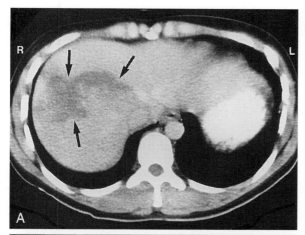

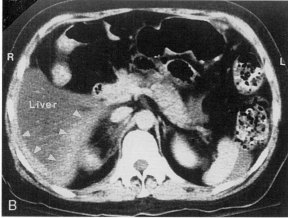

FIGURE 6–26. **Hepatic laceration.** *A,* A computed tomography scan was obtained through the upper abdomen in this patient after a motor vehicle accident. An irregular area of low density *(arrows)* due to hemorrhage within the parenchyma of the liver is seen. A computed tomography scan in another patient *(B),* who was drunk and in a motor vehicle accident, shows fatty infiltration of the liver and acute hemorrhage around the edge of the liver as an area of increased density *(arrowheads).*

percent of patients with cirrhosis and 10% of patients with chronic hepatitis B develop hepatoma. Hepatocellular carcinomas are solitary 25% of the time, multiple 25% of the time, and diffuse 50% of the time.

Metastatic lesions of the liver are quite common. Forty percent of hepatic metastases are from cancer of the colon, 25% from stomach, 20% from pancreas, 15% from breast, and 15% from lung. Metastatic lesions may be small or large and single or multiple. The visibility of hepatic metastases on a CT scan varies greatly, depending on the technical factors used when the filming is done from the computed data. If a CT scan is done with wide windows (wide-contrast scale) and without using intravenous contrast agent, it may be difficult to see the lesions.

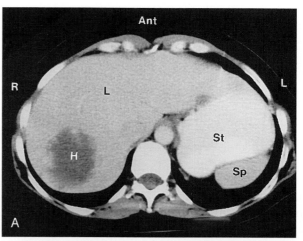

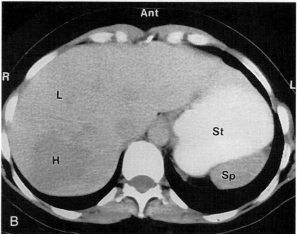

FIGURE 6–27. **Hepatic hemangioma.** On an initial image *(A)* of the contrast-enhanced computed tomography scan of the upper abdomen, hemangioma (H) appears as a low-density area with irregular margins in the posterior aspect of the liver (L). This was an unexpected and incidental finding in this young woman. A scan through exactly the same level obtained 20 minutes later *(B)* shows that the lesion has almost completely disappeared. In this particular patient, no further work-up is indicated. St = stomach; Sp = spleen.

pears as an area of increased or bright echoes within the liver. Hemangiomas are also discovered incidentally on noncontrasted CT scans of the abdomen in which the lesion appears as a rounded area of low density (dark area) within the liver. A hemangioma can look like a malignant primary tumor or even a metastatic lesion. One way to differentiate a benign hemangioma from other lesions is to do serial CT scans as intravenous contrast material is administered. Usually, in approximately 10 to 15 minutes, the hemangioma fills in with contrast material and looks like normal liver, whereas most malignancies will not do this (Fig. 6–27).

The most common primary malignant hepatic tumor is a hepatoma. On CT scans, this appears as an irregular dark area within the liver; however, a contrasted CT scan done during the arterial phase will show increased vascularity (Fig. 6–28). Five

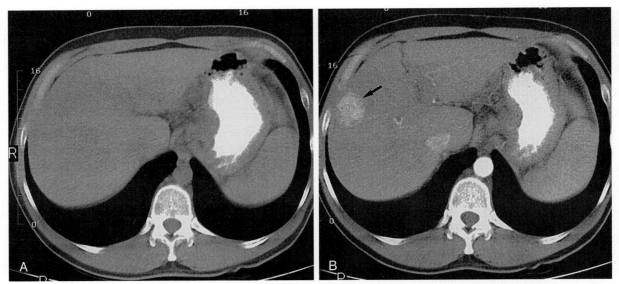

FIGURE 6–28. **Hepatoma.** In this patient with chronic hepatitis, the noncontrasted computed tomographic scan *(A)* shows a subtle low-density lesion in the lateral aspect of the right lobe. With contrast-enhanced CT *(B)* in the arterial phase the hepatoma *(arrow)* is quite obvious.

The best detectability is achieved by using intravenous contrast agent and narrow window settings.

Hepatitis

There is usually no need to image the liver in a patient with known infectious hepatitis. The diagnosis is best made by serum antibody evaluation. If there is hepatomegaly by physical examination, the antibody tests are negative, and there is no known history of hepatotoxins (e.g., alcohol, niacin, sulfa, rifampin, tetracycline, estrogens, acetaminophen), an ultrasound study is indicated to exclude biliary obstruction or occult masses.

Liver Abscess

Abscesses suspected anywhere in the abdomen are best imaged by CT with both intravenous and oral contrast material. Most hepatic abscesses are visualized with CT scanning as low-density masses, darker than the liver. Unless they have gas within them, their differentiation from neoplasm can be quite difficult. Usually, the clinical presentation of an extremely sick, febrile patient is enough to suggest the correct diagnosis. If not, CT scanning can be used to direct a needle aspiration and place a drainage catheter. Ultrasonography can also be used to diagnose a hepatic abscess; however, it is more difficult to appreciate extrahepatic or retroperitoneal complications on an ultrasound study.

■ GALLBLADDER AND BILIARY SYSTEM

Imaging Techniques

There are two common ways of visualizing the gallbladder depending on the clinical presentation. If you suspect gallstones (cholelithiasis) or biliary duct obstruction, the quickest, cheapest, and most efficient imaging test is an ultrasound examination of the right upper quadrant (Fig. 6–29). Endoscopic retrograde cholangiopancreatography (ERCP) can be used to evaluate the cause of biliary duct obstruction, but it is not a primary diagnostic examination in this setting.

Acute Cholecystitis

The diagnosis of acute cholecystitis should be suspected when there is the combination of biliary colic, right upper quadrant pain, and fever or elevated white blood cell count. Either ultrasound or nuclear medicine scans can be used to aid in the diagnosis. Ultrasound imaging may show gallbladder wall thickening and pericholecystic fluid with focal pain, which is produced when the ultrasound transducer is pressed on the right upper quadrant over the gallbladder (sonographic Murphy's sign). Unfortunately, gallbladder wall thickening is nonspecific and can occur with other entities, such as hypoproteinemia, and may be mimicked by ascites around the gallbladder. Associated cholelithiasis is easy to detect.

If the ultrasound is nondiagnostic, a nuclear medicine hepatobiliary scan (iminodiacetic acid

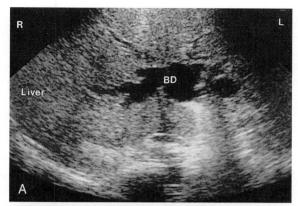

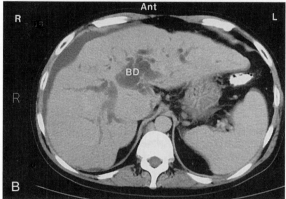

FIGURE 6–29. **Biliary ductal dilatation.** *A,* A transverse ultrasound image through the liver shows a central branching area without echoes that represents dilated bile ducts (BD). A computed tomographic scan of the same patient *(B)* also demonstrates the intrahepatic dilated biliary system. As a screening test, ultrasonography is cheaper and just as effective. Computed tomography scanning is more useful to localize the cause of obstruction, such as a pancreatic carcinoma.

[IDA]) can be performed. Failure to visualize the gallbladder when imaging is carried out to 4 hours has an extremely high specificity for acute cholecystitis. The reason is that in acute cholecystitis there is usually blockage of the cystic duct, and the radioactive tracer cannot get into the gallbladder. Note that cardiac ischemia can mimic biliary pain; patients at high risk for coronary artery disease should have this etiology excluded.

Chronic Cholecystitis and Cholelithiasis

The primary imaging mode for diagnosing chronic cholecystitis is ultrasonography. Gallstones are readily visualized, and the common biliary duct diameter can be easily measured. Intrahepatic lesions may also be identified. On a nuclear medicine hepatobiliary scan, chronic cholecystitis is apparent as delayed gallbladder filling.

Biliary Obstruction and Jaundice

When jaundice is present and there is a question of whether it is due to parenchymal liver disease, such as hepatitis, or to an obstructive lesion of the common bile duct, the initial examination should be ultrasound imaging. When complete ductal obstruction has been present for more than 24 hours, dilatation of the common and intrahepatic ducts is relatively easy to visualize in an ultrasound. The upper portion of the common duct (which is what is normally measured in ultrasonography) is usually less than 4 mm in diameter. It becomes slightly dilated with age and can be up to 7 mm in some patients younger than 60 years. In normal persons older than 60 years, the common duct diameter should be less than 10 mm. The common duct diameter can also be larger than 4 mm (up to 6 to 7 mm), if the patient has had a cholecystectomy.

Although a CT scan provides information on ductal dilatation, because it uses ionizing radiation and is much more expensive, its role is usually limited to a follow-up examination (e.g., if there is suspicion of a pancreatic head neoplasm).

The fine architecture of both the biliary and pancreatic ducts can be visualized by ERCP. To do this, a large endoscopic tube is passed down the esophagus and through the stomach to the duodenum. The ampulla of Vater is then cannulated. Contrast agent is injected into the pancreatic and common bile ducts. ERCP is a useful way to assess the diameter and length of a stricture. During ERCP, it is also possible to do a papillotomy and remove stones from the common biliary duct. If there is jaundice with acute abdominal pain, history of fever, prior biliary surgery, or known cholelithiasis, ERCP is indicated.

Intrahepatic obstruction of the common biliary duct is usually due to cholangitis, Caroli's disease, or an intrahepatic neoplasm (hepatoma compressing the ducts or a rare biliary neoplasm). Extrahepatic biliary obstruction usually occurs distally in the intrapancreatic portion of the duct. Common causes are gallstones, pancreatic cancer, and pancreatitis.

Sometimes, after a cholecystectomy and removal of stones from the common duct, a T tube is left in place. This is done to allow bile drainage through the abdominal wall, while edema related to surgery and prior stones resolves. Before the tube is pulled, contrast material is injected into the T tube to look for possible retained stones.

Occasionally, as a result of surgery, air from the GI tract refluxes into the biliary system. This may be visualized on a plain film of the abdomen (KUB). Air in the biliary tract is usually centrally located in the region of the porta hepatis, and the air is prevented from going very distally into the smaller bile ducts by flow of bile toward the porta hepatis. It is crucial to be able to differentiate this relatively benign finding from that of air in the portal venous system. Air in the portal venous system is usually seen as branching air collections near the periphery of the liver. The air goes peripherally because that is the direction of the flow of blood in the portal veins. Visualization of branching lucencies in the outermost 2 cm of the liver is considered presumptive evidence of portal venous air. This is seen in patients with diabetes and is associated with a high mortality (Fig. 6–30).

Postcholecystectomy Complications

Typical complications include hematoma, retained stones, infections, and bile leak. Ultrasound imaging should be performed for investigating obstruction or retained stones. A nuclear medicine hepatobiliary scan is the procedure of choice for a suspected bile leak, and a CT scan is indicated if a hematoma or abscess is clinically suggested.

■ PANCREAS

Pancreatitis Complications

Seventy percent of cases of pancreatitis are caused either by alcoholic pancreatitis or by ob-

struction due to a gallstone in the distal common duct. The diagnosis is usually made by clinical findings of epigastric or lower abdominal pain accompanied by elevated levels of serum amylase and lipase. Unfortunately, about 30% of patients with pancreatitis have a normal serum amylase level, and about 35% of persons with hyperamylasemia have a disease other than pancreatitis. Serum lipase is more sensitive and specific.

The most sensitive imaging method for a patient with pancreatitis is CT. In rare patients who have sudden-onset pancreatitis, the pancreas may be of normal size but the serum amylase value may be elevated. Most patients with acute pancreatitis have an enlarged pancreas with peripancreatic inflammation, thickening of the perirenal fascia, and peripancreatic fluid collections (Fig. 6–31). Occasionally, there may be one or a few dilated loops of small bowel over the central abdomen caused by a focal ileus from the adjacent inflammation in the pancreas.

With fulminant pancreatitis, there may be an abscess formation. This is seen on CT scan as a large soft tissue mass in the region of the pancreas that contains air bubbles. This condition has a high mortality rate, and usually a percutaneous drain is placed to try to drain the abscess. Another complication is progressive pancreatic necrosis due to digestion of tissue (a phlegmon); it is seen on CT as

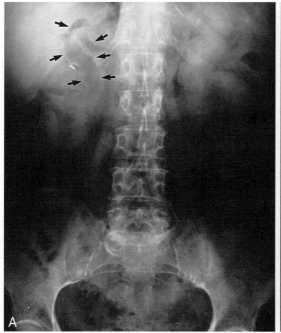 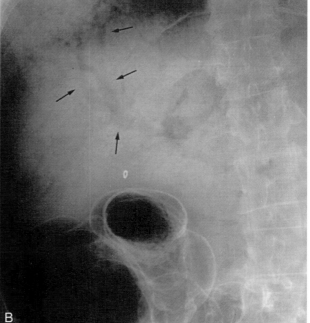

FIGURE 6–30. **Air within the liver.** A branching or serpiginous collection of air is seen within the right upper quadrant *(arrows)* on a supine examination *(A)*. This air is in the region of the porta hepatis and represents air within the biliary system. This is a common finding following gallbladder surgery and has little clinical significance. In contrast, branching collections of air *(arrows)* seen peripherally in the liver *(B)* of a different patient represent air within the portal venous system, and this has a high associated mortality.

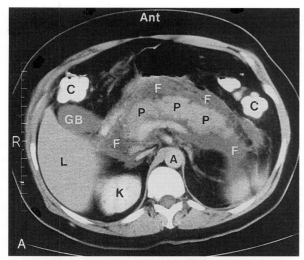

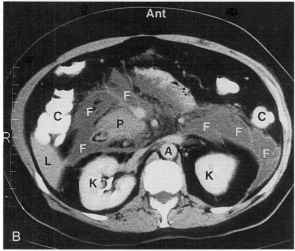

FIGURE 6–31. **Acute pancreatitis.** *A,* A computed tomography scan in this young woman with hyperlipidemia shows the body of the pancreas (P) and surrounding fluid (F). The liver (L), kidney (K), gallbladder (GB), and colon (C) are also identified. Another image in the same patient obtained slightly more inferiorly *(B)* shows a marked amount of fluid (F) around the uncinate portion of the pancreas (P) and fluid extending around into the left paracolic gutter with associated thickening of Gerota's fascia. A = aorta.

multiple areas of low attenuation (dark area) within the pancreas. This condition also has a high mortality rate.

Late complications of acute pancreatitis are pancreatic duct obstruction and pseudocyst formation. A pseudocyst usually takes approximately 6 weeks to fully mature. At this time, a CT scan shows a well-defined cystic area, and CT can be used to perform percutaneous drainage if indicated. Pseudocysts are not necessarily located in the pancreas itself. They can present as focal fluid collections anywhere in the abdomen and occasionally even in the pelvis or thorax.

Ultrasonography can be used to image the pancreas. Often there is an overlying ileus, and the gas in the bowel makes imaging the pancreas difficult or impossible. An ultrasound is useful to follow resolution of a known pseudocyst. The interval between follow-up imaging studies is a matter of clinical judgment. New or worsening symptoms such as pain, fever, increased white blood cell count, or weight loss should be primarily evaluated by CT, although ultrasonography can also be used. ERCP is useful primarily for evaluation of the biliary and pancreatic duct anatomy or obtaining a biopsy. ERCP is indicated in patients with acute pancreatitis for whom no apparent cause can be determined.

Tumor

Adenocarcinoma accounts for 95% of all pancreatic cancers. It has an extremely poor prognosis, with a 1-year survival rate of 10% or less. Clinically, the patients present with jaundice, weight loss, and, occasionally, a dilated, nontender gallbladder. CT is the imaging mode of choice, assessing not only the tumor size and location but also the possibility of hepatic and nodal metastases.

■ SPLEEN

Splenomegaly

Imaging of the spleen is sometimes done to assess splenic size. The spleen is usually about 10 cm in length, and up to 13 cm may be normal. Causes of splenomegaly are leukemia (especially chronic lymphocytic leukemia [CLL]), lymphoma, infection (mononucleosis), storage diseases (amyloid, Gaucher's diseases), portal hypertension, and hematologic abnormalities (anemias, thalassemia, myelofibrosis).

Trauma

Following blunt trauma, the spleen is the most commonly injured intra-abdominal organ; a splenic fracture or hematoma can occur. Although some surgeons try to manage these injuries conservatively, there can be splenic rupture even a week to 10 days after the initial injury. If splenic trauma is suspected, a CT scan is the test of choice. Hemorrhage and hematoma usually appear as areas of lower density than the spleen (Fig. 6–32). Dark areas that are round or irregular represent intrasplenic hematomas or lacerations, and abnormal crescentic areas at the edge of the spleen represent subcapsular hematomas. Occasionally, with conservative management, a splenic abscess may subsequently form and can be identified as such on a CT scan because it contains gas.

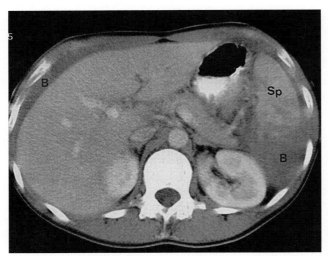

FIGURE 6–32. **Splenic laceration.** The computed tomography scan done without intravenous contrast material through the upper abdomen in a patient who was involved in a motor vehicle accident demonstrates low-density areas of bleeding (B). The spleen (Sp) is intact only in the anterior portion.

Abscess, Infarct, and Malignancy

Other focal splenic lesions can easily be seen on a CT scan. These can be due to splenic abscesses, infarcts, tumors, and, occasionally, cysts. The sensitivity of CT for detection of these is high, but the specificity is poor. Often the clinical history is necessary to narrow the differential diagnosis.

■ SMALL BOWEL

The small bowel can only be effectively imaged through use of plain films and barium contrast studies. An isolated detailed study of the small bowel can be performed using barium and is called *enteroclysis*. With this, a long nasogastric tube is passed to the ligament of Treitz area, and barium and methylcellulose solution are instilled while taking spot film radiographs. This is the preferred procedure for evaluation of suspected small bowel polyps, strictures, and aphthous ulcers. Endoscopy is essentially useless for jejunal or ileal problems. CT can be used to visualize lesions that displace or extrinsically involve the small bowel.

Some small bowel abnormalities can be recognized by examining the gas pattern on plain film of the abdomen. Small bowel can be identified by its central location and by its rather thin mucosal markings (valvulae conniventes) that extend like stripes across the entire lumen. One of the most common remarks that you hear made when a physician is examining a small bowel film is that air-fluid levels are present. The implication is that this is abnormal. In fact, it is quite normal, because

small bowel contents are mostly fluid, and any air or carbon dioxide that is swallowed and passes through the stomach will cause an air-fluid level in the small bowel.

Obstruction vs. Ileus

A common question in a patient with abdominal pain is whether there is either a small bowel obstruction or paralytic ileus. This question can usually be resolved with a stethoscope rather than a radiograph, because if bowel sounds are present and relatively frequent, a paralytic ileus is unlikely. On a plain film radiograph of the abdomen, the diameter of the small bowel should not exceed 3 cm; if it does, it suggests that either an obstruction or an ileus is present.

If the small bowel dilatation is greater than 4 cm, an obstruction is most likely, because in a paralytic ileus there is only mild dilatation. The upright film is used to look at the nature of the air-fluid levels. As mentioned earlier, air-fluid levels can be normal, but if they are seen in the presence of small bowel dilatation, an upright film for a single loop of small bowel may be used to determine whether the air-fluid levels at either end of the loop are at the same level or at differential levels. If they are at different levels in a given loop of small bowel, an obstruction is likely. This is because there is muscle tone within the small bowel causing the differential levels, and this should not be present with a paralytic ileus (Fig. 6–33). A long-standing bowel obstruction can ultimately result in a paralytic ileus; however, the common causes of a paralytic ileus are a postoperative state, vascular ischemia, nearby inflammatory processes (such as pancreatitis and appendicitis), electrolyte imbalance, and drugs (morphine and its derivatives). Small bowel obstructions are mostly due to adhesions, tumors, hernias, and inflammatory strictures.

In the setting of obstruction, if dilated small bowel extends to the lower portion of the abdomen, it indicates that the obstruction is at least in the distal small bowel or perhaps in the proximal colon. If air is seen distally in the colon or in the rectum, either a partial small bowel obstruction or an acute complete small bowel obstruction (the air distal to the obstruction site not yet having been expelled) may be present. Sometimes, as the lumen of obstructed small bowel fills with fluid, small bubbles of air are trapped in the most superior part of the lumen between the valvulae conniventes. This leads to the appearance of a "string of pearls."

The cause of a small bowel obstruction is often difficult to identify on a plain radiograph. Look carefully for gas in the inguinal region to exclude a

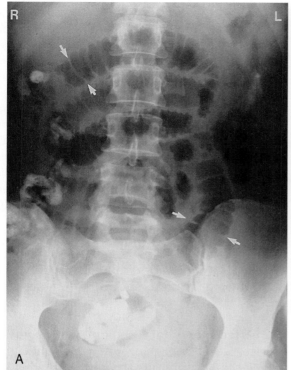

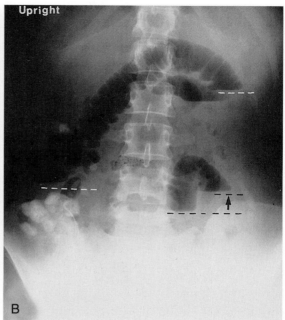

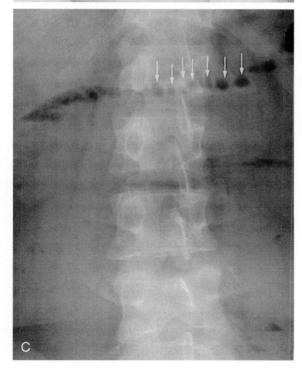

FIGURE 6–33. **Small bowel obstruction.** *A,* On a supine film of the abdomen (kidneys, ureter, bladder [KUB]), there is a large amount of dilated small bowel. This can be recognized as small bowel by the regular mucosal pattern of the valvulae extending across the lumen and looking like a set of thick stacked coins *(arrows).* The small bowel normally should not exceed 3 cm in diameter. *B,* On an upright film of the abdomen, it can be seen that the air-fluid levels within the same loop of bowel are at different heights (dashed lines). This indicates an obstruction rather than a paralytic ileus. A close-up view of the right midabdomen in another patient *(C)* shows the "string of pearls" air bubbles *(arrows)* that indicates a fluid-filled and obstructed small bowel.

strangulated hernia (Fig. 6–34). Dilatation of the small bowel in a child older than a few years should suggest appendicitis (Fig. 6–35).

If a proximal or middle small bowel obstruction is suspected on the basis of plain imaging, a CT scan should be ordered next. A small bowel barium study might give the answer, but it takes longer to do, and the residual barium may interfere with subsequent diagnostic studies. If a distal small bowel obstruction or colon obstruction is suspected, the procedure of choice is a Gastrografin or barium enema. If a colonic or distal small bowel obstruction has been excluded and obstruction still remains clinically suggested, then a barium GI contrast study of the stomach and small bowel should be performed. In patients with a history of abdominal malignancy, a palpable mass, a suspected abscess, or an inflammatory process (e.g., appendicitis,

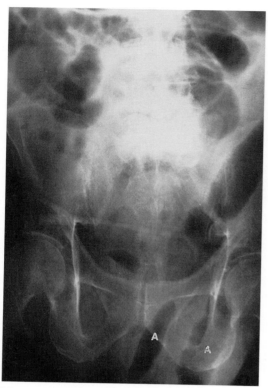

FIGURE 6–34. **Strangulated inguinal hernia.** A film of the pelvis demonstrates some dilated loops of small bowel in the upper abdomen. Over the left groin, two air collections (A) are seen, which represent loops of small bowel descending into the scrotum.

enteritis). Lesions of regional enteritis are most common in the terminal ileum, and about half the patients also have involvement of the colon. Patients have weight loss, recurrent abdominal pain, and diarrhea. Extraintestinal manifestations include skin, eye, joint, and liver abnormalities. Characteristic features are areas of relatively fixed narrowing in the terminal ileum (the string sign) (Fig. 6–36), sinus tracts, and fistulas. In the colon, areas of stricture and ulceration with skip areas have normal mucosa in between. The imaging procedure of choice is a barium small bowel series, although a CT scan is often helpful to look for extraluminal abscesses.

Occasionally, there can be collections of air or gas in the wall of the small bowel (pneumatosis intestinalis). In adults, this is often a benign finding, whereas in children it may be associated with necrotizing enterocolitis or ischemia. In adults, the benign form can occur in patients with chronic obstructive pulmonary disease who have air dissecting down from the chest into the abdomen and along the mesentery of the bowel. This may also be associated with asymptomatic pneumoperitoneum.

GI bleeding can occur as a result of Meckel's diverticulum in the small bowel. Because this is most common in children, it is discussed in Chapter 9.

Crohn's disease, diverticulitis), a CT scan may be indicated.

Benign Diseases

There are a wide variety of diseases that can affect the small bowel and can be visualized on a barium study of the small bowel. The finer points of radiologic differential diagnosis of small bowel disease are beyond the scope of this text, but important findings include mucosal thickening, nodules, dilatation, and areas of stricturing. Fold thickening is assessed by looking at the mucosal pattern. The valvulae conniventes should not measure more than 2 to 3 mm in thickness. The differential diagnosis of small bowel fold thickening includes Whipple's disease, amyloid, giardiasis, cryptosporidiosis, lymphoma, eosinophilic gastroenteritis, and *Mycobacterium avium* complex. Dilatation without fold thickening occurs with sprue, obstruction (or ileus), scleroderma, and other causes (medicines and vagotomy).

There are some diseases and conditions that result in areas of stricturing. The most common are prior surgery, tumor, and Crohn's disease (regional

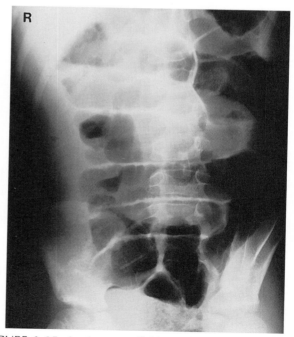

FIGURE 6–35. **Acute appendicitis.** In this supine film of the abdomen of a young child, dilated small bowel loops are seen centrally. No definite gas is seen in the colon. Dilated small bowel loops in a young child should suggest appendicitis as well as intestinal obstruction.

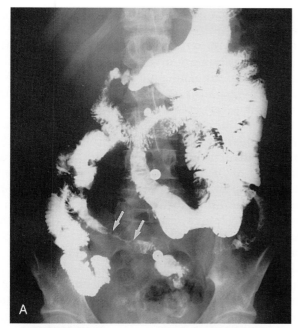

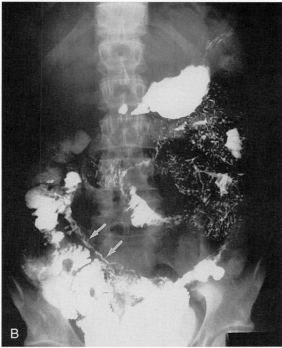

FIGURE 6–36. **Crohn's disease of the small bowel.** *A,* A film obtained midway through a contrast study of the small bowel demonstrates a narrowed segment of distal ileum *(arrows). B,* Another film obtained at the end of the study shows that most of the barium has passed into the colon, but the previously identified area of narrowing *(arrows)* remains and, therefore, represents a stricture rather than peristalsis.

Tumors

Tumors of any sort in the small bowel are rare. Tumor incidence in the colon is about 40 times higher. The most common benign growths of the small bowel are leiomyomas, lipomas, adenomas, and polyps. Malignant tumors tend to be adenocarcinomas and, to a lesser extent, carcinoids and lymphomas. Any tumor in the small bowel can cause obstruction and bleeding.

■ COLON

All of the colon can be directly visualized with endoscopy. This procedure allows biopsy of lesions, but it requires sedation and is expensive.

Radiographic examination of the colon is begun by examining the plain film, but it is best performed by barium or water-soluble contrasted enema. It is imperative that the colon be cleansed before the examination; otherwise, residual fecal material can be mistaken for polyps or malignant lesions. The diagnostic enema can be done under fluoroscopic control either by filling the colon completely with barium (single-contrast examination) or by putting in a small amount of barium to coat the wall of the colon and then using air to distend the bowel (double-contrast examination). The double-contrast examination is generally believed to have a higher sensitivity than the single-contrast examination but it is slightly more uncomfortable. On a barium enema, a number of different views and projections are obtained. This is essential, because otherwise one loop of bowel would overlie another and lesions would be obscured. The ascending, transverse, and descending colon as well as portions of the sigmoid can be appreciated on the anteroposterior or PA views of the abdomen. Lateral views are usually obtained of the rectum; steep oblique views are of the hepatic and splenic flexures.

It is important to be sure that patients are well hydrated after a barium enema. If the barium remains in the colon for several days, water is reabsorbed, and the patient has difficulty in evacuating the barium. Occasionally, barium gets into the appendix during a barium enema. This is a normal finding. It may, however, stay in the appendix and colonic diverticula for months after the remainder of the barium is excreted. This can present a somewhat unusual and confusing appearance on a plain film of the abdomen.

Colonic Obstruction vs. Paralytic Ileus

The key to the differentiation of colonic obstruction and paralytic ileus on a plain abdominal film is whether there is dilatation of the cecum. The cecum is the most dilated segment of the colon in obstruction compared with the rest of the colon. Colonic obstruction is most frequently due to a cancer (65%), but it can also be due to diverticulitis (20%) or a volvulus (5%). If the transverse colon is more dilated than the cecum, a diagnosis of ileus is most likely. The term for an abnormally distended transverse colon is a *megacolon*, and this refers to dilatation greater than 6 cm in diameter. A toxic megacolon can result from ulcerative colitis, Crohn's disease, or infectious causes.

When there is acute colonic distention (cecum >9 cm), a risk of perforation is present. The likely causes are tumor obstruction, volvulus, and paralytic ileus. A number of patients have a chronically distended colon, and they have only a small risk of perforation. In such cases, chronic distention may be a result of chronic laxative abuse, neuromuscular disorders (including diabetes), psychogenic problems, or metabolic problems (electrolyte imbalance, hypothyroidism, opiate use).

Appendicitis

Acute appendicitis is usually diagnosed clinically. Because the differential diagnosis can include acute gastroenteritis, cholecystitis, intestinal obstruction and perforation, urinary tract infection or female pelvic pathology, and other conditions, some confusion may be apparent as to which imaging tests are indicated. Appendicitis should be suspected if there is a combination of abdominal pain; symptoms including nausea, vomiting, constipation, and diarrhea; the physical findings of guarding, rebound, rectal tenderness, and fever; and an elevated white blood cell count with a left shift.

The initial imaging test is usually a three-way view of the abdomen (PA chest, supine, and upright abdominal radiograph). This is useful to look for free air, dilated bowel, abnormal gas collections in an abscess, and possibly an appendicolith. As mentioned earlier, dilated small bowel in a child should suggest appendicitis.

Both CT and ultrasonography can exclude other causes of abdominal pain as well as implicate the appendix. CT gives a more comprehensive view of the abdominal structures. In appendicitis, inflammatory changes or abscesses around the cecum or appendix can be easily seen. Ultrasonography can be used to image the appendix, but the test is harder to interpret. An ultrasound may be used instead of a CT scan when the differential diagnosis includes either cholecystitis or pelvic pathology, because those areas are easily evaluated with an ultrasound, and it is cheaper and does not require use of intravenous or oral contrast material. If the ultrasound image is nondiagnostic, a CT scan is usually needed.

Diverticulosis and Diverticulitis

Chronic lack of fiber in the diet causes herniation of mucosa outward through the bowel wall (diver-

ticula). Fifty percent of individuals older than 50 years have acquired diverticula. Of this group, 15 to 30% present with rectal bleeding and pain. Ninety-five percent of diverticula are located in the region of the sigmoid and descending colon (Fig. 6–37). *Diverticulosis* simply refers to the presence of multiple diverticula.

Diverticulitis is an inflammatory process often caused by extravasation of bowel contents from the tip of the diverticulum. It is confined to the sigmoid colon in 90% of patients, and there is usually significant resultant bowel wall thickening or formation of intramural abscesses (Fig. 6–38). Patients present with left lower quadrant pain 70% of the time, and they may also have diarrhea or constipation, fever, and leukocytosis.

In diverticulitis, a plain film of the abdomen is usually the first imaging test performed for symptomatic patients and may show extraluminal gas shadows, irregularity, or narrowing of the colon. CT can be used to confirm the diagnosis of acute diverticulitis and can identify associated abscesses. CT is also used for patients suspected of having diverticulitis who fail to respond to antibiotic therapy or those who have a high fever, palpable abdominal mass, signs of peritonitis, or marked toxicity.

A contrasted enema can also be used. However, in the acute phase of the disease, care must be taken to avoid bowel perforation. Water-soluble contrast material rather than barium should be used, and the study should be performed with minimal

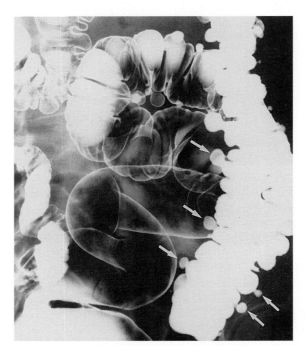

FIGURE 6–37. **Diverticulosis of the colon.** An oblique view of the sigmoid colon during a double-contrast barium enema shows multiple outpouchings *(arrows)* that represent diverticula.

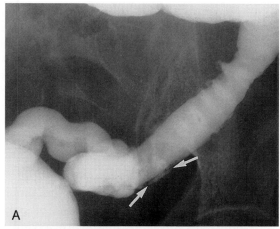

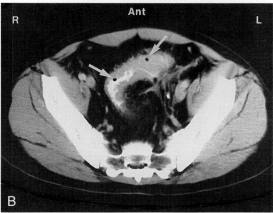

FIGURE 6–38. **Diverticulitis.** *A,* A view of the sigmoid colon obtained during a single-contrast barium enema shows tracking of the barium within the wall of the colon *(arrows).* *B,* A transverse computed tomography scan in the same patient shows the sigmoid colon with a markedly thickened wall. Several gas bubbles *(arrows)* are seen within the wall of the colon, representing abscess formation.

pressure. Endoscopy may also be used. However, because of the risk of bowel perforation, both of these tests are often deferred until symptoms have subsided. If bleeding is identified or if there is a change in bowel habits to suggest a neoplasm, endoscopy is the procedure of choice. If the site of significant blood loss cannot be localized by endoscopy, a nuclear medicine labeled red blood cell scan is indicated.

Ulcerative Colitis

Ulcerative colitis is associated with arthritis and arthralgia, and the patients have diarrhea and rectal bleeding. The disease is confined to the mucosa and submucosa of the colon. It begins in the rectum and spreads from the distal to the proximal colon. There may also be backwash ileitis with involvement of the terminal ileum. Patients are at a 5- to 30-fold higher risk for colonic malignancy compared

with the general population. Because of this it has been recommended that those patients with extensive disease (pancolitis) have annual colonoscopy beginning 8 years after their first attack and that those with left-sided colitis have the procedure annually beginning 15 years after their first attack. The barium enema features of this disease are a short colon with granular mucosa and shallow, confluent ulcers (Fig. 6–39). The barium enema is useful when a colonoscopy cannot be performed or is incomplete and can reveal the extent of disease, strictures, or carcinoma.

Crohn's Disease

Crohn's disease can affect the colon and the small bowel. In contrast to ulcerative colitis, it is transmural and rarely involves the rectum. On a barium enema, aphthous erosions, ulcers, cobblestone fissures, fistula, and strictures can be visualized. Characteristically, the disease is noncontiguous and skips areas of the colon. Thus, there are diseased areas of the colon with segments of normal colon in between.

Ischemic Colitis

Ischemic colitis can result from thrombosis of the superior or inferior mesenteric artery, hypercoagulable states, small vessel disease, or obstruction of the colon. Initial symptoms are usually vague and nonspecific. This is followed by abdominal pain that seems out of proportion to clinical findings, and often by rectal bleeding. The goal is to make the diagnosis without causing perforation or other complications. A plain abdominal film may reveal free air or "thumbprinting" from mucosal edema or intramural hemorrhage. A patient without signs of peritonitis and in whom the plain film findings are nonspecific may have endoscopy or a single-contrast barium enema. In either case, the distension of the colon should be kept to a minimum during the procedure.

Infectious Colitis

Pseudomembranous colitis and a number of other infections caused by *Campylobacter, Shigella,* and *Salmonella* can produce a radiographic pattern similar to that of ulcerative colitis. Cytomegalic virus colitis usually occurs in immunocompromised persons and has variable radiographic features, including ulceration, which can be either localized or pancolonic.

Ulcerative colitis and, less commonly, other forms

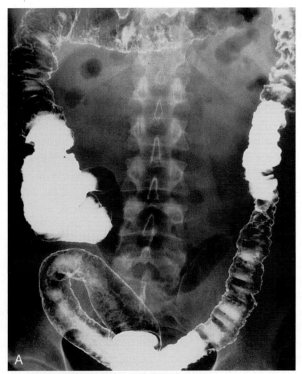

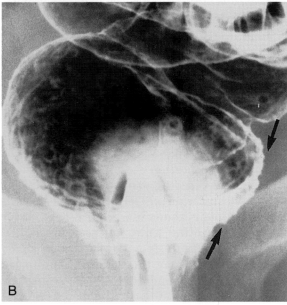

FIGURE 6–39. **Ulcerative colitis.** *A,* A double-contrast barium enema shows small irregular ulcers extending back from the rectum to at least the hepatic flexure. *B,* A spot view of the rectum shows the tiny ulcers in better detail. (Case courtesy of Michael Davis, MD.)

of colitis, can result in a toxic megacolon. A barium enema should not be ordered on a patient in whom a toxic megacolon is suspected, and proctoscopy should be performed. The radiographic features of toxic megacolon are a dilated colon with a deformed bowel wall, most evident in the transverse portion of the colon. The wall may be nodular, irregular, or have haustra that look like thumbprints of soft tis-

sue extending into the colonic lumen. This thickened fold appearance can also be due to ischemia of the colon, but it is usually limited to a specific vascular distribution, that is, proximal to the splenic flexure for the superior mesenteric artery and distal to the splenic flexure for the inferior mesenteric artery distribution.

Polyps

About 90% of polyps are hyperplastic and non-neoplastic. Of those that are neoplastic, adenomas are the most common. Of the adenomatous polyps, 50% are multiple; although many are asymptomatic, they can cause diarrhea, pain, and bleeding.

The larger the polyp is, the more likely it is to be malignant. Of polyps less than 1 cm, only 1% are malignant; between 1 and 2 cm, 25% are malignant; and more than 2 cm, 40% are malignant. A benign polyp is usually less than 2 cm in diameter, has a thin stalk and a smooth contour, is single, and has a smooth underlying colonic wall. Malignant polyps are usually more than 2 cm, have no definite stalk, are often irregular or lobulated, and can be multiple (Fig. 6–40).

There are a number of syndromes with multiple polyps, including familial polyposis, Gardner's syndrome, Peutz-Jeghers syndrome, and juvenile polyposis. Most of the polyposis syndromes have adenomas as the underlying histology, but familial-type Gardner's syndrome and Turcot's syndrome have an extremely high rate of malignancy. In familial polyposis, the rate of malignancy is so high that screening of family members begins at puberty, and treatment often involves a prophylactic total procto-colectomy.

Colon Carcinoma

Colon cancer is the second most common cancer in men and the third most common in women. The most common cancer in men is lung, and in women, breast and lung cancer. Fifty percent of colon cancers occur in the rectum or sigmoid, and about 10% each in the cecum, ascending colon, transverse colon, and descending colon. The clinical presentation is most commonly colonic obstruction or rectal bleeding. There is a debate as to whether colonoscopy or barium enema is the appropriate method of work-up. Barium enema is relatively inexpensive compared with colonoscopy, and it has about the same accuracy rate. The advantage of colonoscopy is that if a lesion is identified, a biopsy can be performed immediately. Screening for polyps and colon cancer is commonly done by an FOBT and sigmoidoscopy. An FOBT has a high incidence of

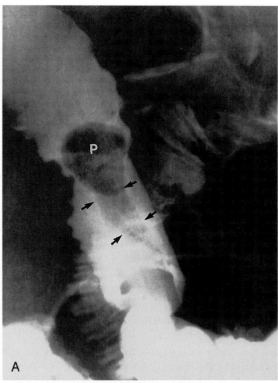

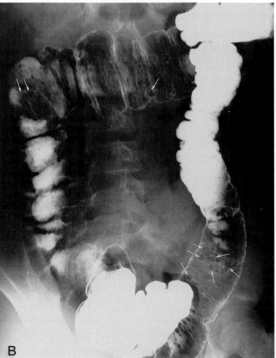

FIGURE 6–40. **Colonic polyps.** *A,* A magnified spot view of the sigmoid during a barium enema outlines a single polyp (P) as well as its stalk *(arrows)*. *B,* In a different patient, a barium enema reveals multiple tiny polyps extending throughout the colon.

false-positive results from a diet high in red meat or peroxide-containing vegetables (e.g., broccoli, turnips, cauliflower). Sigmoidoscopy provides only very limited visualization of the colon. After a positive FOBT, colonoscopy is usually performed. If colonoscopy is not available or if there is inadequate visualization of the entire colon, a double-contrast barium enema is usually performed.

The recommendations for colon cancer screening in asymptomatic persons vary among organizations. For persons older than 50 years, the American Cancer Society, American College of Physicians, and National Cancer Institute recommend an annual FOBT and a flexible sigmoidoscopy every 3 to 5 years. The American Cancer Society also recommends annual digital rectal examination beginning at age 40. The U.S. Preventive Services Task Force has concluded that there is insufficient evidence to recommend either for or against screening in asymptomatic persons. In 1994, the Canadian Task Force on the Periodic Health Examination reported that there is insufficient evidence to support inclusion or exclusion of FOBT, sigmoidoscopy, or colonoscopy for screening in persons older than 40 years.

There are asymptomatic individuals who are at a higher than average risk for colorectal cancer. These include persons with ulcerative colitis; Crohn's disease, familial polyposis syndromes; a personal history of colorectal, breast, ovarian, or endometrial cancer; hereditary nonpolyposis colorectal cancer (HNPCC); and a history of adenomas or colorectal cancer in first-degree relatives. For such individuals older than 40 years, the American College of Physicians recommends a double-contrast barium enema or colonoscopy every 3 to 5 years and an annual FOBT. The American Cancer Society recommends colonoscopy or double-contrast enema every 5 years beginning at the age of 35 years. Recommendations of the U.S. Preventative Services Task Force has concluded that it is prudent to offer screening tests to such persons older than 50 years.

The radiographic appearance of a colon cancer may be a polypoid lesion extending into the lumen of the colon or a mass on one wall of the colon; if more advanced, the lesion may present as a circumferential constriction, resulting in an "apple core" appearance (Fig. 6–41). In about 5% of patients, there is a second colon cancer present at the same time. The radiologist does not usually put a lot of barium retrograde past a high-grade obstructing lesion because the barium stays there. The colon absorbs the water from the barium, and it may almost turn to concrete. At surgery, however, one must look for second tumors.

CT is usually performed to assess the extent of disease locally and in the lymph nodes and liver. Accuracy for detection of lymph node metastases is poor (approximately 60%). If the nodes are enlarged, they probably have a tumor within them, but nodes can be of normal size and still contain tumor. A CT scan with intravenous contrast material of the liver often shows multiple low-density metastases.

Gastrointestinal Bleeding

Bleeding is a common presentation of GI pathology. Although bright red blood from the rectum usually implies a rectal or colonic lesion (98% of the time), this is not necessarily the case; distal small bowel lesions can rarely present this way. Blood in

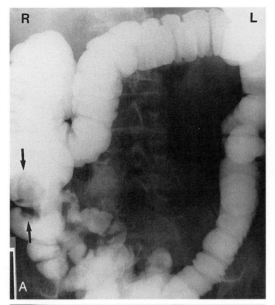

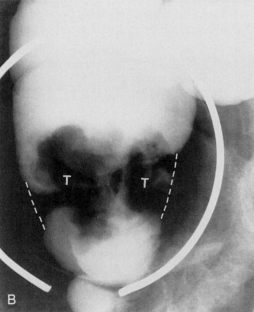

FIGURE 6–41. **Colon carcinoma.** *A,* A single-contrast view of the colon demonstrates a filling defect in the cecum *(arrows).* *B,* A compression ring was applied, and a spot view was taken of the cecum. This shows that the tumour (T) has encircled the lumen, producing a typical apple-core lesion with overhanging edges (dashed lines). This is characteristic of a cancer.

the stool in a person younger than 40 years is usually due to an upper GI source. In such patients with upper GI symptoms and a positive FOBT, a medical trial of ulcer therapy is usually performed before imaging studies. Iron deficiency anemia is most commonly caused by chronic blood loss. Often the site is predicted by symptoms. Endoscopy shows lesions to be about one third in the upper GI tract, one third in the lower GI tract, and nondiagnostic in the other third of patients.

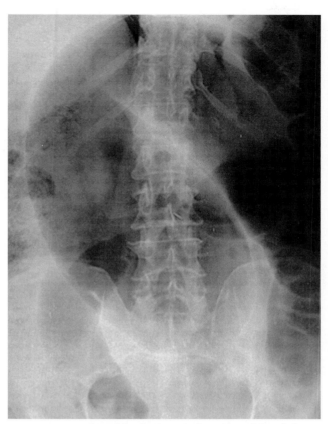

FIGURE 6–42. **Sigmoid volvulus.** A plain film of the abdomen shows the massively dilated "inverted U" of colon pointing toward the right upper quadrant. (Case courtesy of Michael Davis, MD.)

When the source of GI bleeding cannot be found by colonoscopy, it is often valuable to perform a nuclear medicine GI bleeding study. This is done by labeling the red blood cells with radioactive material and then doing sequential imaging over the abdomen to look for abnormal extravasation and pooling. This examination should be ordered before an angiogram or a barium enema. A nuclear medi-

cine study should be ordered only when the patient is having active bleeding, and it is capable of localizing the bleeding site with bleeding rates as low as 0.5 mL/min. In contrast, an angiogram cannot identify a bleeding site if blood loss is slower than 4 mL/min. A nuclear medicine scan is also helpful to direct the radiologist as to which vessels to catheterize if an angiogram is needed. Occasionally, bleeding and other symptoms may be due to a foreign body.

Volvulus

Twisting of the colon can cause either a sigmoid or a cecal volvulus. This obstruction causes severe colicky pain, nausea, abdominal distention, and vomiting. Sigmoid volvulus is about 3 times more common than a cecal volvulus. A sigmoid volvulus is seen on the KUB film as a massively dilated loop of colon that looks like an inverted U (also called the *omega loop sign*) projecting up out of the pelvis toward the right upper quadrant (Fig. 6–42). There is usually air seen in the proximal colon. With a cecal volvulus, there is a dilated loop of colon pointing toward the left upper quadrant, and there is usually associated small bowel dilatation. The diagnostic study of choice for both these entities is a barium enema.

GENERAL SUGGESTED READINGS

Davis M, Sullivan L, Ketai L: The Abdomen and Gastrointestinal Tract, Section III. *In* Juhl JH, Crummy AB, Kuhlman JE (eds): Paul and Juhl's Essentials of Radiologic Imaging, 7th ed. Philadelphia, Lippincott-Raven, 1998, pp 491–615.

Eisenberg RL: Gastrointestinal Radiology: A Pattern Approach, 3rd ed. Philadelphia, Lippincott Williams & Wilkins, 1995.

Margolis AR, Burhenne HJ: Practical Alimentary Tract Radiology. St. Louis, Mosby–Year Book, 1993.

7

GENITOURINARY SYSTEM

■ ANATOMY AND IMAGING OF THE URINARY TRACT

There are a number of methods to image the urinary system. The initial study of choice for many suspected clinical problems is shown in Table 7–1. The most common radiographic method is intravenous injection of an iodine-based contrast agent, which is rapidly cleared by the kidneys. This is called an *intravenous pyelogram* (IVP). In patients receiving glucophage therapy, there is a danger of lactic acidosis after use of intravenous contrast agent. Glucophage should be withheld from the time of intravenous contrast agent administration until 48 hours later. The normal anatomy is shown in Figure 7–1. Initially, a plain film of the abdomen (kidneys, ureter, bladder [KUB]) is obtained. Of particular interest are those calcifications that project or overlie these regions.

The kidneys should be examined for size, shape, position, and axis. The length of kidneys on a radiographic study is typically about 13 cm. On an ultrasound examination they are smaller, being only about 10 to 11 cm in length. The reasons for this discrepancy are that (1) there is magnification on the radiographic images, and (2) the intravenous contrast being excreted during an IVP causes the kidneys to enlarge 1 to 2 cm in length. Normally, the left kidney is somewhat higher than the right; the long axis of the kidneys should be tilted slightly

inward, with the superior pole of the kidney being more medial than the lower pole. There should be uniform thickness of the cortex relative to the calyces of the collecting system. The shape of the kidneys should be relatively smooth in outline, although occasionally there is a slight lump (referred to as a *dromedary hump*) on the lateral margin of the kidneys.

On the IVP, there is normally a dark area surrounding the collecting system of the kidneys, and this represents fat in the hilum of the kidney. The calyces should be quite sharp and pointed (not blunted) at their outer corners. The renal pelvis and ureters should be examined for any intrinsic or extrinsic defects that might be apparent. The ureters should course inferiorly and medially from the kidneys and anterior to the psoas muscles at the L3–L5 level. On the anteroposterior projection, the ureters typically are most medial and project over the lateral aspect of the transverse processes at L3, L4, and L5. As the ureters pass over the sacrum, they deviate laterally and then enter the bladder from the posterolateral aspect.

Renal ultrasonography is a simple noninvasive examination (Fig. 7–2). Remember that all ultrasound images are slices and that the easiest view to understand the kidney is the longitudinal view. The right kidney is easily visualized by transmitting sound through the right lobe of the liver. Because bowel and stomach gas prevents ultrasound

TABLE 7–1 Initial Imaging Studies for
Common Clinical Problems

Clinical Problem	Imaging Study
Ureteral calculus	KUB, IVP, or noncontrasted CT
Hematuria	IVP, CT
Infection	
recurrent in a female	Cystoscopy
first time in a male	IVP
Abscess	CT
Renal trauma	CT
Hydronephrosis	IVP initially, US for follow-up
Probable cyst on IVP	US
Probable mass on IVP	CT
Bladder rupture	Cystogram
Urethral obstruction or tear	Retrograde urethrogram
Bladder cancer	Cystoscopy, CT
Suspected renovascular hypertension	Nuclear medicine captopril renogram
Testicular torsion	Nuclear medicine testicular scan or Doppler US
Testicular or scrotal mass or trauma	US
Pelvic mass (female)	US
Pelvic pain (female)	US
Cervical cancer	CT
Ovarian cancer	CT
Uterine cancer	CT
Uterine fibroids (initial, enlarging, painful, or bleeding)	Pelvic US
Prostate cancer	PSA measurement and biopsy (not imaging), bone scan (to exclude metastases)
Infertility	Physical examination, hormone levels, US
Vaginal bleeding	
Premenopausal, physical examination normal	US
Postmenopausal, not taking hormone currently or taking it for >6 mo	US

KUB = kidneys, ureter, and bladder; IVP = intravenous pyelogram;
CT = computed tomography; US = ultrasound; PSA = prostate-specific antigen.

transmission, the left kidney is usually visualized from the patient's back. The kidney is bean shaped and has bright central echoes owing to the fat surrounding the collecting system. Ultrasonography is poor for evaluation of the ureter and the bladder wall, but it may be preferred as the initial upper urinary tract study in patients who are at a higher than normal risk from contrast material. This would include pregnant women, patients with impaired renal function (creatinine >2 mg/dL), proteinuria, diabetes, congestive heart failure, or prior contrast reaction.

Although the bladder is seen on the IVP (Fig. 7–3), the contrast medium is heavier than urine and therefore layers posteriorly in the bladder, resulting in only limited visualization of the bladder lumen. A cystogram allows specific evaluation of the bladder. A Foley catheter is placed directly into the bladder, the urine drained, and the bladder refilled with contrast material. On a cystogram, images of the bladder are obtained in several different projections. When the catheter is removed, the patient may be asked to void. In males, this gives a good demonstration of the urethra. The male urethra can also be studied in a retrograde fashion by inserting a small tube in the tip of the penis and injecting the contrast material. This is usually done only in cases of suspected urethral trauma or stricture.

Computed tomography (CT) is a commonly used secondary imaging mode of the urinary system. There are a few circumstances in which it is used as the initial imaging mode, such as after major trauma in which other organs may be affected or as an alternative to an IVP for suspected obstructive stone disease. Magnetic resonance imaging (MRI) or CT may be used in cases of renal cell carcinoma to exclude renal vein or inferior vena cava thrombus. Nuclear medicine techniques are used when function or other parameters need to be quantitated. Common indications for radioisotope techniques include evaluation of renal transplants to determine whether a dilated collecting system is obstructive or nonobstructive and to detect renovascular hypertension.

▨ HEMATURIA

Hematuria can be traumatic or nontraumatic and visible or microscopic. In cases of trauma and visible hematuria, a CT scan is indicated. In cases in which there is trauma, microscopic hematuria (<50 RBCs per high power field [HPF]), and little suspicion of injury to other organs, many physicians do not do any imaging but rather wait 48 hours to see if the hematuria clears.

Of patients with nontraumatic visible hematuria, about 25% have cancer, 25% have infection, and 15% have calculi. About 5% of patients with nontraumatic microscopic hematuria (5 RBCs/HPF) have a urologic cancer. Obviously, the presence of unilateral flank pain suggests calculi that are discussed later. If there are red blood cell casts in urine immunologic studies, renal biopsy is usually

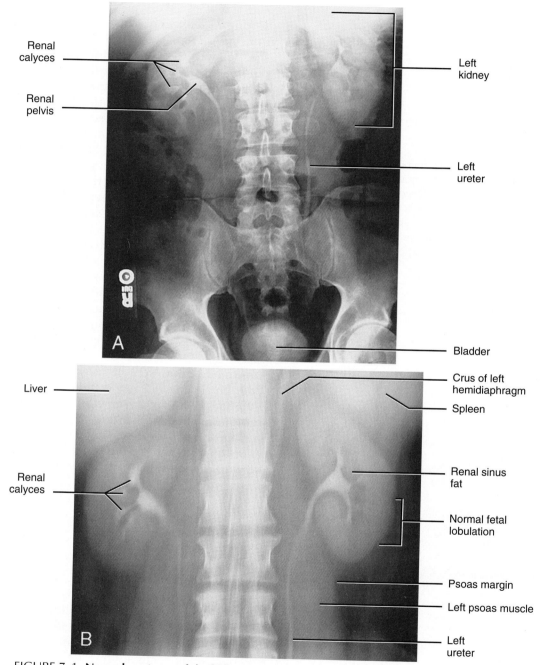

FIGURE 7–1. **Normal anatomy of the kidneys, ureters, and bladder on an intravenous pyelogram.** *(A).* Normal anatomy is also shown on the computed tomographic image *(B)* taken during an intravenous pyelogram.

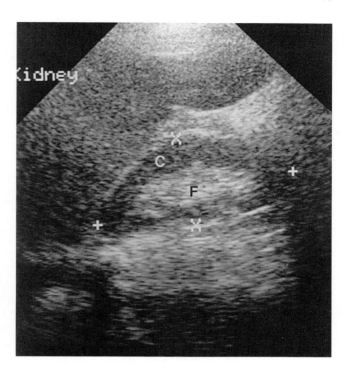

FIGURE 7–2. **Normal renal ultrasound.** A longitudinal view of the right kidney was obtained by passing the sound beam through the right lobe of the liver. The kidney is seen behind this, outlined by the markers. The central bright echoes in the kidney are due to fat (F) around the collecting system. The cortex (C) is seen more peripherally.

performed. Neither an IVP nor an ultrasound examination can completely exclude a urologic malignancy, because an IVP can miss small parenchymal renal tumors, and ultrasound is poor for detection of small urothelial tumors. Both are poor for evaluation of bladder tumors. The best evaluation of painless, nontraumatic hematuria often begins with cystoscopy and possibly retrograde pyelograms at the same time. If this is negative, a CT scan is indicated.

KIDNEYS

Congenital Abnormalities

Congenital abnormalities of the urinary tract occur quite frequently. Embryologically, the ureter buds and grows superiorly from the bladder to meet and to connect with the renal parenchyma. The ureter can divide as it ascends, causing a person to have two partially duplicated or completely sepa-

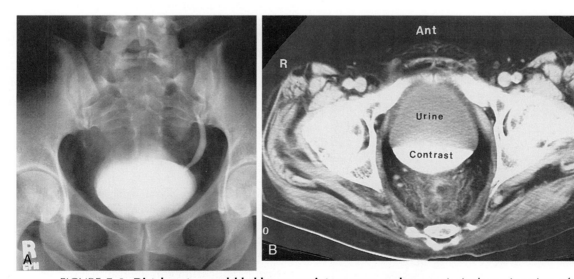

FIGURE 7–3. **Distal ureters and bladder on an intravenous pyelogram.** A single supine view of the pelvis during an intravenous pyelogram (A) shows the distal left ureter and what appears to be the bladder. A computed tomography scan obtained on this patient at the same time at the level of the bladder (B) shows that the contrast material from the intravenous pyelogram is layering only in the dependent portion of the bladder. Thus, on an intravenous pyelogram, when you think you are looking at the bladder, you are simply seeing a puddle of contrast material in the back of the bladder.

rate collecting systems for one kidney. If there is complete ureteral duplication, the ureter that supplies the upper half of the kidney often becomes obstructed. If the obstruction is not severe, this can be seen filling with contrast material on an IVP. If the upper pole collecting system is completely obstructed, all that is visualized is the normally draining lower pole collecting system, and it looks like a drooping lily. The duplicated ureter that supplies the upper pole may often have an ectopic insertion into the bladder, urethra, or vagina.

A number of other anomalies occur in the course of the normal embryologic ascent of the kidneys out of the bony pelvis. These anomalies include one kidney rising normally and the other kidney remaining in the pelvis. It is quite rare to have a unilateral kidney, and thus if there is only one kidney in normal position, an ectopic kidney (Fig. 7–4) must be looked for elsewhere. Another common variant is fusion of the inferior aspect of both kidneys (a horseshoe kidney). This is relatively easy to identify because the axis of the kidneys is abnormal—the superior aspect of the kidneys is tilted outward instead of inward.

Renal Cysts

Renal cysts are quite common, and their incidence increases with age. Most persons older than 60 years have one or more simple renal cysts. These are often found incidentally on an IVP, and they are frequently seen on CT scans ordered for other reasons. An ultrasound examination is a good, inex-

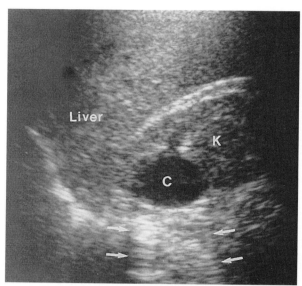

FIGURE 7–5. **Simple renal cyst.** A longitudinal ultrasound image shows the normal liver and renal parenchyma with a cyst (C) in the upper and posterior aspect of the right kidney (K). Notice that there are no (white) echoes within the cyst and that there is increased transmission of sound through the fluid of the cyst, producing a posterior-enhanced echo pattern (arrows).

pensive initial test to characterize a suspected renal cyst found on an IVP. The margins of a benign simple cyst should be well defined, and there should be increased echoes on the posterior aspect of the cyst owing to good transmission of sound through the fluid in the cyst (Fig. 7–5). If a cyst has septa or internal echoes, a CT scan is indicated to further evaluate for a possible cystic neoplasm.

Polycystic renal disease presents a difficult imaging problem. In the adult form of this heritable disorder, progressive renal failure often occurs. A CT scan demonstrates lumpy kidneys, but the cysts may not be well defined because of hemorrhage within them. Cysts are also usually identified in the liver and sometimes in the pancreas.

Renal Stone Disease

Calcification can occur within the substance of the kidney or within the collecting system. Calcification within the substance of the kidney (nephrocalcinosis) may be cortical (near the periphery of the kidney) or medullary (near the ends of the calyces). Cortical calcification can be due to chronic glomerulonephritis, cortical necrosis, or acquired immunodeficiency syndrome–related nephropathy. Medullary calcification may be idiopathic or caused by papillary necrosis, medullary sponge kidney, or other hypercalcemic states (including hyperparathyroidism) (Fig. 7–6).

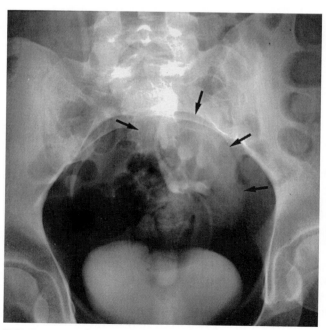

FIGURE 7–4. **Pelvic kidney.** An incidental finding on an intravenous pyelogram is a left pelvic kidney (arrows).

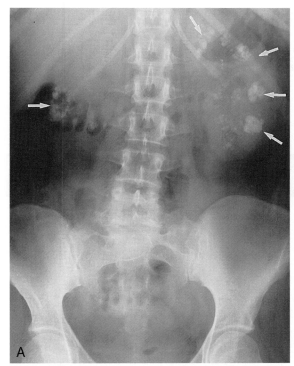

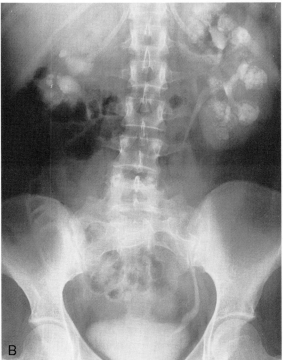

FIGURE 7–6. **Nephrocalcinosis.** A plain film of the abdomen (A) shows multiple calcifications (arrows) within the left kidney. On an intravenous pyelogram (B), the calcifications are located near the ends of the calyces (medullary) rather than in the cortex. This particular patient had medullary sponge kidneys.

At least 80% (and perhaps up to 90%) of renal calculi are radiopaque and appear dense (or white) on a routine radiograph. Occasionally, renal stones become quite large and essentially fill the collecting system of the kidney. These are referred to as *staghorn calculi.* If calculi are overlying the kidneys or are within the course of the ureter, they are usually fairly easy to see. Sometimes it can be difficult to visualize a small stone in the region where the ureter passes anterior to the sacrum. Stones smaller than 4 mm are likely to cause obstruction and often require surgery or lithotripsy. A large number of vascular calcifications occur low within the bony pelvis and to the sides of the bladder. These phleboliths typically can be recognized because they are round, have a lucent (dark) center, and are more lateral and lower in the pelvis than the normal course of the ureter.

The most common clinical and radiographic presentation of renal stone disease is intense unilateral flank pain with hematuria. If the patient is having a first presentation of renal stone disease, an IVP or spiral noncontrasted CT scan is indicated even if no calculus is seen on the plain film of the abdomen. If there is a prior history of renal stones, imaging is not always needed. Imaging may be reserved for those patients who have pain uncontrolled by medication, those with continued flank pain for more than 5 days, those who have continued hematuria 2 weeks after passing a stone, those with microscopic hematuria for more than 1 month, and those who have acute flank pain and are known to have a solitary kidney or pelvic tumor.

On an IVP, the obstruction of the ureter by a stone may cause delayed visualization of the affected kidney and ureter. When it does visualize, the ureter is usually dilated, and the renal calyces are blunted (Fig. 7–7). On delayed radiographs, although the normal kidney is completely clear of contrast material, the affected kidney and ureter are seen retaining contrast material. Delayed images are often necessary to determine the exact level of the ureteral obstruction.

Occasionally, back pressure caused by an obstructing ureteral stone can rupture a renal calyx or renal pelvis. When this occurs, there is extravasation of urine and contrast material outside the kidney into the perirenal space.

When there is an obstructing lesion of the ureter, the urologist may perform cystoscopy and then put a little tube into the distal ureter and inject contrast material (a retrograde pyelogram). The ureter, renal pelvis, and calyces are usually visualized. Because there is pressure being exerted during the injection, minimal blunting of the calyces may result, which is normal under these circumstances. As mentioned earlier, an ultrasound study can be used for stone evaluation but it is poor for stones that are smaller than 5 mm or in the ureter. Spiral noncontrasted CT scanning is often used as an alternative to an IVP because it is much faster and, unlike an IVP,

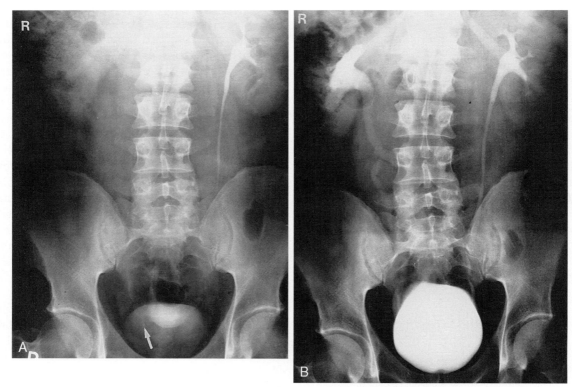

FIGURE 7–7. **Ureteral calculus.** This young male had intense right flank pain and hematuria. *(A),* An x-ray film taken at 5 minutes during an intravenous pyelogram shows good function of the left kidney, and the left ureter is well seen. The right kidney is faintly seen, and a small calcification is seen at the ureterovesicular junction *(arrow).* A delayed image, 20 minutes later *(B),* now shows a dilated right renal collecting system and right ureter due to obstruction by the distal ureteral calculus.

does not require contrast material. Many hospitals have specific CT protocols that result in a CT scan and an IVP costing approximately the same amount.

Renal Failure

Imaging is indicated in patients with unexplained oliguria or new onset of renal insufficiency or failure (serum creatinine level >2 mg/dL). Most imaging studies of the kidneys rely on normal function. The most common clinical question is whether renal failure is due to obstruction or medical renal disease. Because the intravenous contrast material used for an IVP or a CT scan can reduce renal function, the imaging examination of choice in these circumstances is ultrasonography. Normally, the cortex of the kidney has the same ultrasound echo density as the liver or has fewer echoes than the substance of the liver. In cases of medical renal disease, there are more echoes within the renal cortex than within the liver. This is probably the result of fibrosis and scarring.

Pyelonephritis and Renal Infection

The clinical findings of pyelonephritis include fever, flank pain, and pyuria. Most patients with pyelonephritis have no discernible findings on imaging studies. Imaging studies are usually not warranted in women unless there are repetitive episodes or persistent, worsening pain after 3 days of appropriate antibiotic therapy. In patients who have severe acute pyelonephritis, enough edema of the renal parenchyma occurs so that the swelling causes compression of the calyces or renal pelvis, and thus the collecting system is not well visualized on an IVP. Occasionally with acute pyelonephritis, focal areas of edema can be seen on CT scans, although this is usually incidental. In these cases, the real purpose of ordering CT scans should be to look for a renal parenchymal or perirenal abscess.

Patients with diabetes are particularly prone to an unusual form of acute pyelonephritis called *emphysematous pyelonephritis.* In these patients, actual gas is generated by the bacteria within the parenchyma of the kidney. Usually, the kidney is nonfunctional with a dark radiating striated gas pattern seen in the kidney.

Occasionally, inflammatory abnormalities can cause enlargement of both kidneys. This is particularly true in acute glomerulonephritis. The differential diagnosis for bilaterally enlarged kidneys includes bilateral obstruction, leukemia, glycogen storage diseases, lymphoma, polycystic disease, and a number of other conditions (Fig. 7–8).

Renal tuberculosis can affect the kidneys, ureter, and bladder; the infection typically begins in the kidneys and thus first should be looked for there. In the early stages, narrowing or amputation of the infundibulum between a renal calyx and the renal pelvis occurs. In late stages, a nonfunctional shrunken kidney with clumps of calcification is seen. A number of fungal infections can affect the kidney in patients with diabetes and those who are immunosuppressed. Fungal infections often cause large fungus balls within the collecting system that can obstruct the kidney.

Renal Trauma

Blunt trauma, particularly during motor vehicle accidents, can cause a number of renal abnormalities. Significant kidney trauma should be suspected when there is a fracture of the 12th rib or fractures of the transverse processes of the lumbar vertebrae. Another useful sign on the plain film is nonvisualization of the psoas margin on one side. A CT scan

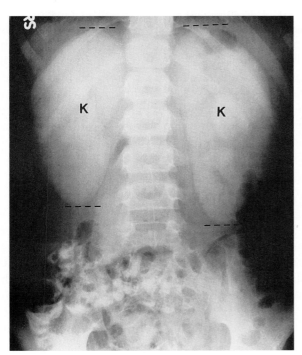

FIGURE 7–8. **Acute glomerulonephritis.** An intravenous pyelogram in this child demonstrates markedly enlarged kidneys (K) bilaterally. The injected contrast material has made the kidneys visible, but the kidneys are unable to excrete the contrast material.

is indicated if there is gross hematuria or suspected injury to other organs. With a renal contusion the kidney is intact, but there is interstitial edema that may lead to reduced blood flow. Lacerations and intrarenal hematomas can be incomplete (not extending into the calyceal system), whereas complete lacerations are usually accompanied by a significant hemorrhage and urine extravasation (Fig. 7–9). Surgical intervention may not be required unless there is major blood loss. Occasionally there may be avulsion of the renal vascular pedicle with disruption of the blood supply. Minor blunt trauma with microscopic hematuria and a low suspicion of injury to other organs is usually treated conservatively.

Renal Tumors

Renal cell carcinoma constitutes about 85% of all primary renal malignancies. It usually occurs in the sixth decade, and males are affected twice as often as females. The classic clinical triad consists of gross hematuria, flank pain, and a flank mass, although this triad is seen in only approximately 10% of patients. Typically, gross or microscopic hematuria is what suggests a urinary malignancy. Large mass lesions within the kidney displace the collecting system and produce an irregular contour of the kidney on an IVP, but extremely small tumors or pedunculated neoplasms can be difficult to appreciate. CT with and without intravenous contrast material (with thin cuts through the kidneys) is the imaging procedure of choice in a patient with persistent painless hematuria, a normal IVP, and normal cystoscopy.

Most renal cell carcinomas are relatively solid, but some are quite cystic, and it is sometimes difficult to differentiate a cystic neoplasm from a benign renal cyst. On a CT scan, the findings of a thickened wall or a mural mass within a cystic abnormality are criteria for malignancy (Fig. 7–10). CT or MRI scans can be used to evaluate potential extension into the renal vein, inferior vena cava, and nearby nodes. Metastases from renal cell carcinoma tend to go either to local nodes, the lung, or the bone. Periodic chest x-ray examinations and CT scans are both indicated for follow-up, even in asymptomatic patients. On the chest radiograph, the metastases are usually nodules ranging from 0.5 cm to several centimeters in size. When the metastases are in the bone, they tend to be quite aggressive, expansive, and lytic (destructive).

Renal Artery Stenosis

Less than 5% of patients with hypertension have renal artery stenosis as the cause. Imaging is usu-

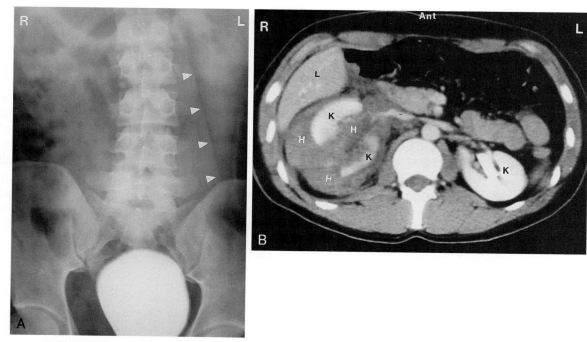

FIGURE 7–9. **Renal laceration.** A radiograph of the abdomen *(A)* in a young male involved in an automobile accident shows a well-defined left psoas margin *(arrowheads)*. The right psoas margin is not identified, and a contrast-enhanced computed tomography scan *(B)* at the level of the kidneys shows a fracture through the midportion of the right kidney. The kidney (K) can be seen in two separate pieces with intervening and surrounding hemorrhage (H). L = liver.

ally reserved for those hypertensive patients who are uncontrolled by two medications or who are uncontrolled by medication and have increasing levels of serum blood urea nitrogen or creatinine. In those circumstances, a nuclear medicine captopril renogram is performed. Evaluation of the patient while giving captopril temporarily reduces function on the affected side.

Obstruction of the Renal Collecting System

Obstruction of the ureter is easily visualized by an IVP, which affords a detailed view of the anatomy. For other clinical indications, however, ultrasonography may be more useful. Although it is difficult or impossible to visualize the full length of the ureter by an ultrasound, it is quite easy to determine whether there is dilatation of the collecting system within the kidney itself (Fig. 7–11). This is seen as an area with relatively few echoes splaying the high intensity echoes (caused by fat) around the renal collecting system. For follow-up of a patient with known hydronephrosis, ultrasonography is the best test. It is also the test of choice to differentiate hydronephrosis from medical renal disease in a patient who has presented with renal failure.

Occasionally, there is dilatation of the renal pelvis that is not caused by obstruction. This may have a congenital basis or may be the result of a flaccid collecting system. A simple way of differentiating the two is to order a nuclear medicine furosemide (Lasix) renogram. The patient is injected with a radioactive material that is rapidly cleared by glomerular filtration. This gives an image of both kidneys that looks like a miniature IVP. However, the advantage of this study is that the patient can be injected with Lasix approximately 15 minutes into the study; using computer analysis, the degree of washout from the collecting system can be measured. If there is rapid clearance of activity from the kidney and renal pelvis, it indicates a flaccid system rather than an obstructed one.

Ureter

Duplication of the ureter and collecting system has already been discussed. Sometimes the ureter has an abnormal entrance into the bladder, with dilatation of the ureter as it passes through the bladder wall (ureterocele) causing a *cobra head deformity* (Fig. 7–12). Ureteroceles are not of much clinical importance and generally do not require treatment.

The ureter normally has peristaltic waves; therefore, on any single film, some portions of the ureter and not others are usually visualized. Because an IVP is done with the patient supine and contrast material is heavier than urine, the most anterior

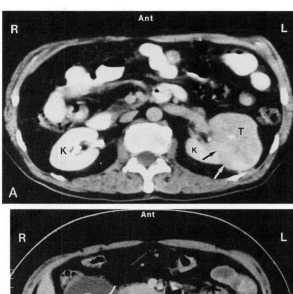

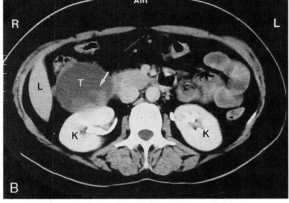

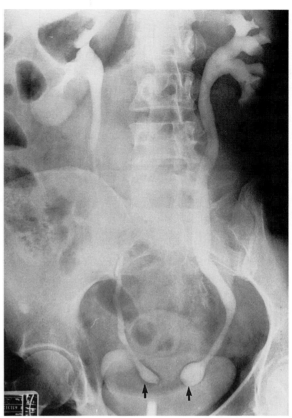

FIGURE 7–10. **Renal cell carcinoma.** A transverse contrast-enhanced computed tomography scan *(A)* in a patient with hematuria shows significant replacement of the left kidney (K) by tumor (T and *arrows*). The left renal vein exiting the K is also quite thick, indicating tumor extension into the renal vein. A cystic renal cell carcinoma is shown in a computed tomography scan on a different patient *(B).* In this patient, a pedunculated cystic lesion is seen projecting off the anterior aspect of the right kidney. The fact that there is a mass projecting within the generally cystic lesion *(arrow)* as well as an irregularly thickened wall makes this highly suspicious for a cancer. L = liver.

FIGURE 7–12. **Bilateral ureteroceles.** This intravenous pyelogram demonstrates a congenital variant with dilatation of the distal ureter as it enters through the bladder wall. This produces a typical *cobra head deformity (arrows),* which is usually of little clinical significance.

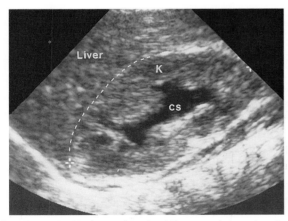

FIGURE 7–11. **Hydronephrosis.** Ultrasound imaging is the simplest and most cost-effective way of determining whether hydronephrosis is present. Here, a longitudinal image of the right kidney (K, outlined by the *dashed line*) demonstrates a dilated collecting system (cs).

portions of the ureters (as they pass over the sacroiliac joints into the pelvis) are usually quite difficult to see. Sometimes the radiologist orders a prone film to rectify this situation.

Dilatation of a ureter is diagnosed when the ureter is seen to be greater than 8 mm in diameter and when contrast material is backed up in the ureter without peristaltic waves. In an acute obstruction, calyceal blunting is almost always present. However, dilatation can be due to a number of causes, including obstruction, ureterovesicular reflux, infection, and congenital megaureter.

Common intraluminal abnormalities of the ureter are renal calculi (as discussed earlier), blood clots, transitional cell carcinomas, and, occasionally, fungal lesions. A clot within the ureter is not visible on a plain film. On an IVP, it is a filling defect that can look like a nonopaque stone. Remember that most renal calculi (80%) are radiopaque and should be visible on plain films. A clot should be suspected following trauma and in patients who are taking anticoagulants.

Transitional cell carcinomas can occur either in the renal collecting system or in the bladder. In the renal collecting system, they can form a mass that spreads the renal sinus fat and can cause obstruction (Fig. 7–13). In the ureter, a renal cell carcinoma may look like a lesion in the wall of the ureter, or it may cause an apple core deformity with encirclement of the lumen.

In addition to lesions that are entirely contained within the lumen, there may be lesions that project into the lumen or are the result of extrinsic pressure. In some patients, there are indentations across the upper one third of the collecting system caused by vascular impressions of blood vessels as they cross over the ureter. Collateral vessels may cause ureteral notching. In patients who have an infection, there may be small fluid-filled cysts in the ureteral wall that project into the lumen (pyelitis cystica). Occasionally, even metastases can indent the ureter at multiple locations. This is most often the result of metastatic melanoma. If there appears to be a ureteral lesion on an IVP, this should be confirmed by the urologist, who may perform cystoscopy and retrograde ureterography.

Deviation of the ureter can signal nearby pathology. In the region between the lower pole of the kidney and the sacrum, the normal course of the ureters on an anteroposterior or a posteroanterior film is over the transverse processes of the spine. Lateral deviation of a ureter can be the result of retroperitoneal adenopathy, retroperitoneal tumors, abdominal aortic aneurysms, and, occasionally, large psoas muscles (in young men or horse riders). Medial deviation can be due to traction caused by fibrosis from chronic leakage of an aneurysm or, if only on the right side, by a congenital retrocaval ureter.

■ BLADDER

Anatomy and Imaging Techniques

As the bladder fills with urine, it has water or soft tissue density. The bladder can often be seen on a plain radiograph, because it is frequently outlined by perivesicular fat. As the bladder enlarges with urine, it pushes the small bowel superiorly and laterally. An enlarged bladder can be quite striking (Fig. 7–14), and without having contrast material in the bladder, it is often difficult to tell an enlarged fluid-filled bladder from some other soft tissue mass arising from the pelvis or abdomen. It is unusual for abdominal masses or tumors to grow down into the pelvis, but it is common for pelvic masses to grow up out of the pelvis into the lower abdomen. Thus, a soft tissue mass that involves both the lower abdomen and the pelvis probably arose in the pelvis. The differential diagnosis of a pelvic mass includes uterine enlargement, ovarian cysts, and tumor or pelvic sarcomas. If the patient is female and the bladder is displaced to one side, an ovarian etiology is suggested. The primary imaging techniques for the bladder are the production of IVPs, cystograms, and CT scans. These images are adequate for large lesions and are particularly good in cases of trauma in which a tear is suspected. All are quite insensitive to small or infiltrative neoplasms. As a result, cystoscopy should be performed first if malignancy is suspected.

Trauma

Fractures of the pelvis are accompanied by hematomas. These may displace the bladder to one side

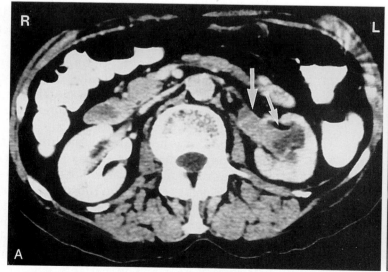
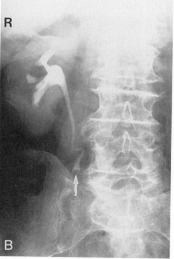

FIGURE 7–13. **Transitional cell carcinoma.** A transverse contrast-enhanced computed tomography scan at the level of the kidneys (A) shows expansion of the left renal pelvis (arrows). This is due to a transitional cell carcinoma within the renal pelvis. In a different patient, an intravenous pyelogram (B) demonstrates an upside-down goblet deformity in the right midureter (arrow). This is a sign of a ureteral transitional cell carcinoma.

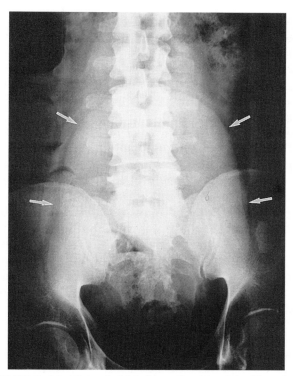

FIGURE 7–14. **Distended bladder.** On this plain film of the abdomen, a large soft tissue mass is seen arising from the pelvis *(arrows).* It has pushed the small bowel out of the way. The differential diagnosis includes a pelvic tumor, distended bladder, or cystic abnormality arising from the pelvis.

if they are unilateral. However, more often pelvic hematomas are bilateral, and they compress and elevate the inferior portion of the bladder (Fig. 7–15) so that it looks like an upside-down teardrop. This shape of the bladder can also be caused by pelvic adenopathy, pelvic lipomatosis (mostly in black males with hypertension), and rarely by prominent iliopsoas muscles.

With pelvic fractures or as a result of direct compression of a fluid-filled distended bladder, the bladder can rupture. This is almost always accompanied by hematuria. About 10% of patients who have a pelvic fracture have bladder rupture. The bladder can rupture either extraperitoneally (80%) or intraperitoneally (20%). Intraperitoneal rupture of the bladder is recognized on an IVP or a cystogram because there is contrast extravasation into the peritoneal cavity that outlines loops of bowel. The contrast also layers in the paracolic gutters.

The vast majority of patients with an extraperitoneal bladder rupture have associated pelvic fractures. With extraperitoneal rupture, the extravasated contrast material is in a streaky or sunburst-type pattern (Fig. 7–16). About 10% of patients with ruptured bladders have both an intraperitoneal and extraperitoneal component.

Penetrating trauma of the lower abdomen or pelvis with suspected urinary system involvement requires a retrograde cystogram or a CT scan. If the CT scan is being done for evaluation of other systems, a CT cystogram can be performed at the same time.

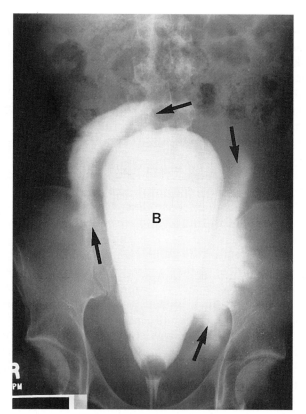

FIGURE 7–16. **Bladder rupture.** A cystogram done in a patient following a motor vehicle accident shows extravasation of contrast agent *(arrows)* into the tissues surrounding the bladder (B). This is an extraperitoneal bladder rupture. With an intraperitoneal bladder rupture, contrast agent would be seen outlining loops of bowel.

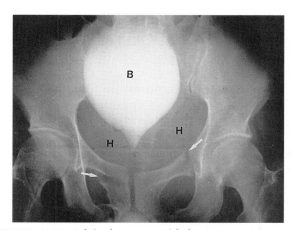

FIGURE 7–15. **Pelvic fractures with hematoma.** This cystogram demonstrates multiple pelvic fractures *(arrows).* The associated bilateral hematomas (H) have elevated and compressed the bladder (B).

Pelvic trauma can also result in injury to the urethra. Because the female urethra is so short, this is rarely, if ever, injured in an accident. In the male, urethral injuries are more common than bladder injuries. The indicated imaging method is a retrograde urethrogram. Because the urethra is fixed at the prostatomembranous junction, tears in this area are secondary to shearing. In a patient with pelvic trauma who has blood at the urethral meatus and who is unable to void or can void only with difficulty, a posterior urethral tear should be suspected. In these cases, a retrograde urethrogram should be done before any attempt is made to catheterize the bladder. The reason is that a small initial tear may be significantly enlarged by any attempt at catheterization. Injuries to the anterior portion of the urethra are much less common. Injuries to the bulbous portion of the urethra are most commonly due to a straddle injury in which the patient falls astride a solid object, such as a beam.

Incontinence

Incontinence in some form affects about 10 million persons in the United States. Inability to hold urine results from a wide number of etiologies. The mechanism of urination involves the bladder wall, sphincters, and pelvic musculature, as well as neurologic control in the bladder, spinal cord, and brain. The work-up is best begun with a thorough medical history, physical examination, urinalysis, and evaluation of postvoid residual volume. There are 4 forms of incontinence: urge, stress, overflow, and mixed.

Urge incontinence can be due to lesions (infection, stones, or neoplasm) of the bladder near the trigone, causing uncontrolled contractions. Stress incontinence occurs with increased intra-abdominal pressure (e.g., coughing, sneezing) and is most common in parous postmenopausal women, as a result of estrogen deprivation and relaxation of the pelvic musculature with loss of the normal ureterovesicular angle. Imaging is not usually indicated, and most women are treated conservatively with exercise of the pelvic muscles. In men, stress incontinence is usually secondary to prostatic surgery. Other causes that should be considered include multiple sclerosis or other neurologic abnormalities. Overflow incontinence is due to large volumes in an atonic bladder secondary to spinal cord injury, diabetes, hypothyroidism, chronic alcoholism, or collagen vascular disease. In patients with incontinence and suspected urologic abnormality, urodynamic studies should be conducted before imaging procedures.

Neurologic Abnormalities

If trauma compromises the spinal cord, the bladder may become either flaccid or spastic. On a contrasted study, a spastic bladder has the shape of a Christmas tree, with little outpouchings along the lateral margins. These outpouching areas of contrast material or urine are pseudodiverticula caused by hypertrophy of the bladder musculature. A hyper-reflexive bladder usually occurs when the spinal cord lesion is at the level of T5 or higher. These patients are prime candidates for urinary infection, calculi, and bilateral collecting system dilatation. Hyporeflexive bladders are usually the result of a herniated disk, multiple sclerosis, diabetic neuropathy, or lower spinal cord tumor. Although these patients may demonstrate a large bladder, the upper urinary collecting systems are usually within normal limits, and vesicoureteral reflux is rare.

Infections

There is little reason to do imaging studies in female patients with uncomplicated cystitis. For women experiencing repeated bouts of infection, an IVP may be indicated to exclude anatomic abnormalities. Because cystitis is rare in males, an IVP is indicated after an initial infection. With severe cystitis, there may be mucosal thickening; however, this should not be diagnosed on a study that has a poorly distended bladder. Once the bladder is fully distended, it may be possible to image thickened mucosa, although this finding rarely changes treatment.

There are a number of unusual bladder infections in which imaging findings are fairly characteristic. Patients with diabetes may develop emphysematous cystitis, in which gas is present in either the wall or the lumen of the bladder. In contrast to emphysematous pyelonephritis, morbidity is not increased with emphysematous cystitis. This condition usually responds well to antibiotic therapy. Air within the bladder itself is more likely due to instrumentation or a bladder-bowel fistula.

Tuberculosis can affect the bladder, but this is extremely rare without strictures and stenosis of the ureters and stenosis of the calyces of the renal collecting system. Schistosomiasis, although quite rare, can produce characteristic bladder wall calcification. A number of inflammatory conditions can cause a bladder of small capacity, including interstitial cystitis, cyclophosphamide cystitis, and radiation therapy. These can also cause calcification within the bladder wall. With the exception of a small capacity, very little is characteristic or disease specific about the imaging findings.

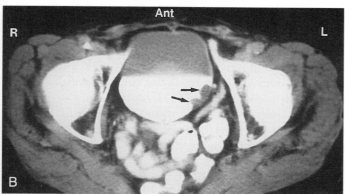

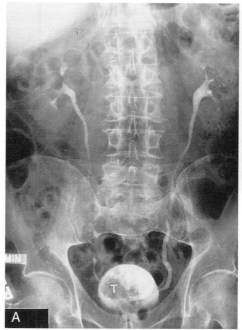

FIGURE 7–17. **Bladder carcinoma.** An intravenous pyelogram *(A)* in a patient with hematuria clearly shows a large irregular filling defect within the bladder caused by a tumor (T). A computed tomography scan *(B)* in a different patient shows a small bladder carcinoma *(arrows)*. This is visible only because the tumor happens to be in the dependent portion of the bladder with the contrast agent. If this lesion had been on the anterior surface of the bladder, it probably would not have been visualized on either a computed tomography scan or an intravenous pyelogram.

Tumors

Ninety-five percent of bladder tumors are transitional cell carcinomas. Transitional cell carcinomas are 4 times more common in men than in women, and a significantly increased incidence has been associated with cigarette smoking. Patients frequently present with hematuria and occasionally with urinary frequency and dysuria. If a bladder carcinoma is suspected, the initial study of choice should be direct visualization using cystoscopy.

Pelvic lymph node extension is relatively common. Hematogenous metastases tend to go to liver, lungs, and, to a much lesser extent, bone. When bone lesions are seen, they are typically lytic. Transitional cell carcinoma of the bladder is associated with upper tract transitional cell tumors, and close follow-up of these patients is essential.

Tumors of the bladder rarely calcify, and the diagnosis of tumors is not obvious on plain films. An IVP may show a filling defect within the lumen of the bladder (Fig. 7–17). On an IVP, a bladder tumor is not visualized unless it is located in the dependent portion of the bladder. CT scanning is useful only to evaluate invasion of adjacent organs and pelvic lymphadenopathy.

Prostate

Enlargement of the prostate causes elevation of the base of the bladder (Fig. 7–18). Prostate enlargement is most often the result of benign prostatic hypertrophy rather than prostatic carcinoma. If the prostate is big enough, there can be outlet obstruction of the bladder. For uncomplicated benign prostatic hypertrophy, no imaging is necessary. Likewise, no imaging is needed for uncomplicated prostatitis.

Prostate cancer is common. There has been a lot of interest in the transrectal ultrasound examination of the prostate as a screening test for prostate

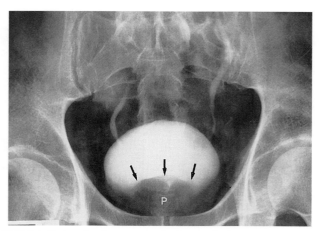

FIGURE 7–18. **Benign prostatic hyperplasia.** A view of the bladder obtained during an intravenous pyelogram shows a smooth defect impressing on the inferior aspect of the bladder *(arrows)* caused by a benign enlargement of the prostate (P).

cancer. At the present time, this is not a useful test by itself, and no screening modality has been shown to reduce mortality. The initial investigation for suspected prostate carcinoma should be by digital rectal examination and evaluation of the serum level of prostate-specific antigen (PSA). Unfortunately, PSA is neither sensitive nor specific for prostate cancer. If the serum PSA value is elevated, ultrasonography may be helpful in locating a suspicious area in which a transrectal biopsy may be performed. There are a number of other indices besides total PSA levels that are being used including age-specific PSA and PSA velocity. In general, the level of PSA in men between the age of 40 and 50 should not exceed 2.5 ng/mL, and in men older than 50 years, it should not exceed 3.5 to 4.0 ng/mL. Notes should be made that patients taking finasteride have a PSA level about 50% lower than the true value.

Ultrasonography, CT, and MRI are not extremely accurate in determining local extension of a tumor. CT or MRI can show metastatic lesions in the rest of the abdomen; however, in a patient with a known prostate carcinoma and a rising PSA level, radionuclide bone scan is the initial test of choice.

Testicular Pain and Masses

The most common lesions of the scrotum that may require imaging are epididymitis, testicular torsion, hematoma, and hydrocele, in addition to evaluation for testicular tumors. In cases in which testicular torsion needs to be differentiated from epididymitis, a radionuclide testicular scan is widely used (Fig. 7–19). Epididymitis is seen as a lesion with hyperemia on the affected side. In acute torsion, an area of decreased blood flow is on the side in which there is pain. In a torsion that has been present for a day or more (missed torsion), there is a lesion without much blood flow centrally but with a hypervascular rim. Doppler ultrasonography can also be used to exclude a testicular torsion, although this is quite operator dependent and more difficult to do. In cases of acute testicular trauma, ultrasonography is the test of choice.

Imaging evaluation of the testicle for either a hydrocele or a tumor should be done using an ultrasound study. In general, any mass within the testicle itself should be considered malignant, whereas those lesions outside the testicle but within the scrotum are usually benign. Ninety-five percent of solid testicular masses are germ cell tumors (seminoma, embryonal carcinoma, choriocarcinoma, and teratoma). Staging of these tumors is done by a chest radiograph and a CT scan of the abdomen and pelvis. Evaluation of a patient for cryptorchidism can be done either by ultrasonography or CT.

■ FEMALE PELVIS

Anatomy and Imaging Techniques

The most common and fruitful imaging methods are pelvic ultrasonography and CT. Ultrasonography is undoubtedly the most widely used method, because it can easily image the uterus and adnexal regions. Because it does not use ionizing radiation, it can even be used during pregnancy. Imaging of the female pelvis with a plain radiograph is usually of low yield, because most significant pathology associated with female pelvic organs does not calcify.

A female pelvic ultrasound is done either transabdominally (by having the transducer on the lower anterior abdominal wall and using a full bladder as a window to image through) or transvaginally. A transvaginal ultrasound has a much smaller field

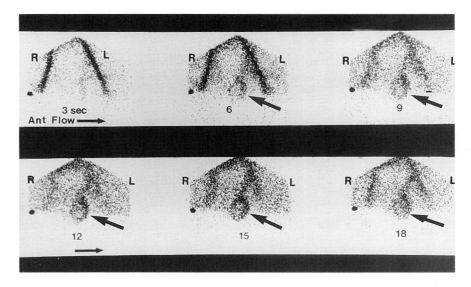

FIGURE 7–19. **Testicular torsion.** Evaluation of blood flow to the testicle has been done by giving an intravenous bolus of radioactive material. The right and left iliac vessels are clearly identified, and sequential images are obtained every 3 seconds. Here, increased flow is seen to the rim of the left testicle (arrows), and there is no blood flow centrally. This is the appearance of a testicular torsion in which the torsion has been present for more than approximately 24 hours.

of view, and orientation with respect to the images is often quite difficult.

Transvaginal ultrasonography is good to look for fine detail of structures low in the pelvis. Typical indications are early pregnancy, suspected ectopic pregnancy, ovarian torsion or cysts, and measurement of the endometrial stripe. With transabdominal ultrasonography, orientation is much easier. Remember that ultrasound imaging gives you a slice picture. The slices are typically either longitudinal or transverse. In the longitudinal plane, the vagina, cervix, uterus, and bladder can be easily seen (Fig. 7–20). Areas of high intensity echoes can be seen in the vagina and sometimes in the center of the uterus as a result of mucus production, hemorrhage, or decidual reaction. Fluid in the bladder, uterus, or cul-de-sac appears as an area without echoes. A small amount of fluid within the cul-de-sac can be a normal finding in the middle of the menstrual period, but in patients in whom an ectopic pregnancy is suspected, this may represent hemorrhage (Fig. 7–21).

Evaluation of the uterus by an ultrasound does not allow determination of patency of the fallopian tubes. A hysterosalpingogram is typically done to assess tubal patency. This is done by putting a cannula in the cervical os and injecting a water-based contrast material. After the uterus is filled, the contrast material normally goes out the fallopian tubes and spills into the peritoneal cavity. In cases in which there is obstruction of the fallopian tubes (hydrosalpinx), the contrast material proceeds to the point of obstruction in the fallopian tubes and then collects in a dilated portion of the fallopian tube without free spill into the pelvis.

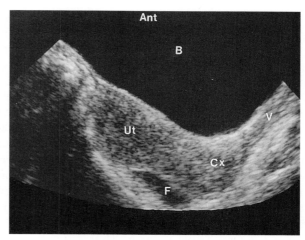

FIGURE 7–21. **Free fluid in the cul-de-sac.** This longitudinal image of the pelvis demonstrates a collection of fluid (F) behind the uterus (Ut). This can be a normal finding during the middle of the menstrual cycle or may represent bleeding from a condition such as ectopic pregnancy. B = bladder; Cx = cervix; V = vagina.

Infertility

Infertility is the inability to become pregnant in 12 months at age less than 30 or in 6 months at age over 30. It may be due to abnormalities of the male or female. In the female, it can be due to absent ovulation from any cause and anatomic factors such as tubal scarring, fibroids, congenital uterine abnormalities, or adenomyomatosis. Initial evaluation includes a complete physical examination, a pelvic examination, and a measurement of serum hormone levels. An ultrasound image can be used to assess follicle development. If ovulation is confirmed and physical examination, complete blood cell count, basal body temperature, thyroid function, and pituitary function are normal, and if the male is normal, a hysterosalpingogram to assess tubal patency is indicated. It is also indicated to assess tubal patency following surgery or in cases of repeated spontaneous abortion.

Vaginal Bleeding

Dysfunctional uterine bleeding is due to a number of causes including hormonal imbalance and tumors. Imaging procedures are not in the initial work-up. An ultrasound examination is indicated in a premenopausal female who has a normal cervix and vagina by physical examination and who has bleeding continuing after three cycles of hormone therapy. Ultrasonography is also indicated in postmenopausal women with bleeding who are not on hormonal replacement therapy or who have been taking daily or cyclical hormonal therapy for more than 6 months.

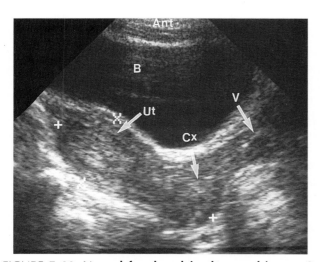

FIGURE 7–20. **Normal female pelvic ultrasound image.** On this longitudinal image obtained in the midportion of the pelvis, the bladder (B), uterus (Ut), cervix (Cx), and vagina (V) are easily visualized. The uterus is outlined by the X and + markers.

Intrauterine and Ectopic Pregnancy

Ultrasonography is the imaging method of choice to evaluate the status of a pregnancy. A routine ultrasound is not indicated, nor should ultrasonography be performed for the sole purpose of determining sex. The common indications for ultrasound during pregnancy are shown in Table 7–2. In very early pregnancy, transvaginal, rather than transabdominal, ultrasonography is the most sensitive. By measuring the fetal crown-rump length and a number of other parameters, the gestational age of the fetus can be determined. The age that is usually quoted refers to menstrual age rather than conceptual age. Thus, a report that indicates a 5-week pregnancy (gestational age) really corresponds to a 3-week pregnancy (conception age).

The first ultrasound sign of pregnancy is the appearance of the gestational sac at 28 to 30 days. A yolk sac can be seen at 5 to 6 weeks, and this is the first reliable sign of an intrauterine pregnancy. A heartbeat is also typically seen at approximately 5 weeks (gestational age) (Fig. 7–22). As the fetus becomes more advanced, it is possible to see decidual thickening and formation of the placenta. A low-lying placenta early in pregnancy does not necessar-

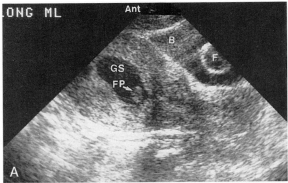
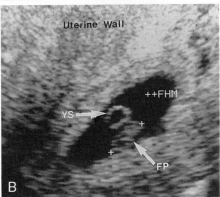

FIGURE 7–22. **Early normal obstetric ultrasound image.** A longitudinal transabdominal ultrasound image *(A)* demonstrates the bladder *(B)* and a Foley catheter (F) within it. Superior to and behind the bladder is the uterus with a gestational sac (GS) centrally and a fetal pole (FP) within it. More detail can be obtained using transvaginal ultrasound *(B)* imaging. In this case, the fetal pole (FP) can be measured; a yolk sac (YS) is also seen. The technician has indicated that fetal heart motion was seen (+ +FHM).

TABLE 7–2 Common Indications for Use of Ultrasound During Pregnancy*

Size/dates discrepancy ≥2 weeks
Multiple gestation
Uterine growth < expected between prenatal visits
Vaginal bleeding
Suspected placental abruption
Suspected congenital anomaly with abnormal estradiol, human chorionic gonadotropin, or alpha-fetoprotein
First-degree relative with congenital anomaly
Assistance in obtaining amniotic fluid
Past obstetric history of congenital anomaly, microsomia (<10th percentile body weight), macrosomia (>90th percentile body weight), or placental structural abnormality
Maternal disease including hypertension, congenital heart disease, diabetes mellitus, renal disease, connective tissue disease, parvovirus, cytomegalovirus, rubella, toxoplasmosis, pre-eclampsia, eclampsia, or human immunodeficiency virus
Follow-up of prior identified abnormalities including oligo or polyhydramnios, intrauterine growth retardation, placenta previa
Suspected fetal demise (no movement or unable to locate heartbeat with Doppler)
Estimate fetal size before elective pregnancy termination
Preterm labor or rupture of membranes <36 weeks

---

* "Routine" ultrasound or ultrasound for the sole purpose of identifying sex of the fetus is not necessary.

ily result in a placenta previa, because significant growth of the lower uterine segment away from the placenta occurs later in pregnancy.

The common emergent clinical question is whether a patient with pelvic pain and a missed menstrual period has an intrauterine pregnancy, an ectopic pregnancy, or an incomplete or missed abortion. An imaging study is not appropriate until the results of a pregnancy test are available. As mentioned earlier, if suspected gestational age is greater than 5 weeks, an intrauterine gestational sac should be identified. In addition, fetal components should be seen within this gestational sac, particularly if transvaginal ultrasound is used.

Patients with an ectopic pregnancy almost always have pain and bleeding, but only 40% have a palpable adnexal mass. On ultrasound examination, a normal-looking uterus and normal adnexal areas do not exclude an ectopic pregnancy. Under these circumstances, a repeat examination in 7 to 10 days may be necessary. If the uterus appears normal and there is a complex adnexal mass, the likelihood of an ectopic pregnancy should be considered high. Sometimes, a gestational sac and fetal heart motion can be seen outside the uterus. In these circumstances, the diagnosis of an ectopic pregnancy (Fig. 7–23) is certain.

If an empty gestational sac is seen within the uterus, it may represent an early intrauterine pregnancy, particularly if the diameter of the sac is 10 to 20 mm. It may also represent a blighted ovum or a pseudogestational sac in a patient with an ectopic pregnancy. A pseudogestational sac is seen in approximately 20% of patients with ectopic pregnancies.

In the second and third trimesters of pregnancy, there can be quite a complete ultrasound evaluation of the fetus. The most common reason for an ultrasound at this stage is to determine placental location, fetal growth, and gestational age. The earlier in pregnancy that gestational age is determined, the more accurate it will be. Dating is done by measuring the biparietal diameter of the head (Fig. 7–24) as well as the length of the femur and other

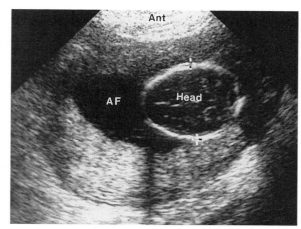

FIGURE 7–24. **Measurement of biparietal diameter.** A transabdominal ultrasound image is done to find and to measure the greatest biparietal diameter. This is one of the measurements used for estimating fetal age. Amniotic fluid (AF) is clearly seen.

structures. At the same time, there should be evaluation of the amount of amniotic fluid, intracranial structures, the heart (to see that it has four chambers), and the abdominal organs (to look for abnormalities, e.g., duodenal atresia, obstructed kidneys, and defects in the spine and anterior abdominal wall). Multiple gestations should be examined to see if there are monochorionic twins, and if so an ultrasound examination is often done at 3 to 6 week intervals to see if there is discordance in fetal growth. This is usually measured by abdominal circumference, estimated fetal weight, head circumference, biparietal diameter, and femur length measurements. The values used are usually those given for singletons (Tables 7–3 and 7–4).

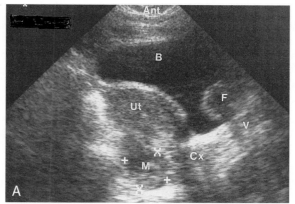

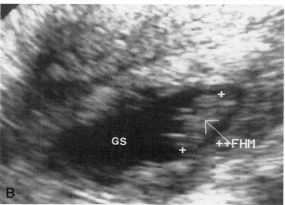

FIGURE 7–23. **Ectopic pregnancy.** A longitudinal transabdominal image *(A)* clearly shows the bladder (B), uterus (Ut), and cervix (Cx). There is a Foley catheter within the bladder. A mass (M) is noted behind the uterus and marked with X and +. A transvaginal ultrasound image *(B)* was performed to get better detail of this abnormality. A gestational sac (GS), a fetal pole, and fetal heart motion (+ +FHM) were identified in this ectopic pregnancy. F = Foley catheter; V = vagina.

TABLE 7–3 Measurements vs. Gestational Age in Early Pregnancy

Sac Size* (mm)	Crown-Rump Length (mm)	Gestational Age (weeks)
10	—	5.0
13	2.0	5.5
17	3.7	6.0
20	5.5	6.5
24	7.4	7.0
27	11.3	7.5
31	14.7	8.0
34	18.2	8.5
—	21.9	9.0
—	30.5	10
—	40.4	11
—	51.7	12

* If sac is not round use the average diameter.

TABLE 7–4 Fetal Measurements vs. Gestational Age

Gestational Age (weeks)	Biparietal Diameter (mm)	Abdominal Circumference (mm) (5th and 95th%)	Femur Length (mm) (50th%)
12	19	—	13.3
14	26	—	14
16	33	105 (85, 126)	17
18	40	129 (108, 150)	26
20	47	152 (132, 173)	32
22	52	175 (154, 196)	37
24	58	197 (176, 218)	42
26	64	219 (198, 239)	47
28	69	240 (219, 260)	53
30	74	260 (239, 281)	57
32	79	280 (259, 300)	62
34	83	299 (279, 320)	67
36	88	318 (297, 339)	71
38	92	336 (316, 357)	76
40	96	354 (333, 374)	80

Radiation During Pregnancy

X-ray examinations may be done during pregnancy but only after careful consideration. There is little, if any, reason to use radiographs in the management of labor. Occasionally radiographs may be needed during pregnancy, for example, x-ray films may be taken to assess potential injuries of the spine, pelvis, or hips after an automobile accident. Under these circumstances, it must be ensured that the same information cannot be obtained by using ultrasonography. If radiographs are necessary, it is prudent to first determine the information that is needed and whether the examination can be tailored or done with less than the normal number of views. If the uterus is not in the direct beam (e.g., a chest radiograph) and the dose is quite low, there is little potential risk to the fetus. If the fetus is in the direct beam and the examination is needed, it should be done, although there is a somewhat increased risk of neoplasm in the child and possibly later in life. Informed consent is usually obtained. A physicist usually calculates the fetal dose, and it is placed in the medical record. The fetal radiation dose from a ventilation/perfusion lung scan is low and should not be cause for concern. Fluoroscopy gives relatively high doses, and pelvic or lower abdominal fluoroscopy should be avoided during pregnancy unless there is no alternative.

Pelvic Inflammatory Disease

Pelvic inflammatory disease is an inflammatory syndrome of the upper genital tract in women and is most commonly associated with *Neisseria gonorrhoeae* and *Chlamydia trachomatis*. The diagnosis is made clinically when there is the combination of lower abdominal tenderness, bilateral adnexal tenderness, and cervical motion tenderness. There may also be associated inflammatory bowel symptoms. Imaging plays a little role in simple pelvic inflammatory disease, but about 15% of patients with acute pelvic inflammatory disease have a tubo-ovarian abscess. This is best detected with ultrasonography, although CT and laparoscopy can also be used.

Pelvic Pain and Masses

Pelvic pain should be classified as acute or chronic. In most cases, patient age, medical history, physical examination, complete blood cell count, pregnancy test, and urinalysis help prioritize the differential diagnosis. An ultrasound examination with Doppler is the imaging test of choice for suspected ectopic pregnancy, tubo-ovarian abscess, and ovarian torsion. It identifies any free fluid in the cul-de-sac. There is no good imaging test for endometriosis, therefore, that diagnosis is usually made laparascopically.

An ovarian lesion is the most common pelvic mass in women, but other etiologies such as uterine, bladder, and intestinal lesions also need to be considered. Most masses are found during routine pelvic examination, and the size, shape, and location are determined. Associated symptoms such as fever, pain, or menstrual abnormalities can provide valuable clues. Laboratory tests such as a complete blood cell count, a urinalysis, and a CA-125 assay are also potentially helpful. In terms of imaging, although an IVP, CT scan, or barium enema can provide some information, the initial imaging test should be a pelvic ultrasound. It provides information about the internal structure and vascularity of the mass. Although there is no imaging test that is quite accurate in differentiating benign from malignant pelvic masses, if there are septations, irregular solid portions, or ascites, malignancy should be considered, and surgery or laparoscopy may be performed.

Tumors

UTERUS

The most common benign uterine tumor is a fibroid. These may be calcified and seen on x-ray examination in the central portion of the pelvis. The calcification is typically somewhat popcorn shaped. This finding is usually incidental, because radiographs should not be ordered to look for uterine fibroids. The most common initial method used to image uterine fibroids and other pelvic masses, as mentioned earlier, is ultrasonography. Routine ultrasound follow-up of fibroids with imaging procedures is not indicated, but it is indicated if the fibroids are enlarging or if the patient develops pain or bleeding. Fibroids enlarge the uterus in a lumpy fashion and make the internal echo pattern inhomogeneous (Fig. 7–25). Although it is difficult to differentiate fibroids from endometrial carcinoma on ultrasound images, this is easily done on clinical grounds, because most endometrial carcinomas are associated with bleeding. There are no adequate screening tests for endometrial carcinoma. Before surgery, CT or MRI can be helpful to locate adenopathy, renal pathology, and other conditions. Dermoid tumors typically contain hair, teeth, and sebaceous secretions. Often a molar type tooth can be seen on an x-ray film of the pelvis.

CERVIX

Carcinoma of the cervix is usually found during annual pelvic examination and with a Papanicolaou smear. Once a cervical carcinoma has been found, CT or MRI scanning can assess the overall size of the tumor and the potential presence of metastases. Often, this cancer obstructs the cervical canal and causes build-up of fluid within the uterus. Cervical carcinomas tend to obstruct the distal ureters, and renal obstruction is the most frequent cause of death from this tumor. Evaluation can initially be done using an IVP; however, in follow-up of these patients, it is probably cheaper and safer to look for potentially obstructed kidneys by means of ultrasound imaging. In contrast to ovarian carcinoma,

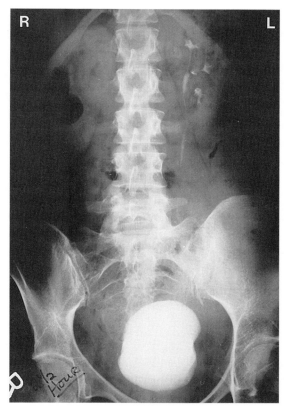

FIGURE 7–26. **Carcinoma of the cervix.** On this intravenous pyelogram, the left kidney is clearly identified and is functional. No contrast material is seen in the collecting system of the right kidney owing to obstruction of the distal right ureter by the cervical carcinoma.

cervical carcinomas often spread locally and involve lymph nodes (Fig. 7–26). Even though CT can detect metastases if the lymph nodes are enlarged, its accuracy for detection of metastases from cervical carcinoma is only 65%, because the nodes may have small metastatic deposits and not be enlarged.

OVARY

For most women there is no effective screening test for ovarian carcinoma. For women known to be at very high risk for ovarian carcinoma, some authors recommend periodic pelvic ultrasound examinations with Doppler to detect ovarian masses. Most ovarian tumors are cystadenomas or cystadenocarcinomas. Both benign and malignant tumors are bilateral in a fair number of cases. When an ovarian tumor is suspected, ultrasound imaging should optimally be done in the first 10 days of the menstrual cycle to minimize the presence of benign ovarian cysts. Cystadenomas and cystadenocarcinomas are usually large cystic adnexal lesions.

One of the most frequent clinical presentations of ovarian carcinoma is increasing weight and abdominal girth due to the presence of ascites. Pleural

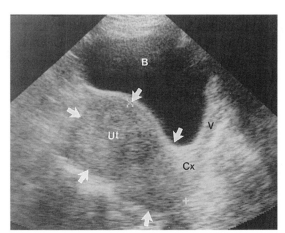

FIGURE 7–25. **Ultrasound image of uterine fibroids.** A longitudinal transabdominal view of the pelvis shows that the uterus (Ut) is enlarged and lumpy *(arrows)*. The echo pattern within the uterus is inhomogeneous; this is the most common appearance of uterine fibroids. B = bladder; V = vagina; Cx = cervix.

effusions are also common. CT scanning is often done for suspected pelvic malignancies to determine the size of the mass, possible involvement of pelvic side walls, and ureteral obstruction as well as to look for metastatic disease. The finding of a pelvic mass on CT or ultrasound study is usually somewhat nonspecific, although if the mass can be traced down into the pelvis and into the adnexa, it is most likely of ovarian origin. Ovarian carcinoma may involve the bowel, particularly the serosa.

■ ADRENAL GLANDS AND RETROPERITONEUM

Retroperitoneum

The adrenal glands are not visualized on a plain film of the abdomen. Many adrenal lesions are found on CT scans of the abdomen done for other reasons. For suspected adrenal pathology, the imaging study of choice is a CT scan (Fig. 7–27). Masses in the adrenal glands are the result of adenomas (50%), metastases (35%), pheochromocytoma (10%), lymphoma, and neuroblastoma (in children <2 years of age). Bilateral masses are usually the result of metastases, bilateral pheochromocytoma, lymphoma, and granulomatous diseases.

At autopsy, about 25% of individuals who died of cancer have adrenal metastases. Lung, breast, stomach, colon, and kidney are the most common primary lesions to metastasize to the adrenal gland. In a patient with cancer and an adrenal mass, there is a high probability that the latter is metastatic (particularly if the masses are bilateral).

An adrenal adenoma usually is low density (dark) on a CT scan and occurs in about 3% of persons. Usually, these are discovered incidentally. An adrenal lesion in excess of 2 to 3 cm in diameter that is not low density on CT is suspected to be malignant. A CT scan may be used to follow these lesions every 3 to 6 months or used to direct a fine needle biopsy. Adrenal lesions larger than 5 cm in diameter should be removed.

Adrenal hyperplasia may be nodular, as in Cushing's syndrome, or smooth, as in 25% of patients with Conn's syndrome. Both these diseases are related to hormone overproduction (cortisol, aldosterone), which may be caused by an adenoma, tumor, or hyperplasia. The primary diagnosis for most of these lesions is made by evaluation of serum or urine hormone levels. Tumors and clinically significant functional adenomas can usually be localized by CT or MRI, but hyperplasia can be difficult to differentiate from normal glands. In these latter rare cases, a nuclear medicine scan with a substance called NP-59 demonstrates increased activity

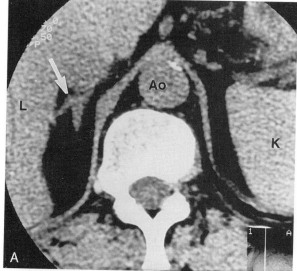

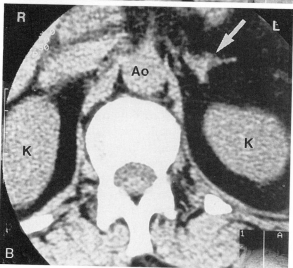

FIGURE 7–27. **Normal adrenal anatomy.** A coned-down computed tomography scan of the upper abdomen above the level of the right kidney (A) shows the right adrenal gland (arrow). It is usually shaped like an upside down V or as a thin line. The left adrenal gland is seen on a slightly lower computed tomography cut (B) and is a triangular structure (arrow) anterior and slightly medial to the upper pole of the left kidney. Ao = aorta; K = kidney.

in an adenoma or hyperplasia. Most pheochromocytomas (90%) occur in the adrenal medulla, and 10% are bilateral. Occasionally, they occur elsewhere in the abdomen. Localization should be done using a nuclear medicine scan with a substance called *metaiodobenzylguanidine* or using MRI.

Retroperitoneal Adenopathy and Neoplasms

CT is the only convenient and practical way to assess patients for retroperitoneal adenopathy. As mentioned earlier in this chapter, patients can have

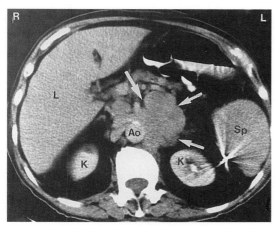

FIGURE 7–28. **Retroperitoneal lymphoma.** In this young patient with suspected Hodgkin's disease, a contrast-enhanced computed tomography scan clearly shows the kidneys (K) and the aorta (Ao). The aorta is surrounded by a lobular soft tissue mass *(arrows)* due to lymphoma. L = liver; Sp = spleen.

normal-sized lymph nodes that contain microscopic metastases. Therefore, one should not automatically assume that if adenopathy is absent, there is no spread of tumor. When there is nodal enlargement in a patient with a known neoplasm, the chances of malignant involvement are high, although not certain, because some patients have hyperplastic lymph nodes without actual tumor involvement.

CT not only can identify adenopathy but also can be used on a serial basis to assess the results of therapy. Unless intravenous contrast agent is given, it can be difficult to differentiate a large mass of lymphadenopathy about the aorta from an abdominal aortic aneurysm. A major advantage of CT is that one can look at the abdominal organs and mesenteric regions for metastatic disease while searching for adenopathy (Fig. 7–28).

Retroperitoneal fibrosis can be confused with an aneurysm or retroperitoneal adenopathy. The distinction is not always easy to make on a CT scan. One differentiating factor is that with retroperitoneal fibrosis, there is usually medial deviation of the ureters because of traction by the fibrotic process. With adenopathy and aneurysms, there is usually lateral deviation of the ureters by a soft tissue mass.

GENERAL SUGGESTED READINGS

Amis ES, Newhouse JH: Essentials of Uroradiology. Boston, Little Brown, 1991.

Besset RAL, Khan AN, Thomas NB, McHugo JM: Differential Diagnosis in Obstetric and Gynecologic Ultrasound. Philadelphia, WB Saunders, 1996.

Davidson AJ, Hartman DS, Choyke PL, Wagner BJ: Davidson's Radiology of the Kidney and Genitourinary Tract, 3rd ed. Philadelphia, WB Saunders, 1998.

Dunnick R, Sandler CM, Amis ES, Newhouse JH (eds): Textbook of Uroradiology, 2nd ed. Philadelphia, Lippincott Williams & Wilkins, 1995.

Kremkau FW: Diagnostic Ultrasound: Principles and Instruments, 5th ed. Philadelphia, WB Saunders, 1998.

Williamson M, Smith A: Fundamentals of Uroradiology. Philadelphia, WB Saunders, 1999.

8

SKELETAL SYSTEM

The majority of skeletal imaging is done with plain radiographs. It is important to get both anteroposterior (AP) and lateral projections for most studies. Additional oblique views are usually necessary for trauma involving joints and hands or feet. Computed tomography (CT), magnetic resonance imaging (MRI), and nuclear medicine all play important roles in skeletal imaging. CT is useful for evaluation of fine bone structure, particularly of the skull, spine, and pelvis. MRI is used most for evaluation of the soft tissues (muscles, ligaments, cartilage, spinal cord, and marrow spaces). Nuclear medicine scans are usually used to evaluate the skeleton for bone metastases, to differentiate cellulitis from osteomyelitis and occult trauma (stress or insufficiency fractures), and to assess prosthesis loosening. Ultrasonography has limited use in skeletal imaging. Myelography is now rarely performed and then usually in combination with a CT scan. Arthrography (direct injection of contrast material into a joint space) has largely been replaced by MRI.

This chapter presents images of the normal skeletal anatomy as well as common variants that should not be mistaken for pathology. Fractures and other osseous abnormalities involving the skull and face are covered in Chapter 2. Initial imaging studies for a number of clinical problems are presented in Table 8–1. Most bone lesions are relatively obvious as a result of the clinical history. More than 95% of bone films are obtained for evaluation of trauma, arthritis, degenerative conditions, or metastases. There are a number of classic fractures

and a few that, if missed, can have dire consequences (especially cervical spine fractures). These are presented in this chapter. The chapter is organized by general skeletal parts, particularly spine, pelvis and hips, and extremities.

■ SPINE

Normal Anatomy

CERVICAL SPINE

The lateral view of the cervical spine is the initial view obtained, particularly in trauma cases. Table 8–2 provides a summary of how to approach a cervical spine examination done for trauma. Initial inspection should be directed toward the contour lines of the cervical spine, which are shown in Figure 8–1. These include the anterior soft tissues, the anterior and posterior spinal lines, the spinal laminal line, and the posterior spinous process line. On the lateral view, the cervical spine should be bowed forward in the middle and have a relatively smooth curve. There should not be a sharp angulation at any level. If the patient is lying on a stretcher when the lateral view is taken, the neck is often flexed, and the cervical spine is straight rather than curved. Whether the straightening is due simply to the supine positioning of the patient or to muscular spasm is not clear. If the trauma was relatively minor, an upright lateral radiograph of the cervical spine usually solves the problem. If major trauma is suspected, a CT or MRI scan may be needed.

Examination of the anterior soft tissues and spaces should be done at several vertebral levels. Evaluation of soft tissue width is typically not a problem unless the patient has an endotracheal tube in place, in which case the normal air/soft tissue interface is obscured, and one has to rely on other findings. The width of the soft tissue immediately anterior to the body of C3 should be between 4 and 5 mm, but on a portable trauma series with significant magnification, a measurement of up to 7 mm may be normal. Below the level of C4, the soft tissue anterior to the lower cervical bodies averages about 15 mm with a range of 10 to 20 mm. If the soft tissue in this region equals or exceeds the anterior to posterior width of the vertebra at or below the level of C4, pathology should be suspected. Another important measurement on the lateral view is the distance from the posterior aspect of the anterior arch of C1 to the most anterior portion of the odontoid. In an adult, this should not exceed 3 mm; in a child, it should not exceed 5 mm.

If there is difficulty in imaging the lower cervical spine, down to C7–T1, a swimmer's view can be ordered. This raises one shoulder and lowers the other, allowing the x-ray beam to more easily penetrate the area of the cervicothoracic junction (Fig. 8–2). There are typically two anterior views that

TABLE 8–1 Initial Imaging Studies of Choice for Various Clinical Problems

Clinical Problem	Imaging Study
Fracture	Plain radiograph
Occult hip fracture	MRI or bone scan
Occult knee fracture	MRI
Stress fracture	Nuclear medicine bone scan
Metastases	Nuclear medicine bone scan, plain radiograph in area of pain
Osteomyelitis	Plain radiograph Nuclear medicine three-phase bone scan or MRI
Low back pain	
without radiculopathy	Bed rest (for several weeks)
with radiculopathy	Noncontrasted CT or MRI
Arthritis (nonseptic)	Plain radiographs
Suspected septic arthritis	Joint aspiration, plain radiograph
Monoarticular joint pain	Plain radiograph, if conservative therapy fails then MRI
Infection or loosening of prosthetic joint	Plain radiograph, if negative nuclear medicine bone scan
Reflex sympathetic dystrophy	Plain radiograph, if negative three-phase nuclear medicine bone scan

MRI = magnetic resonance imaging; CT = computed tomography.

TABLE 8–2 Items to Look for on a Trauma Anteroposterior and Lateral Cervical Spine Examination

Lateral View
- Count vertebral bodies to assure that all seven are seen (if not, consider swimmer's view or shallow oblique view)
- Alignment of
    anterior vertebral body margins
    posterior vertebral body margins
    posterior spinal canal
- Cervical curvature, straightening, or sudden angulation
- Prevertebral soft tissue thickness (see text)
- Widening of vertical distance between posterior processes
- Common fractures
    C1 arch
    C2 odontoid
        arch (hangman's)
        widening between anterior arch of C1 and odontoid
    C3–C7 anterior avulsion
        wedge compression
    C6–C7 posterior process (clay-shoveler's)
- Facets (to exclude unilateral locked facet)

Anterior View
- Odontoid view
    Widening of the lateral portion of C1 relative to C2 (Jefferson fracture)
- General alignment of lateral margins and spinous processes
- Lucent fracture lines

Oblique View (if no major trauma is suspected)
- Neural foraminal narrowing
- Alignment of facet joints

are done after the lateral cervical spine view has been examined by a physician and found to be free of fracture or subluxation. These are an anterior view of the lower cervical spine with the mouth closed (to examine alignment and to exclude oblique fractures) and an open-mouth view of the odontoid (Fig. 8–3) (to show the relationship of the inferior aspect and lateral margins of C1 to the superior aspect and lateral margins of C2). Oblique views of the cervical spine are obtained only when one is quite sure that no major trauma, fracture, or dislocation is present. The value of the oblique view is mostly to see whether impingement or narrowing of the neural foramina by bone degenerative spurs has occurred or to see a unilateral perched, subluxed, or locked facet.

THORACIC SPINE

Plain radiographs of the thoracic spine are taken in AP and lateral projections (Fig. 8–4). The lateral thoracic spine is usually a difficult film to assess. In the upper portion, the vertebral bodies are ob-

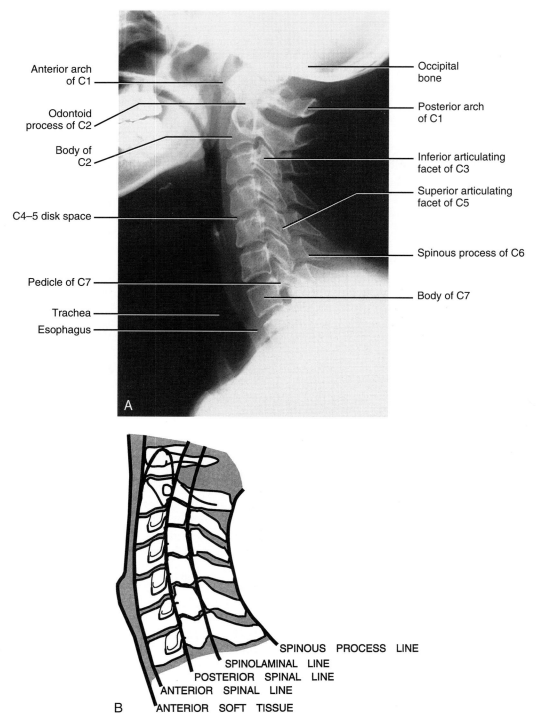

Anterior arch of C1

Odontoid process of C2

Body of C2

C4–5 disk space

Pedicle of C7

Trachea

Esophagus

Occipital bone

Posterior arch of C1

Inferior articulating facet of C3

Superior articulating facet of C5

Spinous process of C6

Body of C7

A

SPINOUS PROCESS LINE
SPINOLAMINAL LINE
POSTERIOR SPINAL LINE
ANTERIOR SPINAL LINE
B   ANTERIOR SOFT TISSUE

FIGURE 8–1. **Normal anatomy of the cervical spine in the lateral projection *(A)* and diagrammatically *(B).***

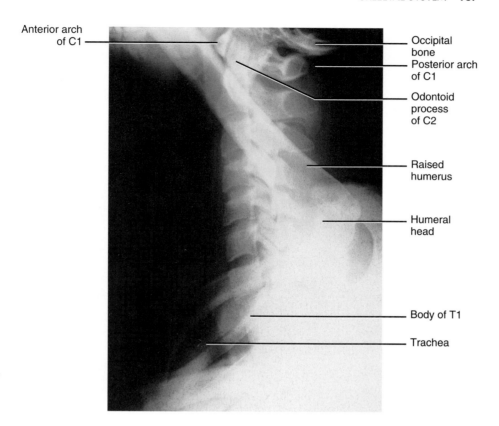

Anterior arch of C1

Occipital bone

Posterior arch of C1

Odontoid process of C2

Raised humerus

Humeral head

Body of T1

Trachea

FIGURE 8–2. **Normal anatomy of the cervical spine on the lateral swimmer's view.**

scured by the shoulders while the middle and lower thoracic spine is usually well seen. When pathology is identified on the lateral view, it is often not easy to distinguish exactly the level of the vertebral body involved. Usually one must go back to the AP view, find the pathology, look at the ribs, and then count up from T12.

A common normal variant seen on the lateral thoracic spine views of children is a bony apophysis that occurs along the superior and inferior anterior margins of the vertebral bodies. This is normal and should not be mistaken for a fracture (Fig. 8–5).

LUMBAR SPINE

The standard views obtained of the lumbar spine are AP, lateral, and a spot view of the L5–S1 area (Fig. 8–6). On the lateral view of the lumbar spine, an analysis is made to see if there is subluxation (displacement) of the vertebral bodies by looking down the contour lines formed by the anterior and posterior margins of the vertebral bodies. The height and shape of the vertebral bodies should be uniform, and the disc spaces should be approximately equal in height. A common normal variant is incomplete fusion of the posterior aspect of L5 or S1 (so-called *spina bifida occulta*). It is of no clinical significance and should be disregarded.

Oblique views of the lumbar spine are useful for examining the facet joints. The typical anatomy on the oblique view is seen as the outline of a "Scottie

dog" (see Fig. 8–6). In this projection, the pedicle is the eye of the dog, the transverse process represents the nose, the superior articular process forms the ears, and the inferior articular process forms the front legs. Postsurgical changes of the lumbar spine involve fusion or laminectomy. Both are seen best on the anterior view.

Trauma

Fifty percent of spine fractures are due to motor vehicle accidents, about 25% to falls, and about 10% to sports injuries. The most common sites are the upper (C1–C2) and lower (C5–C7) cervical spine and the thoracolumbar junction (T9–L2). Twenty percent of spinal fractures are multiple, and about 5% occur at discontinuous levels.

Not all patients require imaging studies to exclude spinal injury. If a patient is fully conscious and there is no neurologic deficit, no pain in the spinal region, no other injuries likely to obscure the injury, and the mechanism of injury is unlikely to have produced spinal injury, further evaluation is unnecessary.

Plain AP and lateral radiographs are the primary screening tool for spinal trauma but are usually indicated in the following situations:

- Recent trauma
- Pain greater than 4 weeks' duration with conservative therapy

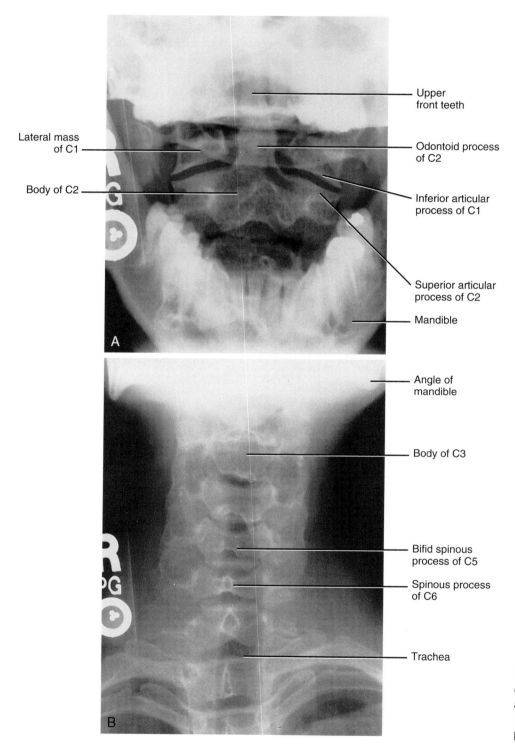

Upper front teeth

Lateral mass of C1

Body of C2

Odontoid process of C2

Inferior articular process of C1

Superior articular process of C2

Mandible

Angle of mandible

Body of C3

Bifid spinous process of C5

Spinous process of C6

Trachea

FIGURE 8–3. **Normal anatomy of the cervical spine on the anteroposterior odontoid view (A) and the standard anteroposterior cervical view (B).**

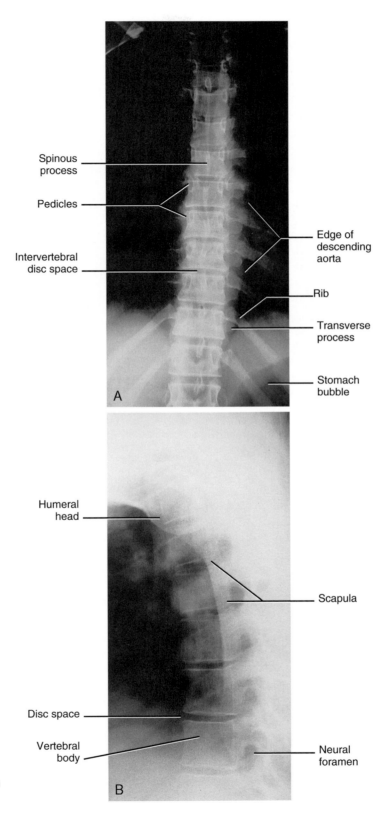

Spinous process

Pedicles

Intervertebral disc space

Edge of descending aorta

Rib

Transverse process

Stomach bubble

A

Humeral head

Scapula

Disc space

Vertebral body

Neural foramen

B

FIGURE 8–4. **Normal anatomy of the thoracic spine in the anteroposterior** *(A)* **and lateral** *(B)* **projections.**

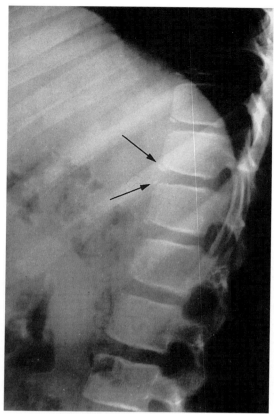

FIGURE 8–5. **Normal spinal apophyses.** In children, a normal apophysis can occasionally be seen on the lateral projection along the anterior superior and inferior margins of the vertebral bodies (arrows). These are normal, are seen on multiple vertebral bodies, and should not be mistaken for avulsion fractures.

- Known osteoporosis or metabolic bone disease
- Infection suspected as a result of fever, increased sedimentation rate, or an elevated white blood cell count
- Known cancer
- Radicular findings including paresthesia or weakness
- Before chiropractic spinal manipulation (to find pathology that may preclude the procedure)

If a patient has severe head trauma requiring CT evaluation, most physicians simply continue the scan into the cervical spine to exclude occult fractures. About 5% of the time, fractures are found that cannot be seen on plain radiographs. In addition, about 50% of the time, plain radiographs are unable to distinguish a vertebral body compression fracture from the more serious burst fracture. MRI is better than CT for detection of the soft tissue and spinal cord components of the injury. Table 8–3 shows the indications for MRI of the spine.

CERVICAL SPINE

Approximately 5% of cervical spine fractures involve C1. Fractures of the atlas can involve any portion of the bony ring. Burst fractures of the ring of C1 are called *Jefferson fractures*. This bursting is usually secondary to axial loading as a result of the skull being smashed down onto the cervical spine (as in diving into a shallow pool) (Fig. 8–7).

Approximately 10% of all cervical spine fractures involve the odontoid process of C2. The most common type of odontoid fracture occurs at the very base of the odontoid process. Often, there is associated soft tissue swelling (see Fig. 8–7). In children younger than 3 years, the odontoid may not be completely fused to the body of C2, and this should not be mistaken for a fracture.

Occasionally, there can be C1–C2 injury of the transverse ligament, causing traumatic atlantoaxial subluxation. This may occur with or without an associated odontoid fracture. If no fracture is present, the subluxation is often fatal, because the odontoid process pushes posteriorly into the spinal cord that is contained within the arch of C1. On the lateral view, the only sign of ligament injury may be some soft tissue swelling anterior to the vertebral bodies. Flexion views sometimes demonstrate increased widening not only of the atlantoaxial space but also of the space between the posterior spinous processes. This type of subluxation also occurs without trauma as a complication of rheumatoid arthritis (Fig. 8–8).

A relatively classic fracture of C2 is the so-called *hangman's fracture*. This involves fracture of the posterior elements of C2, and there is often associated spinal cord compromise. This fracture typically occurs secondary to hyperextension with compression of the upper cervical spine, and there is usually anterior subluxation of the body of C2 relative to

TABLE 8–3 Indications for a Magnetic Resonance Imaging Scan* of the Spine

- Radiculopathy: unchanged after 4 to 6 weeks of limited activity and medications; worsening or extension after 2 weeks of limited activity and medications
- High impact trauma
- New or progressive neurologic deficit
- Neurologic deficit inconsistent with radiographic findings
- Suspected spinal tumor
- Suspected spinal infection
- Acute myelopathy (hyper-reflexia, gait disturbance, clonus, numbness or paresthesia in legs)
- Acute urinary retention or stool incontinence
- Neurogenic claudication (differentiated from vascular claudication by partial relief with back flexion, onset with prolonged standing)
- Cancer elsewhere with new spine pain, new spinal bone lesion on x-ray examination, new neurologic findings

* A computed tomography scan can also be used if a magnetic resonance imaging scan is not available.

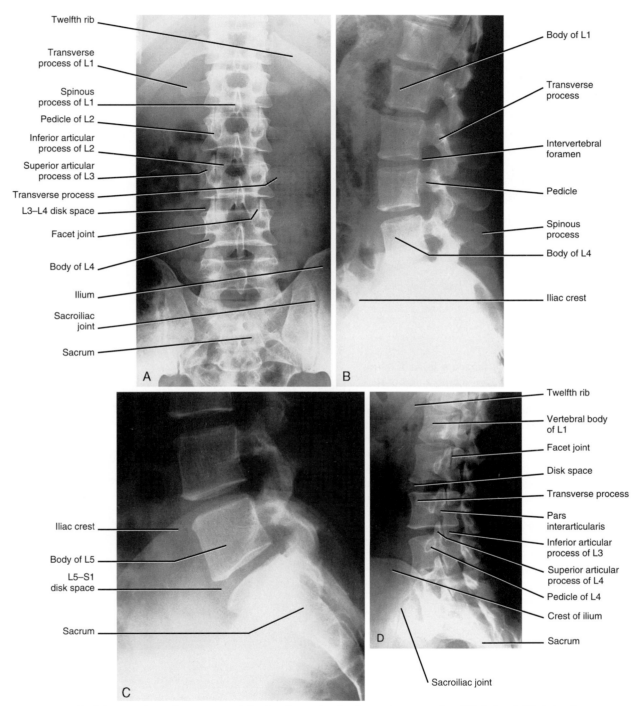

Twelfth rib

Transverse process of L1

Spinous process of L1

Pedicle of L2

Inferior articular process of L2

Superior articular process of L3

Transverse process

L3–L4 disk space

Facet joint

Body of L4

Ilium

Sacroiliac joint

Sacrum

A

Body of L1

Transverse process

Intervertebral foramen

Pedicle

Spinous process

Body of L4

Iliac crest

B

Iliac crest

Body of L5

L5–S1 disk space

Sacrum

C

Twelfth rib

Vertebral body of L1

Facet joint

Disk space

Transverse process

Pars interarticularis

Inferior articular process of L3

Superior articular process of L4

Pedicle of L4

Crest of ilium

Sacrum

Sacroiliac joint

D

FIGURE 8–6. **Normal anatomy of the lumbar spine in the anteroposterior** *(A),* **lateral** *(B),* **lateral sacral** *(C),* **and oblique** *(D)* **views.**

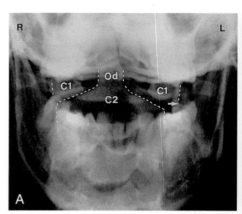

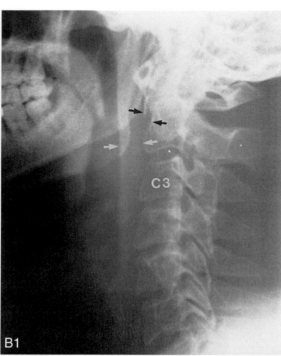

FIGURE 8–7. **A, Jefferson burst fracture of C1.** On this open-mouth anteroposterior view, widening of the space between the odontoid (Od) and the left lateral mass of C1 is evident. The lateral aspect also projects out past the lateral margin of C2 *(arrow)*. **B, Fracture of the odontoid.** In a different patient, the lateral view of the cervical spine *(B1)* shows marked soft tissue swelling in front of the body of C2 *(white arrows)*. There is also discontinuity of the cortex along the anterior surface of C2 *(black arrows)*, indicating an odontoid fracture. A sagittal reconstruction on a computed tomography scan *(B2)* shows the odontoid fracture (od) much more clearly.

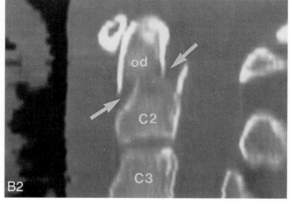

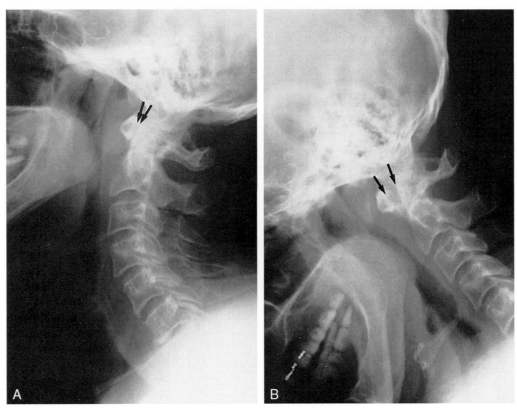

FIGURE 8–8. **Instability of the transverse ligament of C1.** In this patient with rheumatoid arthritis, a lateral view of the cervical spine with the neck extended *(A)* shows little space (which is normal) between the posterior aspect of the arch of C1 and the anterior portion of the odontoid *(arrows)*. With flexion *(B)*, this space markedly widens *(arrows)*, and the odontoid is free to compress the spinal cord, which is posterior to it.

C3 (Fig. 8–9). In spite of the name, this is not the usual fracture that occurs as a result of judicial hangings.

There are two, rather characteristic, fractures of the midcervical spine vertebral bodies. The first of these is caused by hyperextension, which typically tears off either a superior or an inferior anterior corner of the cortex from a vertebral body (Fig. 8–10). A second type of fracture that commonly occurs in the middle cervical spine is a hyperflexion injury. In this, there is compression of the vertebral body, usually with anterior wedging and sometimes with a posteriorly displaced disk fragment. Usually, associated soft tissue swelling is due to the hemorrhage. Evaluation with MRI may show compromise of the neural canal at the level of the fracture (Fig. 8–11).

In addition to fractures associated with subluxation, ligamentous injury can allow the facets of one vertebral body to become slightly subluxed, perched, or locked. This represents a more anterior subluxation of a superior vertebral body on a lower one. Generally these injuries occur in the lower half of the cervical spine and are caused by extreme flexion of the head and neck without axial compression. Occasionally, there may be a fracture or ligamentous injury present that cannot be identified using plain radiographs. If there is a high sugges-

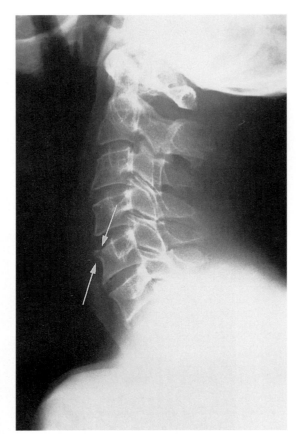

FIGURE 8–10. **Anterior avulsion fracture.** A small avulsed fragment is seen along the superior and anterior aspect of C5 *(arrows)*.

tion of clinical injury in spite of negative plain films, MRI or CT scanning may be useful.

The use of flexion and extension views in the setting of trauma is debated. Some physicians order these after negative plain x-ray examinations to exclude ligamentous injury; however, acute muscular spasm may keep the patient with ligamentous injury from subluxing. Others place the patient in a hard cervical collar and have them return for the examination in 7–10 days.

There are three fractures of the lower portion of the cervical spine that are easily missed. First, occasionally oblique fractures of the lower cervical spine occur, which are only seen on the AP view. The second fracture involves the posterior spinous process at the C6, C7, T1, or T2 level. This is called the *clay-shoveler's fracture*, and it is due predominantly to hyperflexion injury. The third concerns subluxation fractures of C6–C7 that may be easily missed if adequate evaluation of the lower cervical spine is not achieved (Fig. 8–12).

THORACIC SPINE

Fractures of the thoracic spine are typically the result of motor vehicle accidents or osteoporosis. In

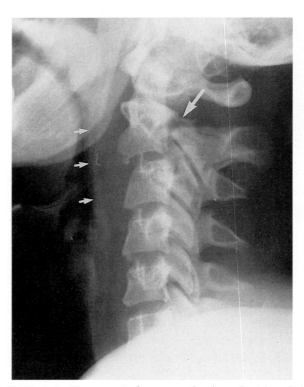

FIGURE 8–9. **Hangman's fracture.** The lateral view of the cervical spine demonstrates marked soft tissue swelling anterior to C1, C2, and C3 *(small white arrows)*. A fracture line is seen just posterior to the body of C2 *(large arrow)*.

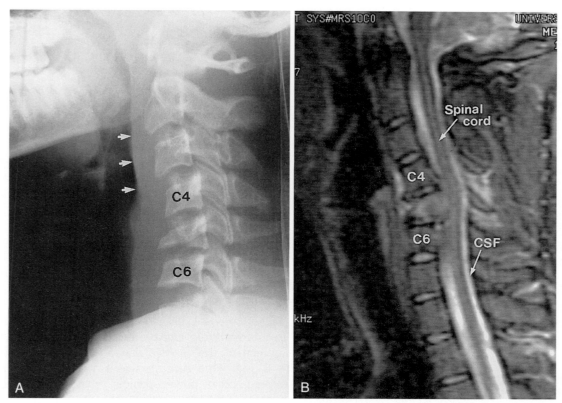

FIGURE 8–11. **Wedge fracture of C5.** A lateral cervical spine view *(A)* demonstrates a reversed normal cervical curvature, anterior soft tissue swelling *(arrows)*, and a wedge fracture of the body of C5. A magnetic resonance imaging scan *(B)*, presented in the same projection, shows the posterior protrusion of C5 into the spinal canal. CSF = cerebrospinal fluid. (Case courtesy of E. Mettler.)

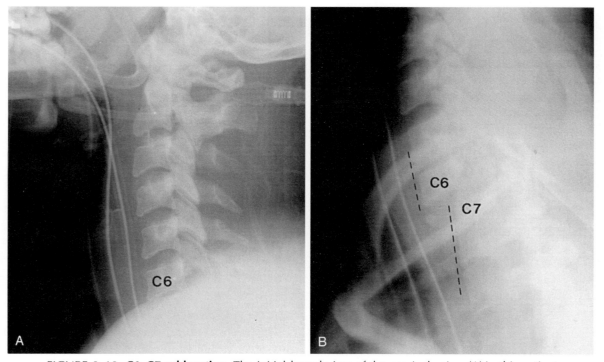

FIGURE 8–12. **C6–C7 subluxation.** The initial lateral view of the cervical spine *(A)* in this patient with paraplegia looked normal; however, C7 was not visualized. When a swimmer's lateral view *(B)* was obtained, it became clear that there was a complete subluxation of C6 forward on the body of C7.

traumatic injuries, the spine is examined on the AP view for malalignment of the posterior spinous processes (Fig. 8–13) and for paraspinous soft tissue swelling. These are both signs that a fracture may be present. Both AP and lateral views should be examined because there can be significant subluxation of one vertebral body forward on another. This is difficult to see on the AP view and usually occurs when there is a hyperflexion injury resulting in a compression burst fracture. Often, there are retropulsed fragments of both disk and bony material that project into the spinal canal that can cause significant compromise of the spinal cord.

In older persons, compression fractures of the middle and lower thoracic spine are common (Fig. 8–14). These are noted as loss of height of the anterior portion of the vertebral bodies. Without prior examinations, it is almost impossible to tell whether any one of these fractures is new or old, but it usually does not make any difference clinically. If there is suspicion of metastatic disease as a cause

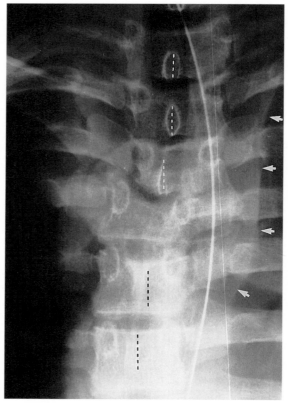

FIGURE 8–13. **Laterally displaced thoracic spine fracture.** An anteroposterior view of the upper thoracic spine in a paraplegic patient who was hit in the driver's side door during a motor vehicle accident shows lateral displacement of the upper thoracic vertebral bodies relative to the lower bodies. This can be assessed by looking at the line formed by the posterior spinous processes *(dotted lines)*. Also note the lateral soft tissue swelling *(arrows)* caused by the paraspinous hemorrhage, which resulted from the fracture. This sort of a fracture is difficult or impossible to visualize on the lateral view.

of back pain in an older patient, a plain radiograph and a nuclear medicine bone scan will usually suffice.

LUMBAR SPINE

The most common fractures of the lumbar spine are wedge compression fractures and compression burst fractures. These are quite similar to those already described in the thoracic spine. Again, the compression burst fractures frequently have fragments that are retropulsed, and CT or MRI is often necessary to evaluate compromise of the spinal canal.

The pars interarticularis of the vertebral body can also be fractured as a result of physical activity (such as gymnastics) rather than external blunt trauma. This injury typically occurs during teenage years at the L4 or L5 level. It can sometimes be seen on the lateral view as a lucency but more commonly is clearly identified as a break in the neck of the Scottie dog on the oblique view (Fig. 8–15). This finding was originally thought to be congenital; however, most of the time it probably is the result of trauma in the early years of life. The term applied to a break in the pars interarticularis is *spondylolysis*. If there is bilateral spondylolysis, the vertebral body can slip forward on the vertebral body that is immediately below. When this happens, it is termed *spondylolisthesis*. The amount of offset caused by the slippage is used to grade the spondylolisthesis. If there is up to one fourth of the vertebral body offset, this is called grade 1. If it is between one fourth and one half, it is called grade 2, and so on to grades 3 and 4 (Fig. 8–16). In a young patient or athlete with low back pain and normal plain x-ray examinations, a nuclear medicine bone scan with single photon emission computed tomography (SPECT) technology may identify otherwise occult spondylolysis (Fig. 8–17).

Degenerative Changes

The main diagnostic challenge is to separate patients who have serious problems from the majority of patients who have nonspecific back pain. Medical history and physical examination usually provide the information needed to do this.

CERVICAL SPINE

In terms of anatomic and mechanical design, the lower aspect of the cervical spine is less than optimal, and by the third or fourth decade of life there are almost always degenerative changes involving C4 through C7. Many cases of neck pain that are seen in an office setting are the result of degenera-

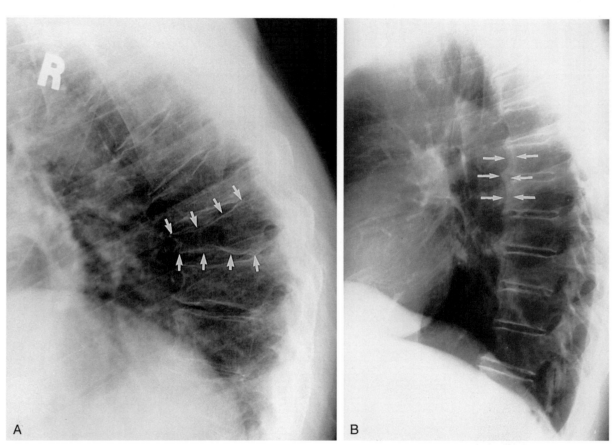

FIGURE 8–14. **Degenerative changes of the thoracic spine.** *A,* With aging and osteoporosis, there can be minimal wedge compression fractures of the middle to upper thoracic spine. *B,* In a different patient, development of calcification of the anterior ligament *(arrows)* is shown.

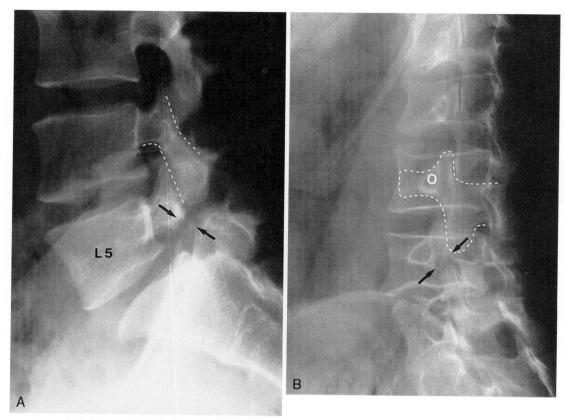

FIGURE 8–15. **Spondylolysis.** On the lateral view of the lower lumbar spine *(A)*, the normal contour of the posterior elements of L4 is outlined by *white dotted lines*. At L5, lysis (fracture) of the posterior elements has occurred *(arrows)*. On the oblique view *(B)*, this is seen as a fracture through the neck of the Scottie dog *(arrows)*. The normal outline for the L4 level is shown.

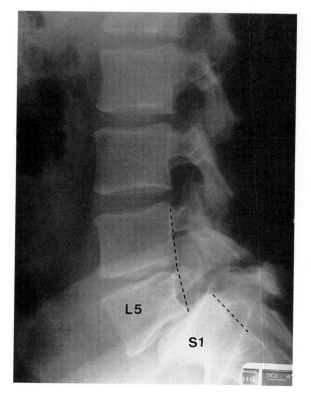

FIGURE 8–16. **Spondylolysis with resulting grade 2 spondylolisthesis.** Discontinuity of the posterior elements of L5 has allowed L5 to slip forward on S1. The degree of slippage is ascertained by looking at the relationship between the posterior portions of the vertebral bodies.

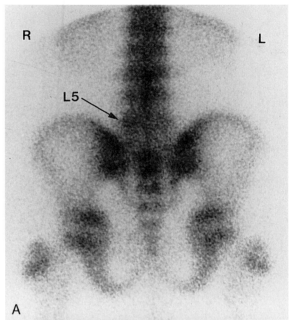

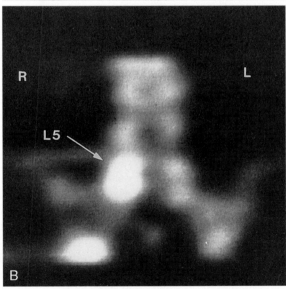

FIGURE 8–17. **Occult spondylolysis.** In this teenage athlete with back pain, plain radiographs were normal. A regular nuclear medicine bone scan (A) was obtained with images over the lower lumbar spine and pelvis. A minimal increase in activity is seen on the right side of L5. An additional tomographic or coronal single photon emission computed tomography (SPECT) image (B) was obtained. It shows markedly increased activity on the right side of L5 due to a traumatic fracture of the pars interarticularis on that side.

tive changes. If conservative therapy fails, plain radiographs with oblique views are usually ordered. Degenerative changes are visualized as decreased disk spaces; sclerosis (increased density) of the vertebral body end plates; and beaking or spurring of the anterior, lateral, and posterior margins of the vertebral bodies. Often patients present with arm pain, and an oblique cervical spine view can easily

visualize hypertrophic osteophytes or spurs projecting into a neural foramen (Fig. 8–18).

If a herniated cervical disk is suspected or there is a neurologic deficit, the plain radiographs are usually followed by an MRI scan. Metastatic disease can also involve the cervical spine with posterior or lateral extension and impingement on the spinal cord or nerve roots. For such patients, MRI is the procedure of choice.

THORACIC SPINE

Three relatively common degenerative findings are seen in the thoracic spine. The first are spurs, or hypertrophic osteophytes, similar to those that are seen in the lower cervical spine. These are almost never a clinical issue and are not an interpretative problem unless they are large, at which point they can cause confusing shadows on the AP or posteroanterior chest radiograph.

A second relatively common degenerative change is calcification along the anterior spinal ligament. This can cross over the length of several vertebral bodies and is sometimes referred to by radiologists as *diffuse idiopathic skeletal hyperostosis (DISH)*. This is of no clinical significance to the patient. The third relatively common degenerative change is calcification of an intervertebral disk. This can occur at almost any level in the spine but is seen most frequently in the midthoracic region. A single calcified disk is usually the result of degenerative change or trauma. If there is calcification at multiple disk levels, one should consider diseases that cause hypercalcemia or rare entities such as ochronosis.

LUMBAR SPINE

As mentioned earlier, degenerative change can result in disk space narrowing, hypertrophic spurs (osteophytes) (Fig. 8–19), or calcification of a disk. In the lumbar spine, loss of the disk space is quite common, as is hypertrophic spurring. Occasionally there is a thin dark line in a narrowed disk space that is referred to as a *vacuum disk phenomenon*. It is not a vacuum but actually nitrogen that is in the joint space. This can appear or be accentuated as a result of hyperextension of the spine, and although indicative of degenerative joint disease (DJD), it is of no special clinical significance.

Very common degenerative changes that occur in the lower lumbar spine are herniated disks and protruded disks. A herniated disk often has a fragment that is asymmetric or loose in the neural canal, whereas a disk protrusion is a posterior central bulge of the disk. Both can be scanned by either CT or MRI (Fig. 8–20). At the present time, MRI is commonly used to make this diagnosis, although

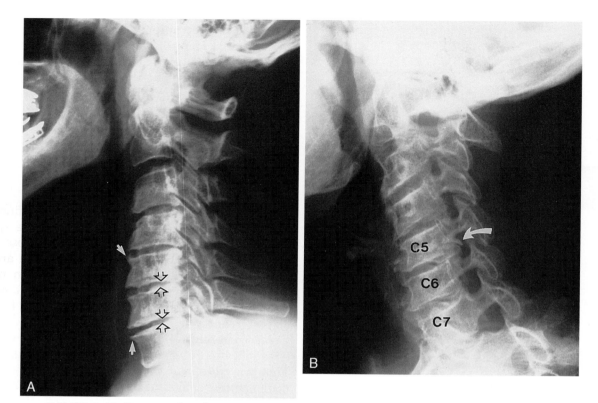

FIGURE 8–18. **Degenerative changes of the cervical spine.** The lateral view *(A)* shows decreased disk spaces *(black arrows)* and hypertrophic spurring along the anterior aspects of the vertebral bodies. These changes are most common at the C4–C7 level. An oblique view *(B)* in the same patient shows that bony spurs are projecting into the neural foramen *(arrow)*. This can cause pain down the arms.

sometimes it is more expensive than CT scanning, and many clinicians simply order a noncontrasted CT scan. If a CT scan is ordered, one should specify thin cuts only through the disk space at which pathology is suspected. Making thin cuts through every disk space in the lumbar spine is time consuming, expensive, and unnecessary.

Management of Low Back Pain

This is probably one of the areas of greatest controversy in medical imaging. Low back pain affects 60 to 80% of the population at some time in their life. The most common cause of low back pain is a herniated or bulging disk. Surprisingly, MRI and CT studies reveal a bulging disk in 25 to 50% of asymptomatic adults. Ninety percent of cases of lower back pain resolve within 4 to 6 weeks as a result of conservative therapy. Unless there is major acute trauma, plain films of the lumbar spine are not of much use. The reason is that a patient can have a herniated disk and totally normal plain films. Conversely, many people who have severe-looking degenerative changes are totally asymptomatic. A herniated disk is usually diagnosed by pain that extends past the knee in a dermatomal

pattern. Foot drop or loss of gastrocnemius strength deserves careful monitoring and not urgent surgery.

In the absence of serious or progressive neurologic deficit, neoplasm, spinal infection, or significant trauma, CT or MRI should not be part of the initial examination. Absence of a reflex or isolated sensory loss is not considered to be a progressive neurologic deficit. If the CT or MRI is nonspecific, a SPECT nuclear medicine bone scan may exclude occult fractures, osteoid osteomas and spondylolysis. Indications for imaging in cancer patients with back pain is given in a following section on neoplasms.

Spinal Infections

Spinal infections usually occur in diabetic and postsurgical patients. If there is a destructive process centered about both sides of a disk space, an infection should be suspected. It is extremely rare for a tumor to involve or cross a disk space. Tumors typically destroy a single vertebral body and then may extend above and below. Evaluation of the bone destruction of a vertebral body is best visualized by a CT scan, but MRI provides more complete evaluation with information on extension

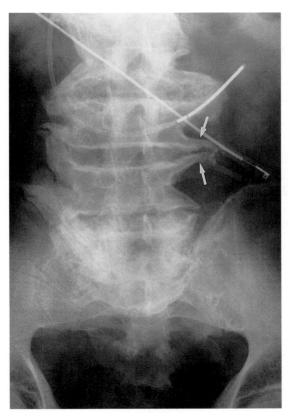

FIGURE 8–19. **Degenerative changes of the lumbar spine.** An anteroposterior view of the lower lumbar spine shows extensive and florid bone spur formation as a result of degenerative change. The extent of these changes does not correlate well with the presence of back pain.

of the pathologic process into the surrounding soft tissues and spinal canal.

MRI is indicated if there is localized pain with an increased sedimentation rate, fever, increased white blood cell count (>10,000), or a positive blood culture.

Spinal Neoplasms and Metastases

Although there can be primary bony neoplasms of the spine, they are rare. The most common neoplastic involvement is from metastatic disease. The metastases may be destructive and cause holes (lytic lesions) in the bone, or they may be dense white (sclerotic lesions). Most neoplasms, including lung, renal, and breast cancer as well as multiple myeloma, cause lytic lesions in bones. Most sclerotic metastases in men are a result of prostate cancer, and those in women, of breast cancer.

Metastases do not begin in the bone cortex but rather in the red marrow, which has filtered the tumor cells out of the blood. As a result, most osseous metastases occur where the red marrow is located (i.e., skull, ribs, spine, pelvis, proximal hu-

merus, and proximal femur). After growing within the marrow space, the lesion becomes large enough to erode the bone cortex. The most sensitive method of finding metastatic disease in the spine is through utilization of MRI. Unfortunately, MRI can look only at limited portions of the body at one time, and it is expensive. Therefore, if osseous metastases are suspected, the most cost-effective imaging study is

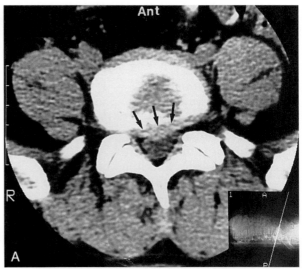

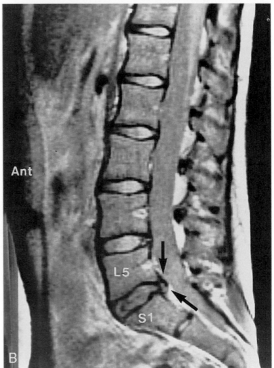

FIGURE 8–20. **Disk herniation and protrusion.** A transverse computed tomography scan *(A)* obtained at the L5–S1 disk space shows posterior protrusion of disk material *(arrows)* into the spinal canal. In a different patient, the sagittal or lateral magnetic resonance imaging view *(B)* of the lumbar spine shows a posterior L5–S1 disk *(arrows)* protruding into the spinal canal.

a nuclear medicine bone scan. If a patient has pain in a specific area, a plain radiograph of the area should be ordered first.

If a patient has a known cancer of the central nervous system, head and neck, lymphoma, ovary, uterus, pancreas, colon, or rectum and if the serum alkaline phosphatase level is normal and there is no bone pain, a nuclear medicine bone scan is not needed for initial work-up. Nuclear medicine bone scans on patients with neoplasms are indicated in the following situations:

Initial staging
    Non–small cell of the lung, breast, or prostate cancer
    Bone pain by history
    Increased serum alkaline phosphatase, calcium, or prostate-specific antigen levels
Follow-up if initial bone scan was positive
    New or worsening pain
    Increased serum alkaline phosphatase, calcium, or prostate-specific antigen levels
    Completion of at least 2 cycles of chemotherapy
    Six weeks after completion of chemotherapy or radiotherapy, negative initial bone scan follow-up and new pain

Ankylosing Spondylitis

A characteristic, but unusual, lesion of the spine is ankylosing spondylitis. It occurs primarily in young males (onset about age 20 years) and sometimes is associated with ulcerative colitis. Ninety-five percent of patients are positive for HLA-B27 antigen. In this disease, calcification bridges the disk spaces. This is easily seen on the lateral plain radiograph of the spine and is referred to as a *bamboo spine*. On the AP view of the pelvis, fusion of the sacroiliac joints may be identified (Fig. 8–21). About 30% of patients have a peripheral arthritis that spares the hands but involves the feet.

Osteoporosis and Mineral Measurements

The accurate measurement of bone mineral density (BMD) using noninvasive methods can be of value in the detection and evaluation of primary and secondary causes of decreased mass. This includes primary osteoporosis and secondary disorders such as hyperparathyroidism, osteomalacia, malabsorption, multiple myeloma, diffuse metastases, and glucocorticoid therapy or intrinsic glucocorticoid excess.

By far the largest patient population is encom-

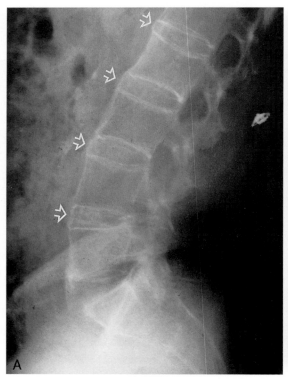
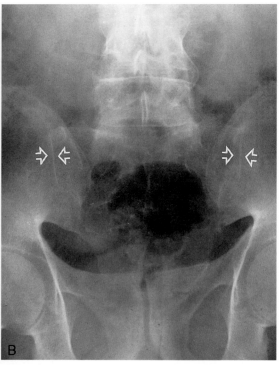

FIGURE 8–21. **Ankylosing spondylitis.** A lateral view of the lumbar spine *(A)* demonstrates calcific bridging across the disk spaces *(arrows)*, causing the typical bamboo spine appearance. *B,* An anteroposterior view of the pelvis shows that the region of the sacroiliac joints *(arrows)* is not easily visualized owing to fusion of both sacroiliac joints.

passed by primary osteoporosis. Osteoporosis is an age-related disorder characterized by decreased mass and by increased susceptibility to fractures in the absence of other recognizable causes of loss. Primary osteoporosis is generally subdivided into type 1 or postmenopausal osteoporosis, which is related to estrogen deprivation, and type 2 or senile osteoporosis, which occurs secondary to aging.

Primary osteoporosis is a common clinical disorder and a major public health problem because of the significant number of related fractures occurring annually. Because the risk of vertebral and femoral neck fractures rises dramatically as BMD levels fall below 1 g/cm², fracture risk in individual patients may be estimated. Furthermore, in estrogen-deficient women, BMD values may be used to make rational decisions about hormone replacement therapy and as follow-up in assessing the success of hormone replacement or specific bone-enhancing therapies.

A number of methods have been devised to permit the accurate and reproducible determination of bone mineral content. Plain radiographs generally require a loss of 30% or more of bone mineral for a change in density to be appreciated and are thus insensitive for the detection of the disease. Presently, bone mineral measurements are made using dual energy x-ray absorptiometry (DEXA) or nuclear medicine techniques. Both are accurate and reliable. Results are usually presented in terms of absolute BMD (g/cm²) as well as percentiles of reference normal young adult and age-matched populations. Normal BMD is defined as being within 1 standard deviation of the young adult mean. Osteopenia is BMD 1–2.5 standard deviations less than the young adult mean. Osteoporosis is a BMD more than 2.5 standard deviations below the young adult mean.

The use of bone mineral measurement has been controversial. Some of this is due to the wide variation of measurements in the normal population. Also, the criteria for selecting the optimal skeletal site for evaluation have not been well defined, because bone mineral loss does not progress at the same rate at different body sites. In any case, the method can be used to determine the presence of osteopenia and to evaluate effectiveness of a therapeutic maneuver by employing serial scans in which the patient acts as his or her own control. Normal results, or bone mineral content in the upper portion of the normal range, defines patients in whom therapy may not be needed. Indications to use DEXA are given in Table 8–4.

■ IMAGING APPROACH TO JOINT PAIN

A reasonable differential diagnosis to joint pain can be made on the basis of history, which can

---

TABLE 8–4 Indications for Using DEXA* to Measure Bone Mineral Density

- Intention to use hormone replacement or other medical therapy if osteoporosis is present.
- Suspect low bone mineral density based on osteopenia on plain radiographs.
- Low impact or nontraumatic vertebral fractures by x-ray examination in a postmenopausal female (see text for additional factors) or premenopausal female or a male with normal serum TSH, serum calcium, alkaline phosphatase, and serum protein electrophoresis levels.
- Loss of height >2.5 inches.
- Risk factors for low bone mineral density include estrogen deficient state, chronic liver or renal disease, thyroxine therapy, steroid therapy for more than 6 months (baseline and 12 month follow-up), hyperparathyroidism, hypogonadism in a male, and nutritional disorder.
- Follow-up hormone therapy (only if a change in management is being contemplated).

* DEXA = dual energy x-ray absorptiometry.

---

indicate whether the problem is acute or chronic and whether it affects one joint or more than one. In this section, joint pain without a suspected fracture is discussed. Fractures of the extremities are discussed later in this chapter.

Monoarticular Joint Pain

Acute monoarticular joint pain is usually due to gonococcal or septic arthritis, or post-traumatic status (occult fracture, ligament, or meniscal injuries or aseptic necrosis). Plain radiographs are indicated. If these are negative and the patient has loss of motion, joint effusion, and acute muscle spasm, an MRI is indicated.

Chronic monoarticular joint pain may be due to degenerative change, aseptic necrosis, chondromalacia, chondral defects, loose body, postsurgical changes, or, rarely, a synovial tumor. For an initial work-up, plain radiographs are indicated. Only if the radiographs are nondiagnostic is there a need to proceed with additional imaging.

Aseptic necrosis is only seen on plain x-ray examinations in advanced stages. If this is suspected on the basis of medical history (e.g., steroid therapy), and 6 weeks of exercise therapy (strengthening and range of motion), and nonsteroidal anti-inflammatory drug (NSAID) therapy is ineffective in reducing pain, MRI is indicated.

With loosening of a joint prosthesis, there is usually pain at rest that increases with activity. Initial management is usually 3 months of NSAID therapy, strengthening exercises, and use of a cane or walker. If pain persists and loosening or infection is suspected, either a nuclear medicine bone scan or an arthrogram is indicated. A ferromagnetic prosthesis may cause too many artifacts for CT or MRI to be of use.

Polyarticular Joint Pain

Acute polyarticular joint pain is usually due to infection (viral) or to an acute exacerbation of a systemic arthritis. Chronic polyarticular joint pain is usually secondary to osteoarthritis, but it may also be due to a number of other arthritides (such as rheumatoid or psoriatic) or to metabolic abnormalities (e.g., gout, pseudogout, and renal disease). Osteoarthritis or DJD is the most common form of joint disease and affects more than 30% of the population. There is degeneration of the cartilage, bone hypertrophy (spurring or osteophytes), and mild inflammation. DJD is mostly due to aging or local trauma. Risk factors include increasing age, female sex, obesity, knee injuries, and chondrocalcinosis. Specific issues related to degenerative arthritis of the shoulder, wrist, hip, and knee are discussed later in the appropriate anatomic sections.

Evaluation of the hands for arthritis can provide some general clues about the type of arthritis, although commonly there are a number of patients whose laboratory findings suggesting rheumatoid arthritis (RA) conflict with the x-ray appearance that looks like degenerative arthritis. The reverse is also true. Thus, the radiographic diagnosis should not be relied on too heavily.

RA occurs most frequently in females who clinically present with morning stiffness, swelling of one or more joints, and subcutaneous nodules. A patient is considered to have RA if four or more of the following criteria are present:

- Morning stiffness (>1 h and >6 weeks)
- Swelling of three or more joint areas for at least 6 weeks
- Swelling of the wrist or hand joints for at least 6 weeks
- Symmetric swelling of the joints for at least 6 weeks
- Rheumatoid nodules
- Positive serum rheumatoid factor
- Radiographic evidence of erosions, osteopenia, or both in the hand and wrist

General radiographic findings of RA include narrowing of the carpal joints, subchondral cysts, and erosion of the bones at the lateral edges of the joints. Patients with clinically obvious RA can often present with normal-looking radiographs of the hand and then undergo rapid progression. In addition to the findings already described, ulnar deviation at the metacarpophalangeal joints is relatively characteristic (Figs. 8–22 and 8–23). Diffuse osteoporosis is mostly seen with RA, but periarticular demineralization is also quite common.

In advanced RA, the patient's hands may develop the so-called *boutonniere deformity*, which is hyperextension of the distal interphalangeal joint and flexion in the proximal interphalangeal joint. Another deformity is almost the reverse of this. The *swan-neck deformity* can also result from hyperextension of the proximal interphalangeal joint and flexion of the distal interphalangeal joint.

Findings of RA in other bones include penciling or erosion of the distal clavicle and narrowing and erosions of the shoulder, hip, and knee joints in addition to atlantoaxial subluxation. There can also be subluxation of the cervical spine at C1–C2, and flexion and extension views are used to monitor the course of the disease. Finally, there can be a widened space between the carpal lunate and navicular bone (the Terry Thomas sign). Remember that patients with RA can also have interstitial lung changes, pulmonary nodules, and various forms of myocarditis.

When an arthritis involves distal interphalangeal joints with relative sparing of the proximal ones, erosive osteoarthritis and psoriatic arthritis become the more likely diagnoses (Fig. 8–24). Pseudogout can cause calcification within cartilage (chondrocalcinosis) (Fig. 8–25).

Gout typically involves the first tarsal-metatarsal joint. There may be soft tissue swelling or calcification of the tophus. Other changes include periarticular erosions without joint space narrowing (Fig. 8–26). The diagnosis is made by serum uric acid determinations or joint aspiration. Imaging studies are not positive until the disease is advanced.

■ BENIGN VS. MALIGNANT BONE LESIONS

It is important to be able to assess bone lesions and the likelihood of their being benign or malignant. Signs that a bone lesion may be benign are as follows: (1) it is small; (2) it does not have associated reaction of the periosteum; (3) it has a narrow (sharp) zone of transition between the normal bone and the lesion; and (4) it has a thin, well-defined sclerotic (white) margin.

In an adult, a lytic (destructive) lesion that does not have a sclerotic margin should be regarded as a malignancy until proved otherwise. Breast cancer, lung cancer, and a host of other neoplasms commonly produce lytic lesions of bone. There are also a number of primary bone lesions that can produce

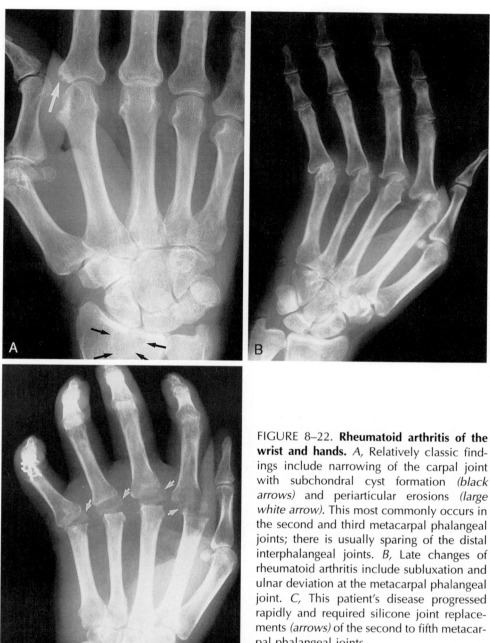

FIGURE 8–22. **Rheumatoid arthritis of the wrist and hands.** *A,* Relatively classic findings include narrowing of the carpal joint with subchondral cyst formation *(black arrows)* and periarticular erosions *(large white arrow).* This most commonly occurs in the second and third metacarpal phalangeal joints; there is usually sparing of the distal interphalangeal joints. *B,* Late changes of rheumatoid arthritis include subluxation and ulnar deviation at the metacarpal phalangeal joint. *C,* This patient's disease progressed rapidly and required silicone joint replacements *(arrows)* of the second to fifth metacarpal phalangeal joints.

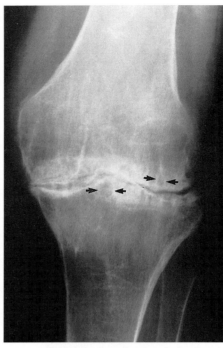

FIGURE 8–23. **Rheumatoid arthritis of the knee.** There is diffuse joint space narrowing with subchondral cyst formation *(arrows)*. A distinguishing feature between this and degenerative arthritis is that in rheumatoid arthritis, degenerative osteophytes or spurs are usually not seen.

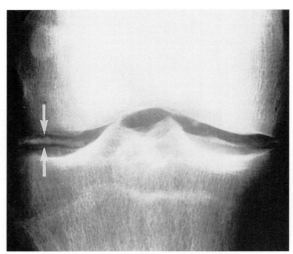

FIGURE 8–25. **Chondrocalcinosis.** Calcification of the cartilage in this knee is seen particularly well in the lateral compartment *(arrows)*. This is due to calcium pyrophosphate deposition disease (CPPD). Calcification is not seen in all patients with CPPD, and not all patients with chondrocalcinosis have CPPD.

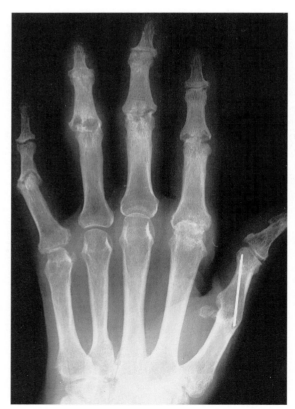

FIGURE 8–24. **Psoriatic arthritis.** Involvement of the distal and proximal interphalangeal joints is most common. Asymmetric changes are also common. Erosions can be aggressive and usually involve the intra-articular joint spaces.

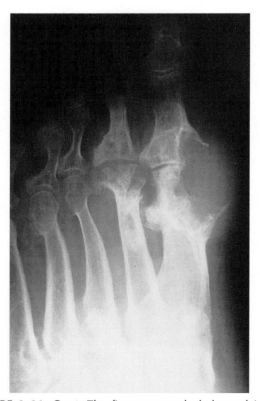

FIGURE 8–26. **Gout.** The first metatarsal phalangeal joint is the most commonly affected. Here, there is a large tophus that has caused erosion at the margins of the joints; in general, however, the joint space itself is reasonably well preserved.

this appearance, including plasmacytoma and eosinophilic granuloma.

■ INFECTION OF BONES AND JOINTS

Osteomyelitis can be acute or chronic. Most are caused by bacteria (*Staphylococcus aureus* or *S. epidermidis*) although tuberculosis, fungi, and, occasionally, viruses and parasites can be involved. Osteomyelitis occurs by three mechanisms: (1) hematogenous (most common in young children and older adults), (2) direct (post-traumatic or postsurgical), and (3) extension from adjacent tissues or organs.

The diagnosis of osteomyelitis is best made by culture. Plain films are also indicated in the at-risk patient. Unfortunately, with osteomyelitis, plain radiographs may be negative for up to 2 weeks. After this, there may be focal loss of calcium, erosion of bone, or periosteal reaction (Figs. 8–27 and 8–28). A three-phase nuclear medicine bone scan or MRI is indicated to localize a site for biopsy if the plain x-ray examinations are negative, the blood culture is positive, the patient has a sedimentation rate greater than 30 mm/hr, and the patient's temperature is higher than 100.4°F or the patient's white blood cell count is greater than 10,000.

Septic arthritis is frequently an acute process. Usually there is localized pain, joint swelling, fever, pain, chills, and arthralgia. Ninety percent of patients have only one joint affected. The knee is involved 50% of the time and the hip 25%, followed by ankle, shoulder, wrist, and elbow. Gonococcus is the leading cause of septic arthritis among young adults. Of the nongonococcal cases, 75% are due to gram-positive cocci (mostly *S. aureus*). The gram-negative infections are usually due to *Escherichia coli* and *Pseudomonas*. The diagnosis is best made by joint aspiration. Plain x-ray examinations of the joint are indicated. CT and MRI are generally not. A whole body nuclear medicine bone scan can be useful to look for other foci of infection.

Infections are quite frequent in the hands as well as the feet. Often, the clinical problem is differentiating between cellulitis, osteomyelitis, and septic arthritis. When the radiograph shows destruction of a single joint space with involvement of the bone on both sides of the joint, septic arthritis should be suspected (Fig. 8–29). Osteomyelitis can be radiographically identified by soft tissue swelling, lucent or destructive areas within the bone itself, or focal periosteal reaction. With cellulitis, there is only soft tissue swelling without radiographic bone or joint changes.

Periosteal Reaction

Periosteal reaction or thickening can be due to either benign or malignant lesions. Obviously, local periosteal reactions are seen about a healing fracture. However, this is normally quite obvious and does not cause any confusion in interpretation. Infections can also cause periosteal reactions. Osteomyelitis that has been present for several weeks can cause minimal periosteal reaction, and chronic

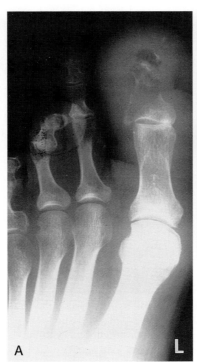 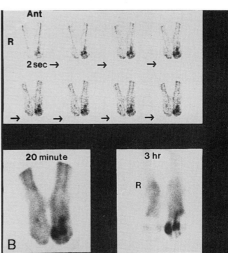

FIGURE 8–27. **Osteomyelitis of the foot.** *A,* In this patient with diabetes, there is a significant soft tissue swelling and destruction of the bony structure of the distal phalanx of the great toe. *B,* When radiographs are normal, there can still be osteomyelitis. A nuclear medicine bone scan is more sensitive and shows increased blood flow in the first seconds after radionuclide injection, increased blood pooling at 20 minutes, and more focal and intense radioactivity on the 3-hour images.

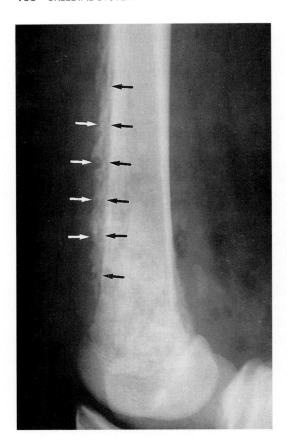

FIGURE 8–28. **Chronic osteomyelitis.** A lateral view of the knee shows florid periosteal reaction *(arrows)*. The periosteal reaction that is dense and extends over a long area suggests chronic osteomyelitis. The bone of the distal femur has a mottled appearance as a result of the infection. Note also that the distal femoral epiphysis is not fused; given the periosteal reaction, the location in the distal femur, and the patient's age, an osteogenic sarcoma must also be considered.

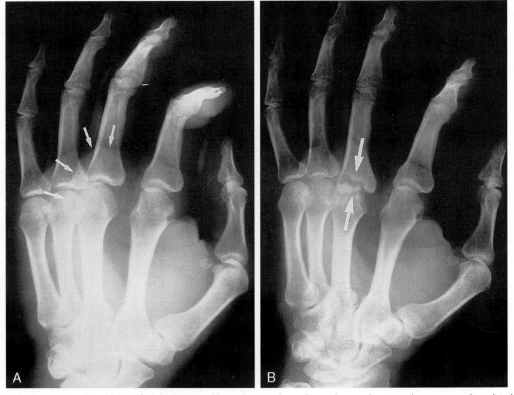

FIGURE 8–29. **Septic arthritis.** *A,* A film obtained 1 day after a human bite over the third metacarpal phalangeal joint shows only some soft tissue swelling *(arrows). B,* Another radiograph 4 weeks later shows that there has been destruction of both the distal metacarpal and the proximal phalanx because of an infection within the joint space.

osteomyelitis that has been present for months and years can cause a florid calcified periosteal reaction. In young patients (between the ages of 5 and 20 years), a periosteal reaction in the midportion (diaphysis) of a long bone should suggest Ewing's tumor; if located around the joint such as the knee, it should raise the suspicion of an osteogenic sarcoma (Fig. 8–30). Sunburst-type (radiating) periosteal reaction is particularly worrisome for malignancy.

Natural History of Fractures

Obvious displaced fractures are easily seen and diagnosed with plain radiographs. More subtle, non-displaced, or hairline fractures may be easily overlooked. A fracture often becomes more apparent a week or so after the initial injury. The reason is that in the early stages of a fracture, hyperemia is accompanied by resorption of calcium along the

FIGURE 8–30. **Osteogenic sarcoma of the knee.** A lateral view of the knee *(A)* in a 19-year-old male shows a sunburst-type periosteal reaction *(arrows)*. Knowing that the distal femur is the most common site of osteogenic sarcoma, that periosteal reaction is a feature, and that this patient is a teenager should make osteogenic sarcoma quite high on your differential diagnostic list. Another common presentation *(B)* is a predominantly destructive central lesion seen here in the distal femur of an 8-year-old girl.

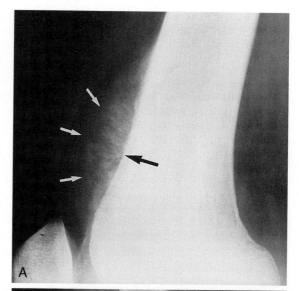

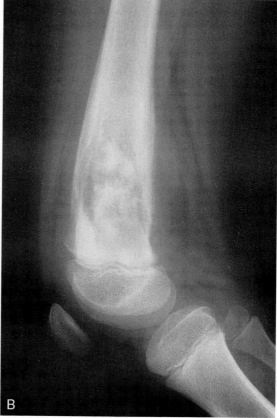

fracture line. This is why radiologists sometimes indicate that although they do not see a fracture on a particular examination, if pain persists, a repeat view in 7 to 10 days may be useful. A second phenomenon is a more general loss of calcium and coarsening of the trabecular pattern in bones around a joint that has a fracture. This process may occur for several weeks and is the result of disuse osteoporosis. Sometimes, even if there is minor trauma to the hands or feet, there can be localized burning pain, swelling, or temperature changes that persist for months with associated vasodilatation. This is referred to as *reflex sympathetic dystrophy* (RSD). The radiographic manifestations are focal osteoporosis and a coarsened trabecular pattern in an articular and periarticular distribution. Usually physical examination and plain radiographs are all that is needed to make the diagnosis. In confusing cases, a three-phase nuclear medicine bone scan can help.

Myositis Ossificans

Calcification can occur in soft tissues. The muscles of the thigh are particularly prone to trauma, and bleeding within the soft tissue can subsequently calcify. This condition is referred to as *myositis ossificans* (Fig. 8–31) and may require surgery after the calcification has matured.

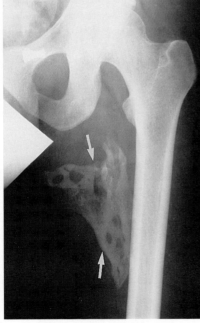

FIGURE 8–31. **Myositis ossificans.** The soft tissues of the thigh are a common location for blunt traumatic injury. In this case, dystrophic calcification has developed within the soft tissue *(arrows)*, significantly limiting the range of motion of this young soccer player.

Plain radiographs may show the calcification, but maturity can be demonstrated by lack of intense activity on a nuclear medicine bone scan.

Foreign Bodies in Soft Tissue

X-ray films are often taken for localization of foreign bodies. The most common are glass, gravel, pencil lead, metallic slivers, and pieces of wood. Glass or gravel is usually somewhat radiopaque. Glass is recognized by its sharp corners or a geometric shape. Metallic fragments are, of course, easy to spot, because they are so dense. Wood, plastic, and pencil lead are typically not visible on a radiograph. Pencil lead is not visible because it is actually graphite and not lead. Even if the object is visible on a plain radiograph, it may be difficult to locate clinically for removal. In these circumstances, concurrent fluoroscopy may be needed.

■ SHOULDER AND HUMERUS

Normal Anatomy and Imaging

The standard view of the shoulder is obtained in an AP or a posteroanterior projection with the arm rotated internally and then externally (Fig. 8–32). When the arm is in internal rotation, the humeral head looks generally smooth and spherical over the upper portion. In external rotation, there is a concavity of the bicipital groove seen in the lateral aspect of the humeral head. In children, the proximal humeral epiphysis and an epiphyseal plate are visualized. This can sometimes be confused with a fracture. If the epiphyseal plate is not parallel to the x-ray beam, several lucent lines traversing the proximal portion of the humerus can be seen, because the epiphyseal plate is tilted off axis relative to the x-ray beam (Fig. 8–33). In adolescents, both on the end of the coracoid process and on the acromion, one should be aware of an apophysis. The clavicle, scapula, and ribs should be examined for fractures and other lesions. Also, look to see whether there is any pathology in the visualized portions of the lung.

There are two other commonly ordered views of the shoulder. The first is called the *Y view*. This is done with the patient rotated somewhat so that the scapular blade is seen on end and projects off the chest wall. The acromion, spine of the scapula, and blade of the scapula form a "Y" (Fig. 8–34). The humeral head should normally project at or near the intersection of the three lines. This view is usually obtained if a shoulder dislocation is suspected and is also useful to look for fractures of the scapular blade.

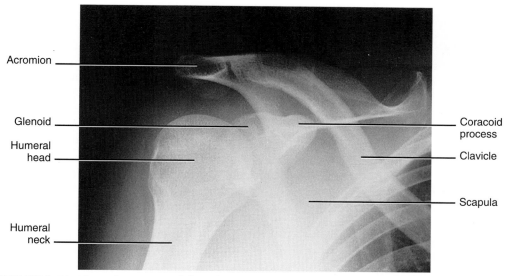

Acromion

Glenoid

Humeral head

Humeral neck

Coracoid process

Clavicle

Scapula

FIGURE 8–32. **Normal anatomy of the adult shoulder in the posteroanterior projection with the humerus in internal rotation.**

FIGURE 8–33. **Normal shoulder of an 11-year-old patient in internal rotation *(A)* and in external rotation *(B).* The epiphy**seal plate of the proximal humerus should not be mistaken for a fracture.

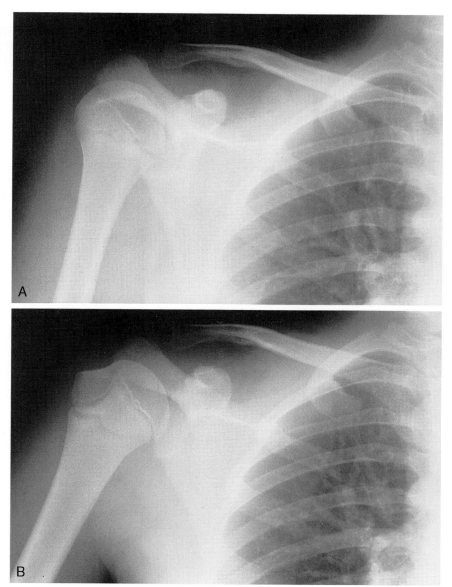

A

B

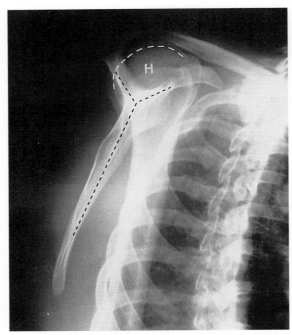

FIGURE 8–34. **Normal oblique or Y view of the shoulder.** On this view, the elements of the scapula form a Y and the humeral head (H) should overlap the intersecting arms of the Y.

Another view that is often obtained is the axillary view, in which the elbow is elevated, and the beam projection is directly up and down through the shoulder. This allows clear visualization of the relationship of the glenoid to the humeral head. Unfortunately, this view is difficult to obtain on patients who have a true dislocation or a fracture. Radiographs of the shoulder are really useful only to define bone anatomy. There are many shoulder injuries that involve soft tissues, and the most useful imaging test for evaluation of these is an MRI.

Fractures

Most clavicular fractures occur either in the midportion or the distal third of the clavicle. Usually, the fractures are clinically obvious. Rarely, there is dislocation of the proximal head of the clavicle from the sternoclavicular joint; however, this is also clinically obvious. Fractures of the scapula are reasonably rare, although they can occur as the result of a direct blow. Often this is apparent on a routine shoulder film and from the clinical history. In many cases the fracture cannot be seen in its entirety as it traverses the blade of the scapula, and if there is any additional question, a Y view or a CT scan may be useful. Fractures of the middle or proximal humerus present few problems in radiographic interpretation.

Acromioclavicular Separation

In this injury, there is superior dislocation of the distal clavicle relative to the acromion (Fig. 8–35). Because the clavicle is slightly anterior relative to the acromion, if the patient is leaning back when the film is taken, it sometimes looks as though there is a separation when there is not. If you have any question, a single view that includes both shoulders for comparison is often useful.

Shoulder Dislocation

More than 95% of shoulder dislocations occur with anterior dislocation of the humeral head relative to the glenoid. This is in contrast to the hip, in which the vast majority of femoral head dislocations are posterior. In an anterior shoulder dislocation on the AP projection, the medial aspect of the humeral

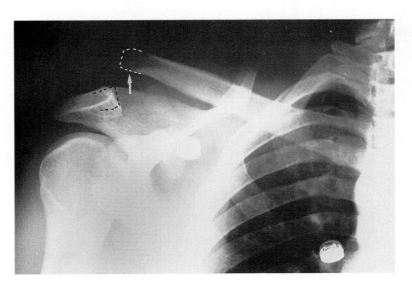

FIGURE 8–35. **Acromioclavicular separation.** The distal end of the clavicle is superiorly dislocated *(arrow)* relative to the acromion.

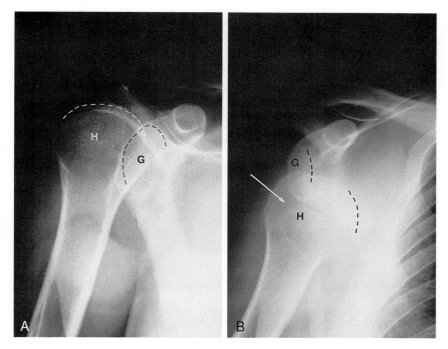

FIGURE 8–36. **Anterior dislocation of the shoulder.** *A,* In the normal anteroposterior view of the shoulder, the humeral head (H) is located lateral to the glenoid (G), but there is a small amount of overlap. *B,* In the same patient with an anterior dislocation, the humeral head (H) goes inferiorly and medially *(arrow)* with respect to the glenoid (G).

head is seen to be inferior and medial to the glenoid (Fig. 8–36). As mentioned earlier, on the oblique view of the shoulder (the Y view), the humeral head should project over the central portion of the Y. A Y view clearly shows the anterior and inferior dislocation of the humeral head (Fig. 8–37).

As a dislocation occurs, there is sometimes a fracture of a portion of the humeral head or of the glenoid. Some physicians relocate a dislocated shoulder without obtaining a prereduction film. If this is done and the postreduction film demonstrates a fracture, the question may occasionally

arise as to whether the fracture occurred during the reduction maneuver. In patients who have had repeated dislocations, chronic trauma caused by interaction of the inferior edge of the glenoid with the humeral head may produce a deformity or groove in the superolateral portion of the humeral head known as a *Hill-Sachs deformity* (Fig. 8–38).

Posterior shoulder dislocations are rare, and they are quite tricky to identify on a standard AP shoulder radiograph. With internal rotation, the humeral head on the AP projection is typically like the top half of a sphere. However, with a posterior shoulder

FIGURE 8–37. **Anterior dislocation on the Y view.** *A,* On the Y view, the humeral head (H) is clearly anterior and inferior *(arrow)* to the intersection of the Y of the scapula. *B,* After relocation, the humeral head overlaps the Y formed by the scapula.

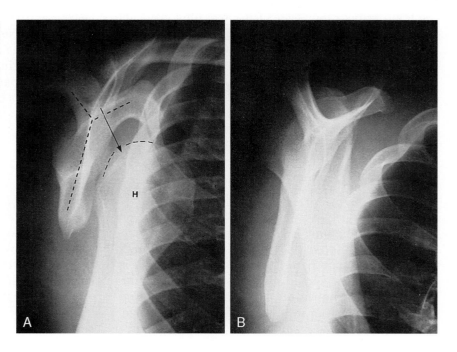

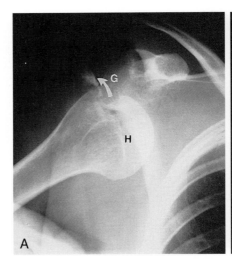
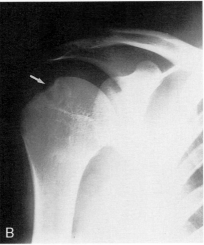

FIGURE 8–38. **Complications of shoulder dislocation.** *A,* In a patient with an anterior dislocation of the humeral head (H), a fracture fragment arising from the humerus *(arrow)* can be identified. *B,* In a different patient chronic anterior dislocations caused a Hill-Sachs deformity seen as a groove in the upper outer portion of the humeral head *(arrow).* G = glenoid.

dislocation, the humeral head does not appear to be rounded (Fig. 8–39), and there is slightly increased space between the humeral head and the glenoid. A Y view clearly shows the posterior dislocation.

Shoulder Pain

Most shoulder pain is due to degenerative change or degenerative arthritis. Because the glenohumeral joint is off the axis relative to an AP x-ray beam, minimal joint space narrowing is not easily evaluated. However, if the changes are severe enough (Fig. 8–40), it is easy to see that the joint is narrowed. Typically, there is associated sclerosis and often spurring and deformity of the humeral head and the inferior aspect of the glenoid.

A degenerative change that is sometimes seen on the plain radiograph is calcification of tendons. This usually appears as amorphous white densities over the superolateral aspect of the humeral head. Degenerative change also includes rotator cuff tears. This is suspected when there is pain with abduction and weakness at more than 60 degrees. If pain persists after 6 weeks of NSAID therapy and supervised physical therapy and if surgery is contemplated, MRI is indicated.

Tumors

Specific malignant lesions develop in the shoulder. Because the scapula is a flat bone, Ewing's sarcoma can occur here. The proximal humerus is the third most frequent site of osteogenic sarcoma in children. The appearance of this particular lesion is discussed further in the section on the knee, because the knee is a more common location.

■ ELBOW

Normal Anatomy and Imaging

Most radiographs of the elbow are done because of trauma. The normal images obtained include AP and oblique views with the elbow extended and a lateral view with the elbow flexed at 90 degrees (Fig. 8–41). The lateral view is the most promising view to look for pathology in the elbow. There is a small dark line seen just anterior to the distal humerus. This is the anterior fat pad, and although it is normal to see this, it should be right up against the bone. A posterior fat pad is never seen normally, and if seen it indicates pathology. In an adolescent, lack of fusion of the normal epiphyses and presence of apophyses can cause confusion. The last areas of fusion include the radial head (5 years), medial epicondyle (7 years), trochlea and olecranon (10 years), and finally the lateral epicondyle (11 years) (Fig. 8–42). Normally, apophyses are distinguished from fractures by noting that apophyses have well-defined margins without sharp edges and that the anterior fat pad is in normal position and a posterior fat pad is not seen.

Trauma

The place to begin looking for traumatic injuries of the elbow is on the lateral view. Anterior displacement of the anterior fat pad or any visualization whatever of the posterior fat pad, should indicate that a fracture is likely to be present, even if none is visible on any of the plain radiographs. Sometimes, repeating the radiograph 7 to 10 days later will allow decalcification of the fracture to occur so that it will be more easily seen.

The most common fracture of the elbow seen in adults is a radial head fracture (Fig. 8–43). Less

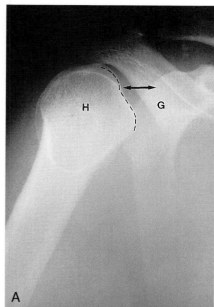

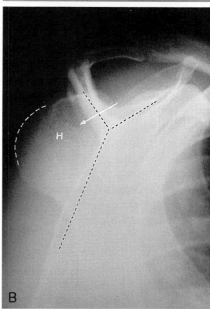

FIGURE 8–39. **Posterior dislocation of the humeral head.** *A,* An anteroposterior view of the shoulder initially looks fairly normal. However, there is an increased space *(double-ended arrow)* between the humeral head (H) and the glenoid (G); the fact that the humeral head is not spherical *(dotted line)* is another clue. *B,* On the Y view of the shoulder, the humeral head (H) can clearly be seen to be posteriorly displaced *(arrow)* relative to the central portion of the Y formed by the scapula.

common are fractures of the coronoid process of the ulna and fractures of the olecranon. Olecranon fractures are typically caused by falling directly on the elbow when it is flexed.

■ FOREARM

Typical normal views of the forearm are obtained in AP and lateral projections. If you suspect trauma

or abnormalities of either the elbow or the wrist, a forearm view alone is not satisfactory. Order forearm views only when the abnormality is in the midportion of either the radius or the ulna, otherwise wrist or elbow views are more appropriate.

Trauma

A traumatic injury is, by far, the most common reason for ordering forearm x-ray examinations. There are three classic forearm fractures. The first is the *nightstick fracture.* This is a single fracture through the midportion of the ulna (Fig. 8–44). It is called the nightstick fracture because it easily occurs when an individual raises his or her arm to protect against being hit with a stick. There are two other classic (although uncommon) fractures of the forearm. The *Monteggia fracture* is a fracture of the proximal ulna with dislocation of the radial head. The dislocation of the radial head can be missed unless one realizes that the radius and radial head should point toward the capitellum of the distal humerus. The *Galeazzi fracture* is a fracture of the distal radius with dislocation of the ulnar head from the wrist joint. The mechanism is somewhat similar

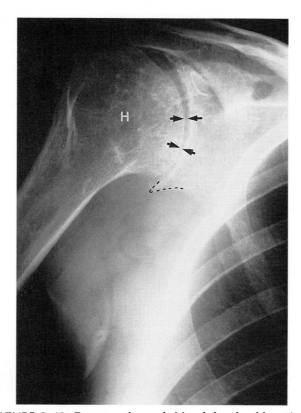

FIGURE 8–40. **Degenerative arthritis of the shoulder.** There has been marked narrowing of the normal joint space *(arrows).* There is flattening of the humeral head (H), and there is spurring deformity *(dashed curve)* of the inferior portion of the glenoid (G).

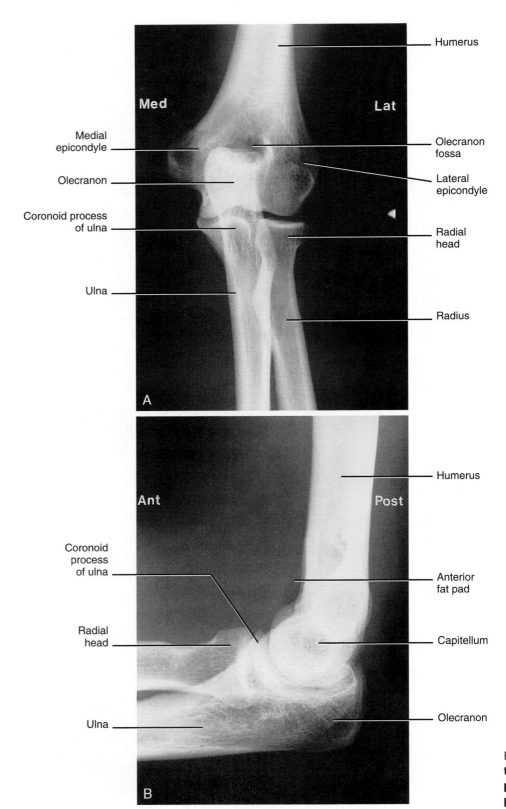

FIGURE 8–41. **Normal anatomy of the elbow in the anteroposterior projection** *(A)* **and in the lateral projection** *(B).*

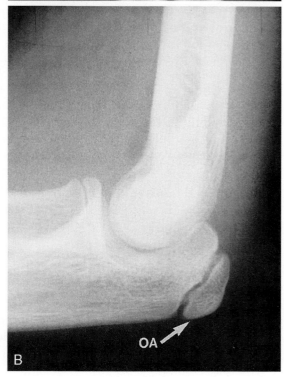

FIGURE 8–42. **Normal apophyses.** On the anteroposterior projection *(A)*, a coronoid apophysis (CA) can be seen along the medial aspect of the distal humerus. On the lateral view *(B)*, an olecranon apophysis (OA) is often visualized in older children. The epiphysis has not yet fused.

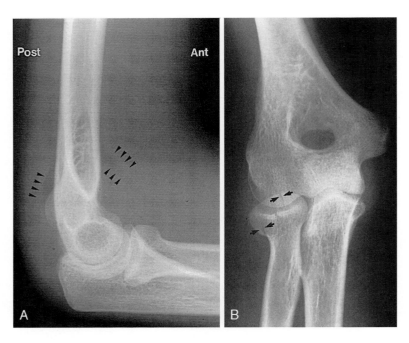

FIGURE 8–43. **Radial head fracture.** The lateral view of the elbow *(A)* shows anterior displacement of the dark stripe of the anterior fat pad *(arrows)*; a posterior fat pad is also seen *(posterior arrows)*. On the anteroposterior view *(B)*, a lucent fracture line is seen going obliquely across the humeral head *(arrows)*.

to that of the Monteggia fracture but with the fulcrum located more distally.

HAND AND WRIST

Normal Anatomy and Imaging

The typical views obtained when either hand or wrist x-ray examinations are ordered include AP, oblique, and lateral (Fig. 8–45). Radiographs of the hand and fingers taken for trauma should also include AP, oblique, and lateral views. If the clinical issue is related to arthritis, an AP view of both hands is all that is needed. There is a relatively common finding in the hand that involves shortening of a metacarpal, typically the fourth. This is usually a normal variant, but the differential diagnosis includes Turner's syndrome, pseudohypoparathyroidism, and a few other much less common conditions.

Wrist Pain

Carpometacarpal osteoarthritis usually occurs at the base of the thumb and patients have pain and swelling or enlargement at the affected joint. Plain radiographs are indicated, and symptomatic patients have abnormal radiographs with sclerosis, joint space narrowing, and spur formation.

Wrist pain can also be due to chronic ligamentous injury usually involving the fibrocartilaginous complex. There is tenderness, dorsal and volar subluxation at rest, and pain with stress. If pain persists after 6 weeks of NSAID therapy and a wrist splint, MRI may be indicated.

Carpal tunnel syndrome is a compression neuropathy with loss of sensation in the tips of the first three digits and forearm and wrist pain. Physical examination and medical history are often diagnostic. Nerve conduction velocity tests are indicated but not imaging. Similarly, imaging is not needed for evaluation or treatment of an uncomplicated dorsal ganglion.

Trauma

Common fractures of the wrist include Colles' fracture. This is a fracture of the distal radius with dorsal angulation of the distal fragment and an associated fracture of the ulnar styloid (Fig. 8–46). The mechanism of injury is typically falling on an outstretched hand with the palm facing down at the time of the fall. A Smith fracture is essentially a reverse Colles fracture, with the distal radial fragment angulated toward the palmar surface (Fig. 8–47). The most common fracture of the carpal bones is a fracture of the midportion of the carpal navicular. The navicular has an unusual blood supply. The arteries first supply the distal aspect of the bone and then circle back to supply the more proximal portion. A fracture through the midportion of the navicular can disrupt the blood supply to the proximal portion and cause aseptic necrosis. When this occurs, the proximal portion of the navicular becomes dense or white relative to the rest of the carpal bones (Fig. 8–48).

An injury that can result from impaction of the distal radius and the carpal bones is disruption of the ligaments between the navicular and the lunate. Sometimes this can be a subtle finding. The

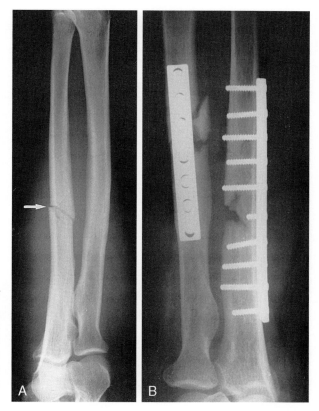

FIGURE 8–44. **Nightstick fracture.** *A,* An anteroposterior view of the forearm demonstrates a single fracture *(arrow)* across the midportion of the ulna. This is called a *nightstick fracture* because it occurs when the person lifts the forearm to protect against being hit with a stick. *B,* In a different patient with a much more severe fracture of the radius and ulna, the fracture has been fixed using a plate and screws. Notice the asymmetric holes in the plate, which allow for compression of the fracture fragments.

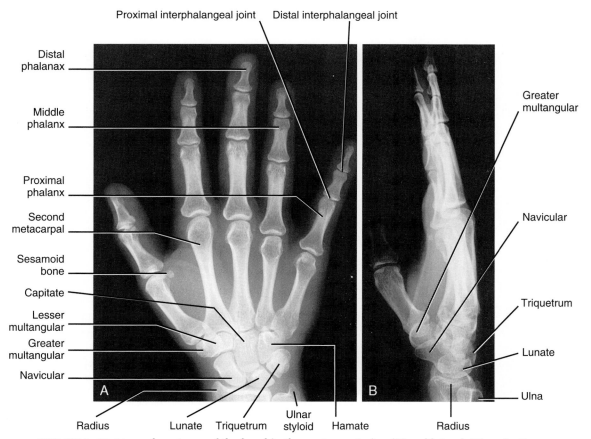

FIGURE 8–45. **Normal anatomy of the hand in the posteroanterior *(A)* and lateral *(B)* projections.**

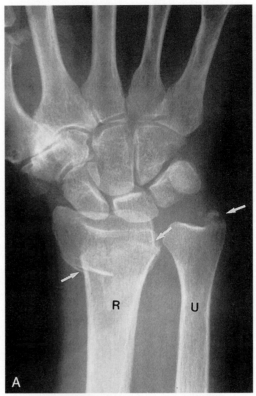

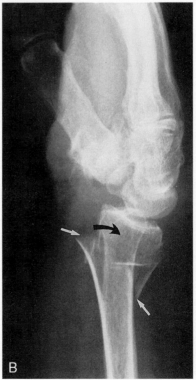

FIGURE 8–46. **Colles' fracture.** *A,* An impacted distal radial fracture (R) and a fracture of the ulnar styloid (U) *(white arrows)* are identified on the posteroanterior view in this patient who fell on the outstretched hand. *B,* The lateral view of the wrist shows that there is dorsal displacement *(black arrow)* and angulation as well as some impaction of the distal radius. If the fracture of the distal radius extends into the joint, this would be termed a *Barton fracture.*

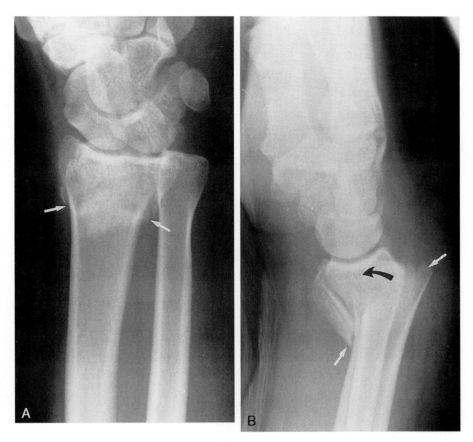

FIGURE 8–47. **Smith's fracture.** *A,* An anteroposterior view of the wrist shows that there is an impacted fracture of the distal radius *(arrows). B,* The lateral view shows that there is volar displacement of the distal fragment *(black arrow).* If the fracture had extended into the articular surface *(white arrows),* this would have been called a *reverse Barton fracture.*

space between the distal radius and the carpal bones should be about the same as the distance between the lunate and the navicular. If there is a question as to whether this space is widened, an AP radiograph of the other wrist can be used for comparison. Tenderness over the dorsal aspect of the wrist should raise the possibility of a triquetral fracture. This fracture is usually seen only on the lateral view and may be just a small avulsion fragment.

Major falls can cause either lunate or perilunate dislocations of the carpal bones. The key to initial recognition of these dislocations on the AP view is the loss of the usual configuration consisting of a distinct proximal and distal row of carpal bones. The lateral view usually makes the type of dislocation reasonably clear. In perilunate dislocation, the lunate is in normal position at the end of the radius, but the remainder of the carpals are dislocated posteriorly and are usually overriding with some shortening of the wrist. In a lunate dislocation, the rest of the carpals remain in a line along the axis of the radius; however, the lunate is usually rotated and dislocated toward the palmar surface.

There are two relatively frequent fracture sites of the metacarpals. The most common of these is a fracture of the distal fifth metacarpal (the so-called *boxer's fracture*). In this fracture the head of the

fifth metacarpal is displaced toward the palmar surface and may be somewhat impacted (Fig. 8–49). The second common location for hand fractures is the base of the thumb. The *Bennett* and *Rolando* fractures refer to triangular fractures of the base of the first metacarpal, with extension into the articular surface. There can be oblique fractures of the first metacarpal base that do not extend into the joint. Another rather classic fracture of the thumb is an avulsion fracture of the base of the proximal phalanx. Although this is called a *gamekeeper's thumb,* the most common mechanism of injury is getting a ski pole caught in the snow with the thumb being pulled backward. Another relatively common fracture of the fingers involves the base of the middle phalanx on the palmar surface. This is a small avulsion fracture referred to as a *volar plate fracture* (Fig. 8–50). It is easily missed unless the lateral view is examined carefully. Of course, fractures of the terminal tuft of the distal phalanges occur quite frequently from people slamming their fingers in doors. These are quite obvious on the radiograph.

Fingers can not only be fractured but also dislocated (Fig. 8–51). All dislocations are clinically obvious, but if there is unusual associated deformity or angulation, it may be useful to get a prereduction radiograph to see if there is an associated fracture.

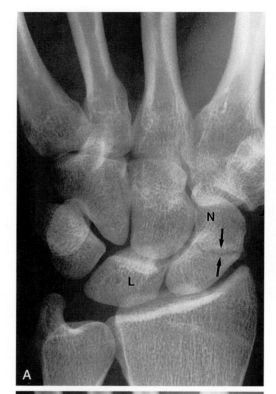

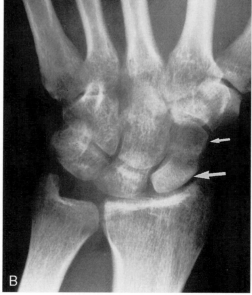

FIGURE 8–48. **Scaphoid or navicular fracture.** *A,* A posteroanterior view of the wrist in a patient who fell on his outstretched hand shows a lucent line (L) extending through the midportion *(arrows)* of the navicular (N). *B,* A later complication in this patient is aseptic necrosis of the proximal fragment *(large arrow).* Note that this fragment has maintained normal mineralization because the blood supply has been interrupted. In contrast, the remainder of the carpal bones and distal navicular fragment *(small arrow)* are demonstrating a loss of calcium caused by hyperemia and by disuse after the fracture.

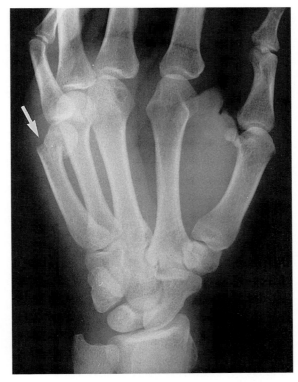

FIGURE 8–49. **Boxer's fracture.** This hand film was obtained on a teenager who had hand pain after punching a wall. The fracture *(arrow)* usually occurs at the neck of the fifth metacarpal, with volar angulation of the distal fragment. Contrary to its name, it is not often seen in professional boxers.

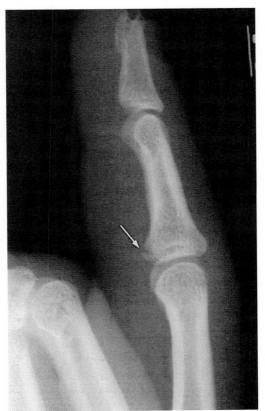

FIGURE 8–50. **Volar plate fracture.** This fracture *(arrow)* is seen only on the lateral view and is a small avulsion fracture, most commonly occurring at the base of the middle phalanx.

Tumors

Tumors of the hand and wrist are quite rare. The most common tumor is a benign enchondroma. This typically occurs in either the metacarpals or the proximal phalanges. It causes a lucent area in the central portion of the shaft with some expansion and inner table thinning of the cortex. There can be pathologic fractures through these areas as a result of the bone thinning.

■ PELVIS

Normal Anatomy and Imaging

Normally only an AP view of the pelvis is obtained. On the AP view, iliac wings, ischium, pubis,

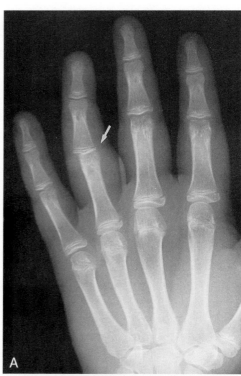

FIGURE 8–51. **Complete dislocation of a proximal interphalangeal joint.** *A,* A posteroanterior view of the hand shows some soft tissue swelling *(arrow)* in what looks like only a narrowing of joint space. *B,* A lateral view clearly shows the dislocation, although this, of course, would be clinically obvious. This case should serve as a lesson in why two views are needed before a conclusion is drawn about the position of various structures on a radiograph.

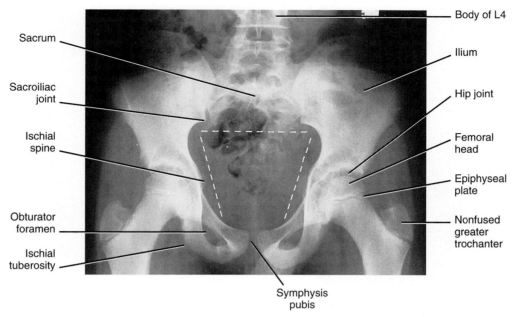

FIGURE 8–52. **Normal anatomy of the teenage male pelvis.** Note the generally triangular (android) shape of the pelvic inlet.

and both hips as well as the lower lumbar spine are clearly demonstrated. The inlet of the male pelvis is generally somewhat triangular (Fig. 8–52), whereas the female pelvis has a much more ovoid shape (Fig. 8–53).

The general age of the patient is ascertained by the presence or absence of degenerative changes in the lower lumbar spine and hip joints. In children, there is incomplete fusion of the acetabulum; in slightly older children, the apophysis of the greater trochanter and the epiphyseal plate of the hip are visualized. In the middle to late adolescent years, an apophysis appears on the iliac crest as well as on the inferior ischium (Fig. 8–54). Although these apophyses can sometimes be mistaken for avulsion

fractures, the symmetry from one side of the pelvis to another and their location are usually enough to clearly identify them. There are several normal variants or benign common conditions that need to be appreciated. These are symmetric sclerotic areas (white) about the symphysis pubis or the sacroiliac (SI) joint. These are essentially normal findings and occur much more commonly in women, probably as the result of pelvic widening during childbirth.

Trauma

A number of traumatic lesions can occur in the pelvis. A relatively common and probably unneces-

FIGURE 8–53. **Normal anatomy of the adult female pelvis.** Note the generally ovoid (gynecoid) shape of the pelvic inlet.

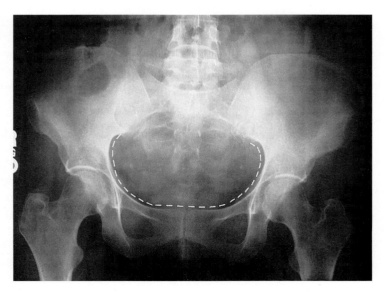

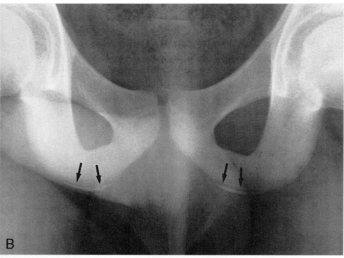

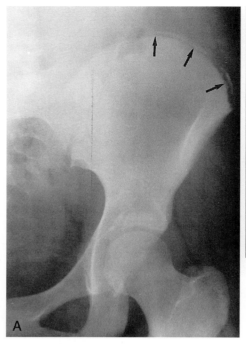

FIGURE 8–54. **Normal apophyses.** During the middle and late teen years, an apophysis *(arrows)* can be seen over the iliac crest *(A)* and along the inferior aspect *(B)* of the ischium *(arrows)*. These should not be mistaken for avulsion fractures.

sary radiograph to order is a view of the coccyx. Demonstration of a coccyx fracture does not change treatment. When a pelvic fracture is suspected, an AP radiograph is the initial view to order. A widening of the symphysis of more than 1 cm is definitely abnormal. If the symphysis is widened, also look for widening of one of the SI joints (Fig. 8–55). The reason is that the pelvis is essentially a fixed bone ring, and it is difficult to widen it or break it in one place without causing a traumatic injury elsewhere.

Many pelvic fractures are accompanied by internal pelvic hematomas. When a fracture in the pubic region is identified, urethral and bladder injuries may have occurred. A contrast cystogram or CT cystogram is often performed to rule out bladder

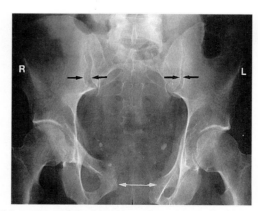

FIGURE 8–55. **Pelvic fracture.** There is marked diastasis of the pubis *(white arrow)* and widening of both sacroiliac joints, but the right is greater than the left *(black arrows)*. Whenever the pelvic ring is interrupted (as in this case), the fracture is unstable.

rupture (Fig. 8–56). Most pelvic fractures can, and should, be visualized on the plain radiograph of the pelvis, although occasionally it is necessary to get a CT scan. This is done when a fracture is suspected but is not identified on the plain radiograph or when there are multiple fragments around the hip or SI joint.

Benign Lesions

Paget's disease is a common benign lesion of the pelvis. Usually there is involvement of only the right or left half of the pelvis. The iliopectineal line becomes thickened; there is coarsening of the trabecular pattern, and the cortex becomes thickened. A generalized coarse trabecular pattern and patchy sclerosis of the whole pelvis and other bones can be a result of renal failure. A diffuse increase in bone density can occur as a result of myelofibrosis, fluoride poisoning, osteopetrosis ("marble bone" disease), or diffuse sclerotic metastases.

Malignant Lesions

Focal lesions of the flat bones of the pelvis are often malignant. The differential diagnosis depends to a large extent on the age of the patient. In a young patient, suspect Ewing's sarcoma. Chondrosarcomas tend to arise in the pelvis of adults. On radiograph, these tumors often have cauliflower or popcorn calcifications extending from the bone. In older patients, multiple lytic or destructive lesions

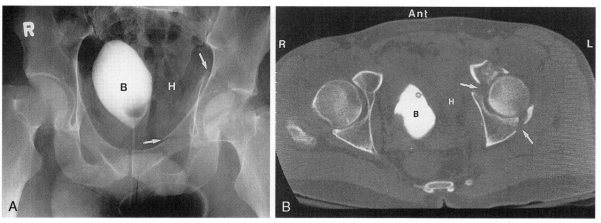

FIGURE 8–56. **Fracture of the acetabulum.** An anteroposterior view of the pelvis *(A)* clearly shows the corners of the fracture *(arrows)* as well as a hematoma (H) displacing the bladder (B) to the right. In order to see the exact nature of the acetabular injury, often a computed tomography scan *(B)* is required; in this case, it shows a complex fracture *(arrows)* involving both the anterior and the posterior portions of the acetabulum.

are often due to metastases from lung, breast, renal cell carcinoma, or multiple myeloma (plasmacytoma). Dense or sclerotic lesions of the pelvis include metastases from prostate carcinoma (Fig. 8–57) and occasionally breast cancer.

■ HIP

Radiographs of the hip are done in the AP and "frog leg" (abducted) projections. Lateral views are usually difficult to obtain and even more difficult to

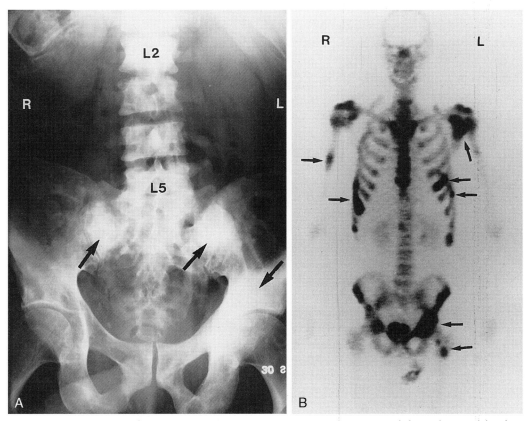

FIGURE 8–57. **Metastatic prostate cancer.** *A,* An anteroposterior view of the pelvis and lumbar spine demonstrates multiple areas of increased density *(arrows)* in a patchy distribution. Vertebrae L2 and L5 are also abnormally white or increased in density. *B,* A nuclear medicine whole-body bone scan most commonly shows the metastatic deposits as areas of increased activity *(arrows).*

interpret. It is important to examine the relationship of the femoral head to the acetabulum, look for cortical discontinuities to suggest fractures, and examine the trabecular pattern to look for potential osseous lesions. In young teenagers, there is an apophysis of both the greater and the lesser trochanter. Children younger than 10 or 12 years do not yet have fusion of the midportion of the acetabulum (Fig. 8–58).

Trauma

Dislocations of the hip are usually the result of motor vehicle accidents. By far the most common dislocation is posteriorly, and on the AP radiograph the head of the femur appears to be superiorly and laterally displaced. When the hip is anteriorly dislocated, the femoral head appears inferior and medial to the acetabulum (Fig. 8–59). With any dislocation, there may be associated fracture fragments from the rim of the acetabulum. CT scanning can be of value in such cases.

Ninety percent of hip fractures occur in the region of the femoral neck (with osteoporosis) and in the intertrochanteric region (post-traumatic). The majority of hip fractures are suspected clinically in patients who were ambulatory and become unable to walk after a fall or develop pain with movement. Fractures of the femoral neck usually have little deformity. Patients with intertrochanteric fractures often have a shortened leg with internal rotation (Fig. 8–60).

Stress fractures of the femoral neck may appear only as an ill-defined sclerotic (white) band extending across the femoral neck. In older persons, a hip fracture may be difficult to see because there is so little calcium in the bone. Nondisplaced hip fractures are best diagnosed by MRI. Nuclear medicine bone scans can also be used, although they may not be positive until several days after the fracture has occurred.

Hip Pain

Acute hip pain can be due to inflammatory arthritis, septic arthritis, trauma, and tumors. These entities have been discussed earlier. Chronic hip pain can result from a number of conditions. The most common is degenerative arthritis. Complaints are typically of groin or thigh pain or loss of mobility. Physical examination initially shows a loss of internal rotation, and as the disease advances, ex-

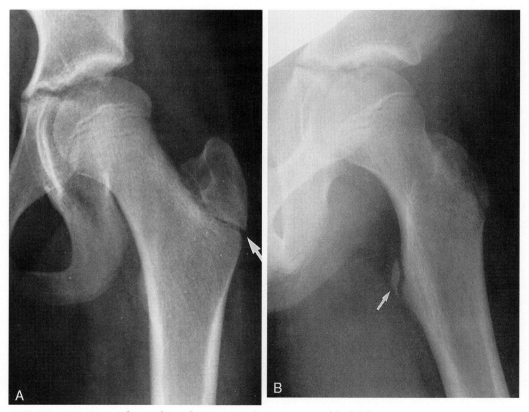

FIGURE 8–58. **Normal apophyseal structures in a 10-year-old child.** *A,* An anteroposterior view of the hip clearly shows the apophysis *(arrow)* of the greater trochanter. *B,* An oblique view shows another apophysis *(arrow)* of the lesser trochanter. Also notice that at this age, the acetabulum is not completely fused.

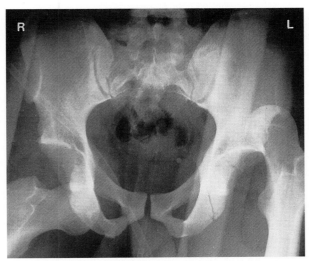

FIGURE 8–59. **Hip dislocation.** In this patient who was in a motor vehicle accident, there is both an anterior and a posterior dislocation of the hips. Posterior dislocation occurs 90% of the time and is seen here on the left, with the femoral head displaced superior and lateral to the acetabulum. On the right, there is an anterior dislocation, with the femoral head displaced inferiorly and medially.

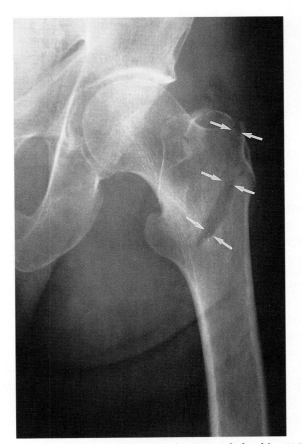

FIGURE 8–60. **Intertrochanteric fracture of the hip.** With extracapsular hip fractures, an intertrochanteric fracture *(arrows)* occurs 70% of the time, whereas a subtrochanteric fracture occurs 30% of the time. Intracapsular fractures most commonly affect the femoral neck.

ternal rotation is lost. The initial work-up should include plain radiographs, even though symptoms may be present before radiographic changes occur. Conversely, about 90% of persons older than 40 years have degenerative changes of the hip, but only about 30% of them have symptoms. Degenerative changes include joint space narrowing, subchondral cyst formation, and bone spurs. Advanced imaging techniques are usually not needed. Follow-up x-ray examinations are indicated if hip rotation has decreased by 20% or more or if function has changed dramatically.

Pain in the upper outer thigh and tenderness in the midtrochanteric region should suggest trochanteric bursitis. A regional anesthetic block eases the pain. If there is not a dramatic response, other etiologies should be considered.

Aseptic necrosis of the hip is most commonly manifested on a plain radiograph by flattening, irregularity, and sclerosis of the superior aspect of the femoral head (Fig. 8–61), but these are late findings. The most sensitive imaging study for early aseptic necrosis is MRI. If this is not available, a nuclear medicine bone scan can be used.

A common problem associated with a prosthetic hip is pain due to loosening, infection, or dislocation. Dislocations are easily visualized on a plain radiograph. Pain may occur with loosening of the prosthesis or infection. If the prosthesis is loose and wiggling, the distal tip moves more than the rest of the shaft. A plain radiograph may show thinning of the bone cortex near the tip of the prosthesis. With loosening, a nuclear medicine bone scan shows increased activity near the distal tip of the prosthesis. A nuclear medicine abscess (labeled *white blood cells*) scan can be ordered to exclude infection.

FEMUR

Normal Anatomy

The normal osseous anatomy of the femur is quite obvious. The normal x-ray projections are AP and lateral. Fractures of the femur are also extremely obvious. As expected, they may be transverse, spiral, or comminuted, with various degrees of angulation and overriding of the fragments.

Benign Lesions

The bones of the leg are favored places for a benign fibrous cortical defect. These are usually located near, but not at, the ends of the bones and are usually well marginated. As the name suggests, they are present predominantly in the cortex of the bone rather than having their epicenter in the

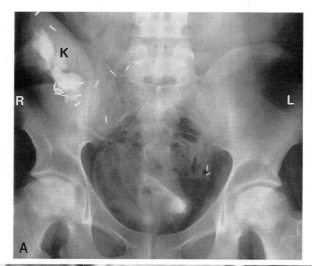

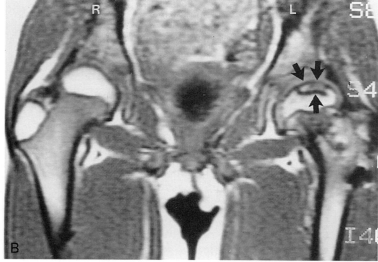

FIGURE 8–61. **Aseptic necrosis of the hips.** *A,* Aseptic necrosis can occur from a number of causes, including trauma and steroid use. In this patient, an anteroposterior view of the pelvis shows a transplanted kidney (K) in the right iliac fossa. Use of steroids has caused this patient to have bilateral aseptic necrosis. The femoral heads are somewhat flattened, irregular, and increased in density. *B,* Aseptic necrosis in a different patient is demonstrated on a magnetic resonance imaging scan as an area of decreased signal *(arrows)* in the left femoral head. This is the most sensitive method for detection of early aseptic necrosis.

marrow space. There is another lesion, called a *non-ossifying fibroma*, with the same characteristics, but it is bigger. Whether these lesions are truly different or simply a spectrum of the same lesion is unknown.

Fibrous dysplasia is usually a lytic lesion that looks like a hole in the bone. Fibrous dysplasia may present as a single lesion (monostotic), or it may be in multiple areas throughout the skeleton (polyostotic). It is centered in the marrow cavity thinning the cortex on the inner margins. Most fibrous dysplasia lesions are found in children or young adults. In addition to the lucent, somewhat cystic, variety, a form can occur in which the bone is diffusely involved and softened. When this happens in the femur, there is deformity with lateral bowing. This is referred to as a *shepherd's crook deformity.*

Amorphous or scattered calcifications projecting within the marrow space are usually the result of benign lesions, such as enchondroma or bone infarcts. Bone infarcts are relatively common in patients with sickle cell disease and can also be a result of decompression sickness from diving.

Malignant Lesions

Chondrosarcomas tend to occur in the femur, pelvis, and ribs. In the femur, they are most common in the metaphysis. They can be quite variable in appearance, from purely destructive to destructive with irregular calcification. They also may be exostotic (projecting away from the cortex of a bone). The mean age for occurrence is 40 to 45 years.

Even if a patient has known metastatic disease elsewhere, it is important to identify metastatic sites in the pelvis and lower extremities. Because these are weight-bearing sites, they are susceptible to pathologic fractures that can disable the patient (Fig. 8–62). Early detection can allow for placement of a medullary rod or radiation therapy, which may allow a terminal patient to ambulate rather than being bedridden for the remaining months of life.

▪ KNEE

Normal Anatomy

The standard x-ray projections of the knee are AP and lateral views (Fig. 8–63). The lateral view

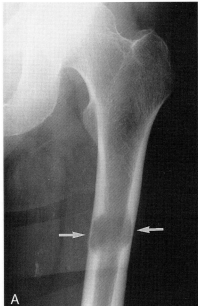

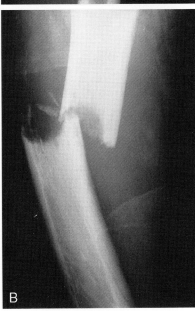

FIGURE 8–62. **Lytic bone metastases.** *A,* A view of the femur in this patient with known lung carcinoma shows a destructive lesion expanding from the marrow space and thinning the cortex *(arrows).* This lesion has no clear margin or white rim to distinguish it from normal bone. Lesions such as this in weight-bearing bones are important to find so that therapy can be undertaken to prevent pathologic fracture. *B,* A view of the femur in the same patient who returned 2 weeks later with a pathologic fracture.

is taken with the knee partially flexed. The AP view is important for assessing whether there is joint space narrowing and whether there is calcification of the cartilage in the joint space. Sometimes the tibial plateaus are at slightly different angulations so that the x-ray beam does not go horizontally through both medial and lateral compartments. This makes them appear asymmetric.

The lateral view is used to evaluate the patella and to determine whether a joint effusion is present. Both views are used to assess degenerative changes; fractures; and the general matrices of the bone of the distal femur, proximal tibia, and proximal fibula. Both views are also needed to see whether there is a bone fragment within the joint space.

There are two special views of the knee that are commonly requested. The first of these is the *sunrise* or *merchant view.* This is a tangential view of the anterior portion of the flexed knee, looking from the top down. The advantage of this view is that the relationship of the patella to the anterior femur is clearly shown. Another view that is available is the *tunnel view.* In this, the knee is flexed more than on the routine lateral view, and the x-ray beam is directed across the tibial plateau through the "tunnel" created by the femoral condyles. This affords an excellent look at the anterior and posterior tibial spines as well as the femoral condyles.

In children, the epiphyseal plate of the distal femoral epiphysis and the proximal tibial epiphysis is well seen, until at least 10 years of age. Complete fusion typically occurs in girls at about the age of 15 and in boys, several years later (Fig. 8–64). In adolescents, it is important to note on the lateral view that the anterior portion of the proximal tibial epiphysis folds down to form the attachment for the inferior aspect of the patellar tendon. It almost looks like a horn projecting downward from the anterior portion of the proximal tibia, and this is normal. A fairly common normal variant is the fabella. This is a small, smooth ovoid or round sesamoid bone in the tendons posterior to the knee joint. It is easily seen on the lateral view.

With MRI, the soft tissues, including the tendons, ligaments, and cartilage of the knee, can be exquisitely visualized. Structures of particular interest on these images are those that are commonly involved in trauma, such as the cruciate ligaments and the medial and lateral menisci. The most common reasons for ordering knee x-ray films involve trauma or degenerative change (Fig. 8–65). Questions about tumor and infections in children are discussed later in the pediatric bone section of this chapter.

Knee Pain

A knee joint effusion may be difficult to see on plain radiograph. It is easiest to identify superior to the patella and anterior to the distal femur (in the suprapatellar bursa). This is only visible on the lateral view. The effusion is basically water or blood, which has the same density as muscle, and

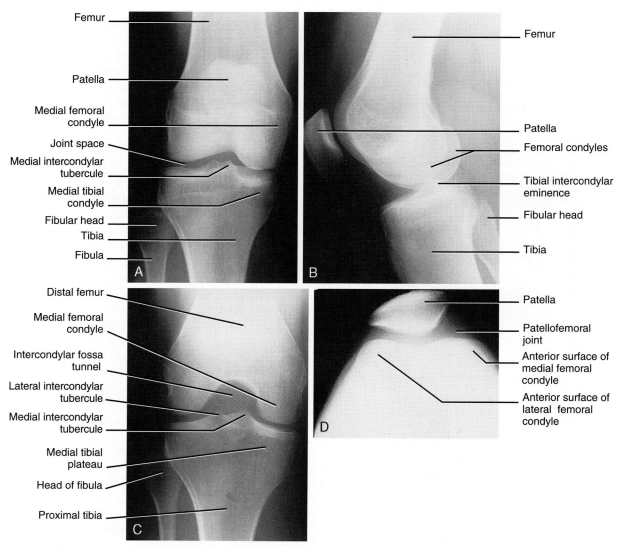

FIGURE 8–63. **Normal anatomy of the knee in the anteroposterior projection** *(A)*, **lateral projection** *(B)*, **tunnel view** *(C)*, **and sunrise view** *(D)*.

it is visualized only because there is anterior displacement of the normal fat line. Clinical examination is much better than a knee radiograph to detect an effusion. Knee effusions are usually identified as an incidental finding in patients who have had bone or soft tissue trauma and for whom the radiograph was ordered because a fracture was suspected.

The two most common soft tissue injuries of the knee involve the cruciate ligaments and the menisci. The diagnosis of collateral ligament injury is often made on clinical grounds and plain x-rays are usually normal. If a meniscal tear is suspected plain films of the knee are indicated to show the degree of joint space narrowing or identify calcified loose bodies within the joint. With MRI, the cruciate ligaments can be well seen, and tears or partial tears of these ligaments can be easily identified. MRI is indicated when the physical examination is inconclusive or equivocal and the physician strongly sus-

pects a tear. If the physical examination is unequivocal, an MRI is not needed.

The diagnosis of chronic meniscal tear is based upon a history of pain, knee catching, locking, giving way, snapping or clicking. On physical examination there may be tenderness along the joint line and reproduction of the clicking sound by manipulation (McMurray's sign). Radiography is indicated to exclude significant osseous injury. With acute meniscal injury there is often loss of motion, joint effusion and acute muscle spasm. Again, radiography is indicated to exclude a fracture. There is a difference of opinion as to whether to then proceed with arthroscopy or to do a magnetic resonance scan. Both approaches are used.

Chronic knee pain may be due to degenerative change. On physical examination there is usually limited motion or pain with motion and, unlike RA, there are no systemic symptoms. There can be red-

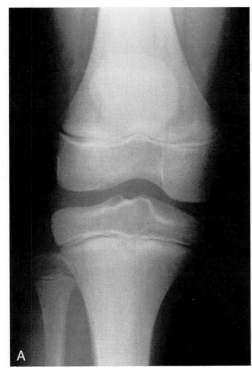

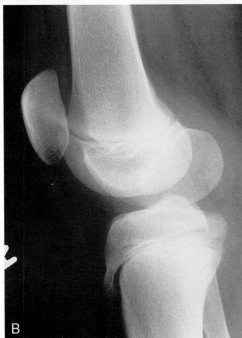

FIGURE 8–64. **Normal knee in an 11-year-old child.** *A,* An anteroposterior view clearly demonstrates the epiphyses of the distal femur, proximal tibia, and fibula. *B,* A lateral view shows the normal downward projection of the proximal tibial epiphysis along the anterior portion of the tibia to form the tibial tubercle.

ness or swelling over the joint as well as deformity. Lab tests are not needed. Plain radiographs are indicated for initial work-up to determine the extent of disease, even though radiographic findings often do not correlate with symptoms. Degenerative

changes of the knee are manifested by joint space narrowing and sclerosis of the bony articular margins. It is quite common to have only the medial or lateral compartment involved while the other compartment appears quite normal (see Fig. 8–65). Other signs of degenerative change are small overhanging spurs at the edges of the joints. No other imaging is indicated unless symptoms significantly progress or surgery is planned and then plain radiographs are again ordered.

Occasionally, degenerative changes of the joint can involve disruption of pieces of cartilage that come loose and are a nidus calcification. These calcifications are often within the joint space and can be single or multiple. If they are single, they are called a "loose body." If they are multiple and extensive, the condition is termed synovial chondromatosis. Internal derangement of the knee is usually suspected on the basis of clinical findings (clicking, locking, giving way, limitation of motion or pain with passive range of motion). An MRI is indicated if plain radiographs are nonspecific and only if some form of therapy is anticipated.

Sometimes, calcification can be seen within the articular cartilage of the knee. This finding is called chondrocalcinosis (see Fig. 8–25); it is usually easy to distinguish from loose bodies within the joint space, because it is calcification that is horizontal and linear within the meniscus. Chondrocalcinosis may be due to degenerative change, hypercalcemic states, and pseudogout as well as some other less common entities.

When degenerative changes of the knee are extensive enough, a prosthetic knee replacement may

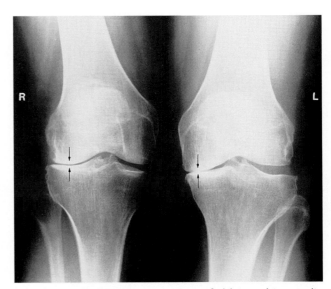

FIGURE 8–65. **Degenerative osteoarthritis.** In this standing view of both knees, significant narrowing and sclerosis *(arrows)* of the medial compartment of the left knee and of the lateral compartment of the right knee are shown.

be required. A number of prostheses are available, but, in general, they have a femoral condylar component as well as proximal tibial and patellar components. Sometimes the patellar component is not installed. On the AP view, these prostheses may look like they are not touching each other when, in fact, they are in contact. This is because of a plastic surface that is not visible on the radiograph. Abnormalities to look for with a prosthesis involve infection and loosening. Both are seen as a lucent space or rarefaction of bone around the screws or the base of the implant.

A palpable popliteal mass may be a Baker cyst or a popliteal artery aneurysm. Initial work-up may be done with Doppler ultrasound but MRI is also indicated because about 50% of persons with a Baker cyst also have intra-articular pathology. Localized pain over a bursa usually implies bursitis. X-ray studies are not necessary for the diagnosis and if done are usually normal. If the pain does not respond to therapy, plain x-ray films are indicated to exclude other causes.

Fractures

Patellar fractures are usually caused by a direct blow to the patella during a fall. The fractures are seen as dark lines across the bone, with sharp corners and edges. Repair of these fractures is done by using fixation pins and wire (Fig. 8–66). A normal variant that is often confused with a patellar frac-

ture is the *bipartite patella*. It is a normal variant of growth and results in a rounded or oval bony fragment in the upper and outer portion of the patella (Fig. 8–67). It is usually not a problem to differentiate from a fracture because of its location (upper outer portion) and its rounded and well-marginated edges.

Tibial plateau fractures are best visualized on the anterior view. They are reasonably common, and one should look for a vertical lucent line, often located slightly lateral to the center of the tibial spines. Sometimes, if the fracture is oblique to the x-ray beam, it can be difficult to see, but you may notice depression (inferior placement) of one of the tibial plateaus, and a step-off in the tibial cortex along the joint surface as clues to the presence of this type of fracture. With tibial plateau fractures, there is often a collection of fluid above the patella. Because lateral knee x-ray examinations are done for trauma with the patient lying down, often a horizontal "fat-fluid" level "above" the patella can be seen (Fig. 8–68) if a fracture is present that allows blood to enter the joint. Because tibial plateau fractures can sometimes be difficult to see, if a fat-fluid level on the lateral knee radiograph is present, an MRI may be needed to detect a subtle tibial plateau fracture.

Tumors

There is a benign tumor, called a *giant cell tumor*, that commonly occurs around the knee, particularly

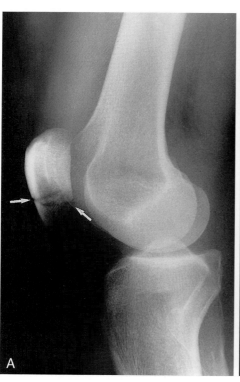 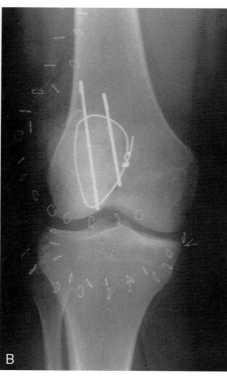

FIGURE 8–66. **Patellar fracture.** A lateral view *(A)* of the knee shows lucent or dark lines with sharp corners along the inferior portion of the patella *(arrows)*. An anteroposterior view *(B)* after surgery shows fixation pins and a tension wire in the patella. Multiple skin staples are also seen overlying the soft tissues.

A

B

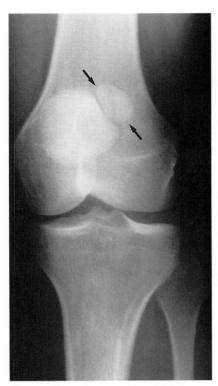

FIGURE 8–67. **Bipartite patella.** On this anteroposterior view of the knee, a fragment can be seen in the upper outer portion of the patella *(arrows)*. Note that this is rounded and that the location in the upper outer portion of the patella indicates that this is a normal variant of no clinical significance; it should not be mistaken for a patellar fracture.

in the proximal tibia. It is a lytic lesion that is often quite large and characteristically occurs in patients between the ages of 20 and 35 years. The tumor appears to arise from the old epiphyseal plate and to extend in both directions. It is not seen before epiphyseal closure, and when it is present, it typically crosses the fused epiphyseal plate. Usually it is not confused with a malignant lesion, because it generally occurs in older adolescents or in young adults. This is beyond the age for most osteogenic sarcomas and before the age for most metastatic lesions. In addition, its single focus and location peripherally in an extremity would be quite unusual features of a metastatic lesion. Osteogenic sarcoma is discussed later in the pediatric section of this chapter. Remember that osteosarcomas in older adults can be produced by malignant degeneration of Paget's disease and may occur at any age as a consequence of radiation therapy.

TIBIA AND FIBULA

Typical plain x-ray views include AP and lateral projections. The x-ray series should include the entire length from the tibial plateau to the ankle joint.

Trauma

Spiral fractures usually involve the distal tibia and often occur as the result of boot-top ski injuries. When a spiral tibial fracture is present and if there is overriding of the fragments an associated fracture of the proximal portion of the fibula needs to be excluded.

Tumors

There are some benign bone tumors that occur in long bones, particularly in the lower extremity. The first of these is simply an outgrowth of bone and is called an osteochondroma. The cortex of the bone typically sticks out on a stalk and ends with a bulbous or mushroom-shaped cartilage cap on it. This growth almost invariably arises near a joint, with the stalk always pointing away from the joint (Fig. 8–69). These lesions are usually asymptomatic unless they stick out far enough to be traumatized easily. If there is enlargement of such a lesion or associated pain without previous trauma, malignant transformation should be suspected. There is also a form of hereditary multiple exostoses. The number of exostoses in a person with this condition may vary from a few to hundreds, but they are usually bilaterally symmetric.

An osteoid osteoma usually occurs along the cortex of a bone. It has a central area of lucency with a little sclerotic (white) nidus within it (Fig. 8–70). About 75% of such cases occur in persons between the ages of 11 and 26 years. This lesion incites a large amount of reaction, causing dense, thickened surrounding cortex, and sometimes local periosteal reaction. It is typically painful, and the pain is more intense at night and relieved by aspirin. On a nuclear medicine bone scan, these lesions are intensely active.

With the exception of metastatic disease, most bone tumors are quite obvious and rare. Because the differential diagnosis depends on the age, location, radiographic characteristics, and clinical history, it is best to seek consultation with a radiologist before assuming that an unusual lesion is benign or malignant.

ANKLE

Normal Anatomy

Standard x-ray projections of the ankle are AP, lateral, and oblique. Although oblique views of most bones and joints are not normally obtained, this is important in the traumatized ankle because many oblique fractures in the ankle are not easily seen

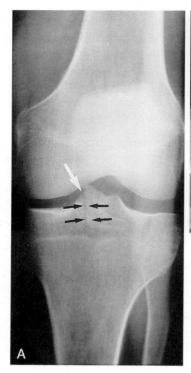

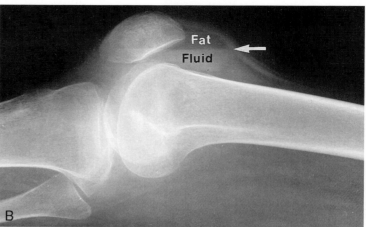

FIGURE 8–68. **Tibial plateau fracture.** An anteroposterior view *(A)* shows a vertical lucent line *(black arrows)* extending into the upper portion of the tibia. A cortical step-off *(white arrow)* is also seen just medial to the intercondylar tubercle. The true extent of these fractures may be difficult to appreciate on plain films. A lateral cross-table view of the knee *(B)* shows a typical fat-fluid level in the suprapatellar region. This actually is settling blood in a hemarthrosis.

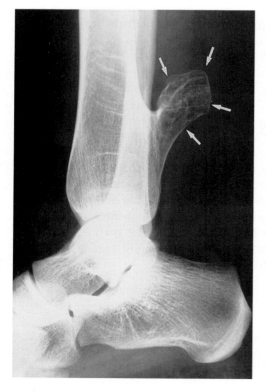

FIGURE 8–69. **Osteochondroma.** On this lateral view of the ankle, a benign osteochondroma is seen projecting posteriorly on a stalk. The end *(arrows)* is often covered with a cartilaginous cap. These lesions always occur near a joint but point away from it.

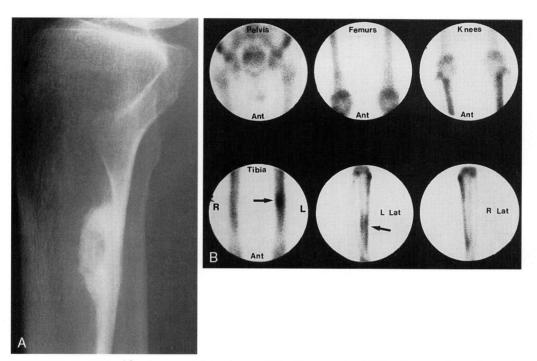

FIGURE 8–70. **Osteoid osteoma.** A lateral view *(A)* of the proximal tibia shows a dense lesion in the posterior cortex. There is a darker central area that contains a white nidus. This lesion in a 20-year-old male caused pain in this area that was relieved by aspirin. Fifty-five percent of these lesions occur in the femur and tibia. *B,* A nuclear medicine bone scan in a different patient with an osteoid osteoma in the left lower tibia shows increased activity *(arrows)* at the site of the lesion.

on the AP or lateral views. The oblique view also allows a better look at the ankle joint (Figs. 8–71, 8–72).

The ankle of a child contains an epiphysis in the distal tibia and fibula. In children between the ages of 7 and 12 years, a calcaneal apophysis is visible on the lateral view. This is seen as a crescentic density over the posterior aspect of the heel, and it should not be mistaken for a fracture (Fig. 8–73).

Trauma

The vast majority of ankle radiographs are obtained to evaluate the effects of trauma. On the lateral view of the ankle, look for an anterior thin dark fat line right in front of the joint space. If it is displaced or bowed forward, there is an effusion in the ankle joint, frequently because of hemorrhage, or an infection. The most common fractures of the

FIGURE 8–71. **Normal anatomy of the ankle in the antero-posterior projection *(A)* and in the lateral projection *(B).***

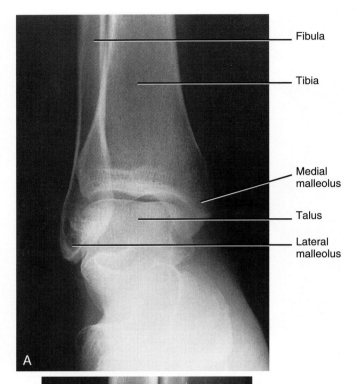

Fibula

Tibia

Medial malleolus

Talus

Lateral malleolus

A

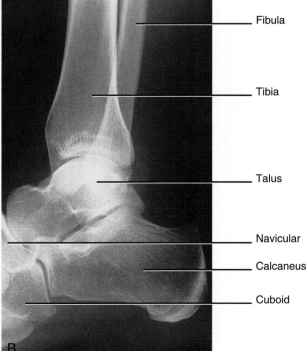

Fibula

Tibia

Talus

Navicular

Calcaneus

Cuboid

B

also of the posterior aspect of the tibia (trimalleolar fracture). Whenever the posterior malleolus is fractured, there is almost always an associated medial or lateral malleolar fracture. The extreme force and disruption necessary to cause a trimalleolar fracture disrupts ligaments, often causing subluxation of the distal tibia relative to the talus.

Just because the bone structures of the ankle look normal on the radiograph does not mean that there is no soft tissue pathology. There may be significant ligamentous disruption that is not appreciated. If clinical suspicion persists about ligamentous disruption and laxity of the ankle, stress views can be performed. These are radiographs taken while the ankle is being manipulated; they can show abnormal widening of the ankle joint when the stress is applied (Fig. 8–75). MRI is rarely indicated for most ankle trauma.

Benign Nontraumatic Abnormalities

There are three fairly common dense bone abnormalities that are seen typically in the distal tibia. These lesions do occur in other bones, but because the ankle is so frequently radiographed, concerns about these come up more often relative to the ankle. The first of these are horizontal dense lines in the metaphysis of the tibia (Fig. 8–76). These are called *growth arrest lines*, and they represent a time when there was some interference with the normal longitudinal growth process of the bone, perhaps periods of sickness during the individual's life.

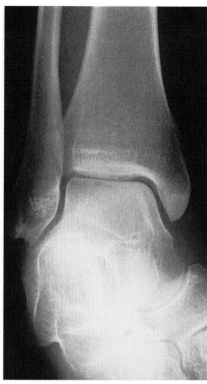

FIGURE 8–72. **Oblique view of the ankle.** This projection is the best one to show the ankle mortise and the relationship of the talus to the medial and lateral malleolus.

ankle involve either the medial or the lateral malleolus. Less commonly, there are fractures of both (Fig. 8–74). With severe trauma, there are fractures not only of both medial and lateral malleoli but

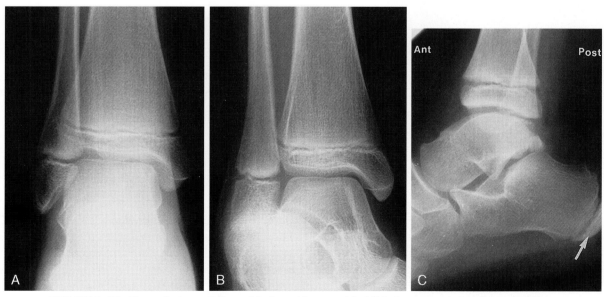

FIGURE 8–73. **Normal view of the ankle in a 10-year-old child.** Anteroposterior *(A)* and oblique *(B)* projections clearly show the distal tibial and fibular epiphyses and the transverse dark epiphyseal plates. The lateral view *(C)* shows a normal calcaneal apophysis *(arrow)*, which is usually denser than the nearby bone.

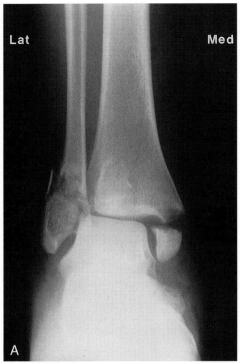

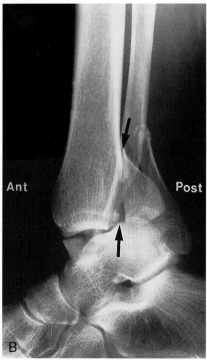

FIGURE 8–74. **Ankle fractures.** *A,* In this bimalleolar fracture the horizontal fracture medially and an oblique fracture laterally mean that this was an eversion injury. With an inversion injury, there would have been a horizontal fibular fracture and oblique fracture of the medial malleolus. *B,* Trimalleolar fracture in a different patient. The lateral view is necessary to show a fracture of the posterior malleolus *(arrows).* Also note that there has been anterior subluxation of the distal tibial on the talus.

Growth arrest lines are of no clinical significance at the time they are seen, because they are a representation of a historical event. Uncommonly, dense lines such as these reflect heavy metal ingestion (lead poisoning or ingestion of bismuth or phosphorus).

Small oval sclerotic or dense lesions can occur in most bones. These are called *bone islands,* and their origin is uncertain. They are completely benign le-

sions and should be regarded as a normal variant. They rarely measure more than 5 or 6 mm in width and 1 cm in length. The long axis of the oval is always in the long axis of the bone or aligned with the trabecular pattern.

Benign fibrous cortical defects and nonossifying fibromas have been discussed in relationship to the femur, but they also occur in the distal tibia and fibula. If the lesions are large they may fracture, oblique. For purposes of an arthritis work-up, AP and lateral views are sufficient (Fig. 8–77). When a fracture of the calcaneus is suspected, a special view is obtained. The foot is flexed, and the x-ray beam is angled down through the posterior aspect of the heel. This provides a good view of at least the posterior half of the calcaneus (Fig. 8–78). A wide variety of small accessory bones are seen about the ankle and tarsal bones (Fig. 8–79). These are variable but can usually be easily distinguished from fractures, because accessory bones are well corticated and typically round or oval.

Trauma

A number of foot x-ray examinations are ordered to look for foreign bodies that the patient stepped on. If the suspected object is metallic, it can normally be visualized. As discussed in the section on the hand, most glass and gravel can also be seen. If the object is not visible externally, a radiologist may operate a fluoroscope while another physician is locating the object. Digging around in the sole of the foot often causes residual painful scars, and the more easily an object can be located, the less scarring there should be. Wooden objects or graphite from pencils are not visualized by radiograph.

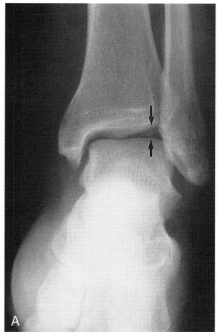
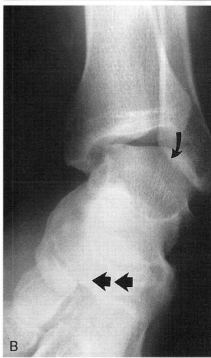

FIGURE 8–75. **Ankle instability.** *A,* An anteroposterior view of the ankle demonstrates slight widening of the lateral aspect of the ankle mortise *(arrows).* *B,* A stress view was obtained by inverting the foot (in the direction of the *large arrows*). This makes the ligamentous injury much more obvious by opening the ankle mortise even further *(curved arrow).*

but many resolve spontaneously during young adult life, leaving behind an area of dense bone.

▪ FOOT

As with the ankle, standard x-ray projections of the foot after trauma include AP, lateral, and

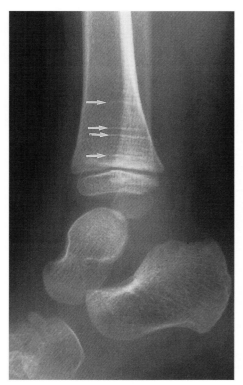

FIGURE 8–76. **Growth arrest lines.** These transverse dense lines *(arrows)* in the metaphysis of a long bone are due to bouts of illness that this child had in the past. Similar horizontal lines can be due to episodic heavy metal ingestion, such as lead poisoning.

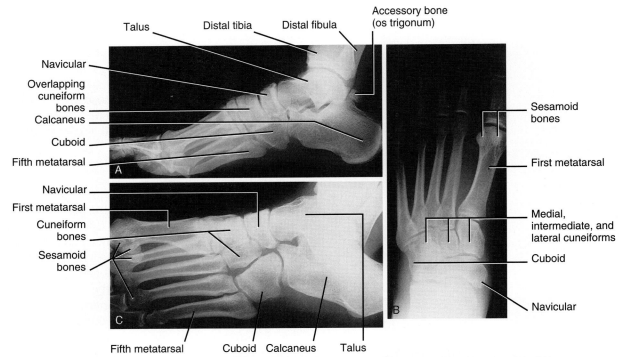

Talus Distal tibia Distal fibula Accessory bone (os trigonum)

Navicular
Overlapping cuneiform bones
Calcaneus
Cuboid
Fifth metatarsal

Sesamoid bones
First metatarsal

Navicular
First metatarsal
Cuneiform bones
Sesamoid bones

Medial, intermediate, and lateral cuneiforms
Cuboid
Navicular

Fifth metatarsal Cuboid Calcaneus Talus

FIGURE 8–77. **Normal anatomy of the foot in the lateral** *(A)*, **anteroposterior** *(B)*, **and oblique** *(C)* **projections.**

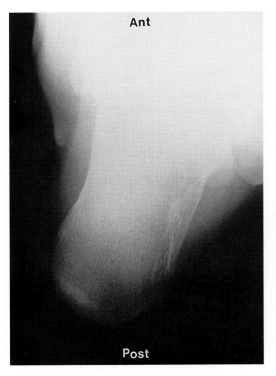

Ant

Post

FIGURE 8–78. **Calcaneal view.** This view is taken to look for subtle fractures of the posterior aspect of the calcaneus. It is taken by placing the foot on a film and shooting down along the backside of the ankle.

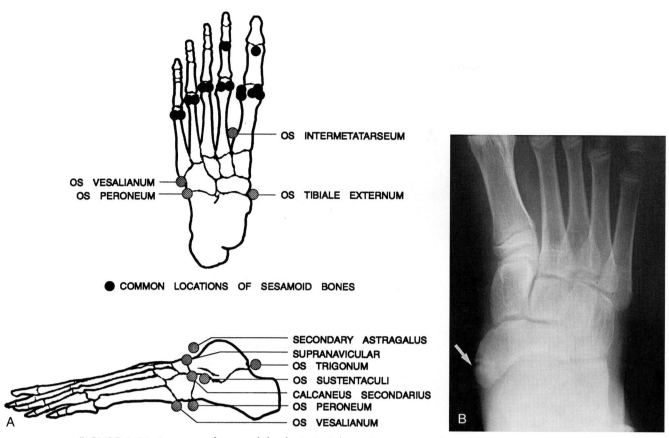

OS INTERMETATARSEUM

OS VESALIANUM
OS PERONEUM

OS TIBIALE EXTERNUM

● COMMON LOCATIONS OF SESAMOID BONES

SECONDARY ASTRAGALUS
SUPRANAVICULAR
OS TRIGONUM
OS SUSTENTACULI
CALCANEUS SECONDARIUS
OS PERONEUM
OS VESALIANUM

A

B

FIGURE 8–79. **Accessory bones of the foot.** A, Schematic representation of normal accessory and sesamoid bones. B, A radiograph of the foot of a child shows an accessory os naviculare (arrow).

Fractures of the foot can involve any bone. Fractures of the talus are rare but almost always involve the neck of the talus (Fig. 8–80). These fractures are often due to motor vehicle accidents. Calcaneal fractures can often be difficult to appreciate on the lateral view and are almost impossible to see on an AP view. For this reason, a calcaneal view should also be ordered (Fig. 8–81). Sometimes there are patients with persistent foot pain who have normal plain radiographs. A nuclear medicine bone scan can often localize an occult fracture.

A common fracture of the foot involves the base of the fifth metatarsal. There is frequently an apophysis on the lateral aspect of the fifth metatarsal base, and this is often confused with a fracture. The way to tell the two apart is by noting that the

FIGURE 8–80. **Talar neck fracture.** A lucent line can be seen extending through the talus (arrows). This is the second most common fracture of the proximal foot, and historically it is referred to as an aviator's fracture.

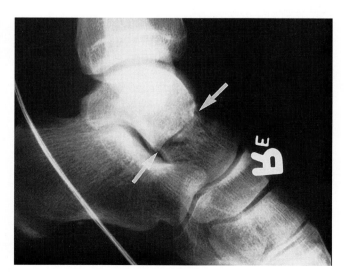

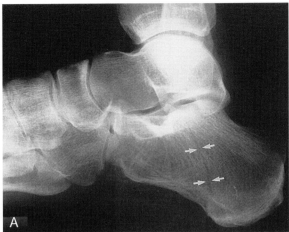

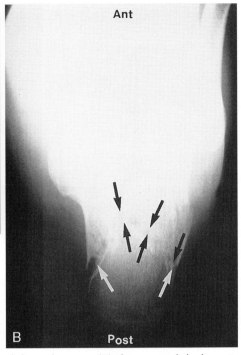

FIGURE 8–81. **Calcaneal fracture.** The lateral view of the calcaneus *(A)* shows a subtle lucent (dark) line *(arrows)* through the calcaneus. This extends into the subtalar joint about 75% of the time. This fracture has also been called a *lover's fracture* (probably from tales of disappointed lovers jumping off buildings or bridges). A calcaneal view *(B)* in the same patient makes the fracture much more obvious *(arrows)* particularly at the lateral margins.

long axis of the apophysis is parallel to the long axis of the metatarsal. Fractures, however, are typically transverse (perpendicular) to the long axis of the bone (Fig. 8–82).

Most fractures of the metatarsals are fairly easy to recognize. Two unique fractures can occur in this region. The first is the so-called *Lisfranc fracture.* This is actually a fracture and lateral dislocation of the second, third, fourth, and fifth metatarsals relative to the tarsal bones. This usually happens as a result of falling out of a saddle while horseback riding and getting a foot caught in the stirrup.

Another classic fracture of the metatarsals is the so-called *march fracture.* This is a stress fracture that typically occurs in army recruits who have to march long distances and are not used to it, but it is also seen in athletes and dancers. The distal third of the second, third, or fourth metatarsal is its usual location. There may be slightly increased sclerosis or periosteal reaction (Fig. 8–83). If the radiograph is normal, a stress fracture may still be present. In this circumstance, it is usually easily visualized as an area of intensely increased activity on a nuclear medicine bone scan.

There is a form of aseptic necrosis that most commonly involves the head of the second metatarsal. This is manifested as flattening of the articular

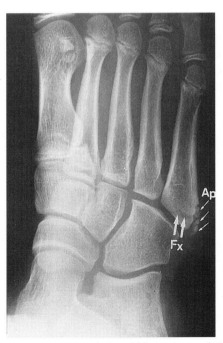

FIGURE 8–82. **Fracture of the fifth metatarsal base.** This fracture usually occurs from inversion of the foot and is transverse across the base of the metatarsal. This should not be confused with a normal fifth metatarsal apophysis, which this patient also has. The fracture (Fx) is always transverse and is referred to as a *Jones fracture.* The apophysis (Ap) is always parallel with the long axis of the metatarsal.

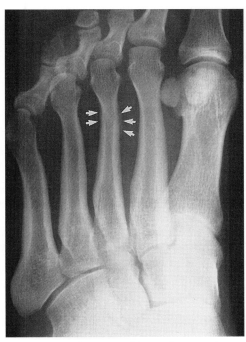

FIGURE 8–83. **Stress fracture.** This Marine recruit complained of foot pain. A small amount of periosteal reaction is seen *(arrows)*, and there is slight sclerosis extending across the medullary cavity. Stress fractures commonly occur at the distal third of the second and third metatarsals. This is also referred to as a *march fracture.* They can be difficult to appreciate even when you know where to look.

surface with associated sclerosis. This is called *Kohler-Freiberg infarction.* The lesion is seen less frequently in the head of the third or first metatarsal. This injury is believed to be a type of stress fracture, and it is often found during late adolescence. DJD is a late complication of this condition.

Foot Pain

Views of the feet obtained for arthritis evaluation are often unrevealing or nonspecific, and if any radiograph is ordered for arthritis evaluation, the highest yield is usually obtained with an AP view of the hands. As mentioned earlier, the radiographic findings, although somewhat characteristic, are not as specific as laboratory findings. The major metabolic abnormality that occurs in the foot is gout (see Fig. 8–26). This is clinically manifested as swelling over the first metatarsophalangeal joint. On x-ray examination, there are erosions in the periarticular region with overhanging edges. These are late findings, and again the diagnosis is best made by laboratory analysis.

Infection

Patients with diabetes may develop peripheral neuropathy as well as vascular insufficiency. The latter is particularly acute in the toes, and often concomitant soft tissue, bony infection, or both may occur. Radiographs of the feet can demonstrate changes of osteomyelitis to help distinguish this from cellulitis. The characteristic signs of osteomyelitis include soft tissue swelling, focal loss of trabecular pattern, periosteal reaction, and frank bone destruction (see Fig. 8–29). The differentiation of osteomyelitis from cellulitis is important because the therapy for osteomyelitis involves many more weeks of antibiotic therapy. Osteomyelitis can be present when there is a normal radiograph, and if clinical suspicion is high, evaluation with a three-phase nuclear medicine bone scan or MRI is often useful, although biopsy may be necessary. Other plain x-ray changes that are characteristic of diabetic involvement of the foot include vascular calcification and occasionally air within the soft tissue due to infection and gangrene.

■ PEDIATRIC MUSCULOSKELETAL RADIOLOGY

Skull

ANATOMY

Standard views of the skull in a child are the same as in adults—AP and lateral. The differences that distinguish a child's skull from an adult's include dark or lucent lines that represent the cranial sutures (Fig. 8–84) and a small face in comparison with the cranium. Cranial sutures usually remain partially open until at least midlife, and it is particularly important that they remain open in the early years of life to allow growth of the brain. The sutures of the skull can close prematurely (craniosynostosis). The sagittal suture is the most commonly involved, and the coronal suture less so. Premature closure of the sagittal suture results in growth of the skull in the areas where the coronal and lambdoid sutures remain open, and the skull becomes much longer than normal (scaphocephaly) (Fig. 8–85). If the coronal suture closes prematurely, growth continues to occur along the sagittal suture, and the skull becomes much wider than normal. A skull film is often not necessary, because the shape of the skull and a ridge of bone over the closed suture are clinically apparent. On a skull film the prematurely closed suture may be dense (white) at the edges or may just be difficult to see.

TRAUMA

Fractures are seen as sharply defined lucent lines that do not correspond to sutures. The margins of the sutures are somewhat wiggly, especially

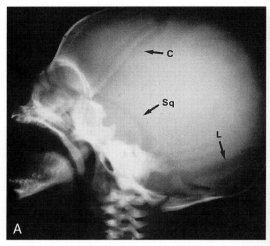
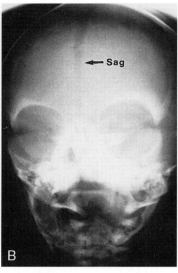

FIGURE 8–84. **Normal newborn skull.** *A,* The lateral view clearly shows the lambdoidal (L), squamous (Sq), and coronal (C) sutures. *B,* An anteroposterior view clearly shows the sagittal (Sag) suture.

as they near closure. Sometimes it can be difficult to differentiate between a fracture and a vascular groove. Most vascular grooves are seen on the lateral view of the skull and radiate superiorly and posteriorly from a position just above the ear. In addition, if one looks carefully, the vascular groove is a branching lucent line that is bounded by a sclerotic (white) margin relative to the normal bone of the skull. A skull fracture will be a lucent line (dark) and then normal skull and without a sclerotic margin.

Occasionally, a fracture line may widen progressively during the first weeks or months after injury. The widening is due to formation of an underlying leptomeningeal cyst, which causes pressure and subsequent atrophy of the bone at the edges of the

fracture line. The dura is torn at the time of injury, allowing this process to occur. Sometimes this lesion is referred to as a *growing skull fracture* of childhood, and it usually does not heal without surgery (Fig. 8–86).

Another common traumatic lesion of childhood is a cephalohematoma. These are caused by traumatic hemorrhage into the neonatal scalp during labor, although they can also occur following cephalic injury during infancy or childhood. With healing, usually a new shell of subperiosteal bone is over the hematoma, which then thickens and calcifies. Clinically, cephalohematomas can disappear in weeks to months, although the x-ray finding may persist long afterward (Fig. 8–87).

Neoplastic lesions of the skull can occur during childhood. Almost all present as multiple lucent holes (Fig. 8–88). Typical malignant lesions in young children are due to histiocytosis X, although with slightly older children, metastatic lesions may occur from neuroblastoma.

SINUSITIS

Many clinicians order sinus views to look for sinusitis. This is often the result of parental concern rather than medical need. You should remember that the sinuses are not developed at birth and are progressively pneumatized over the first 10 years of life. The first sinuses to appear are the maxillary sinuses; the frontal sinuses come much later. For both children and adults, it is inappropriate to order sinus views for what clinically appears to be routine sinusitis (Fig. 8–89).

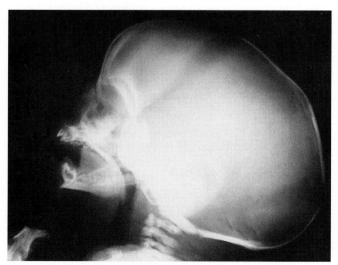

FIGURE 8–85. **Premature closure of the sagittal suture.** Closure of the sagittal suture has allowed growth of the skull only in the anteroposterior direction; here the coronal and lambdoidal sutures can be seen to be widened.

Spine

There are two items that cause confusion in interpretation of cervical spine views in children. The

be found until a scoliosis work-up is done in adolescence or adulthood.

A rather unusual spinal abnormality of childhood is called *diskitis*. This usually occurs in the lumbar spine and appears radiographically as a decreased disk space. On a nuclear medicine bone scan, increased activity of the vertebral bodies on both sides of the affected level is seen. The origin of this entity is uncertain, but it may represent a low-grade infection.

Extremities

In children, fractures about articular surfaces can occur in a variety of ways. They may involve only the epiphyseal plates or various combinations of the epiphyseal plate and the metaphysis. The Salter-Harris classification, shown schematically in

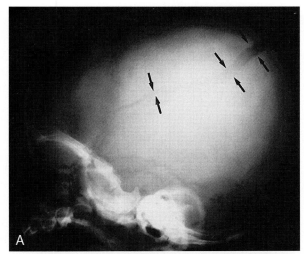
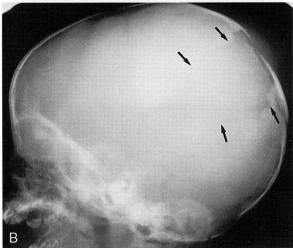

FIGURE 8–86. **Growing skull fracture of childhood.** *A,* A parietal skull fracture is easily seen on this lateral view of the skull *(arrows). B,* Two months later, a repeat skull film shows that the fracture line has become very wide *(arrows).* This is due to a leptomeningeal cyst and continued pressure erosion of the bone.

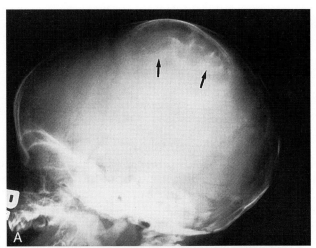
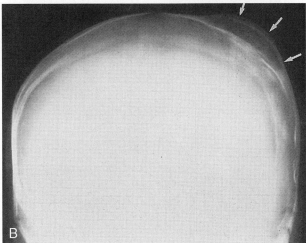

FIGURE 8–87. **Cephalohematoma.** *A,* A lateral view of the skull shows a lucent multilocular and expansile lesion *(arrows). B,* An anteroposterior tangential view of the skull shows that this lesion is primarily bulging out (arrows) from the normal skull cortex because of calcification of the hematoma.

first is that the odontoid process and the body of C2 form as separate ossification centers, and fusion occurs in the first year or so of life (Fig. 8–90). Occasionally, nonfusion can persist into adulthood. The differentiation from an odontoid fracture can be made by the absence of sharp, angulated corners and the absence of soft tissue swelling. Another surprising but common finding in children is a pseudosubluxation at C2 and C3. This is simply a normal variant and occurs when the child has his or her neck slightly flexed. If this occurs in children older than approximately 5 years, a traumatic cause should be suspected rather than a normal variant.

There are a number of congenital spinal abnormalities that occur, including hemivertebra and butterfly vertebra, which often result in scoliosis. Severe abnormalities are usually diagnosed soon after birth, but more minor abnormalities may not

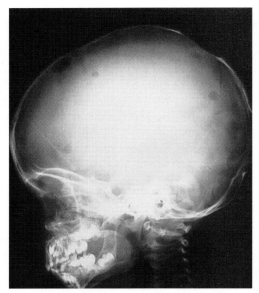

FIGURE 8–88. **Histiocytosis X of the skull.** Multiple lucent holes of varying sizes are seen in this lateral projection of the skull. A large scalloped lesion has destroyed the cortex over the posterior aspect of the skull and has beveled edges, which is characteristic of this disease.

Figure 8–91, is used for describing childhood fractures about most joints.

HUMERUS

Lesions in the proximal humerus that are lytic, somewhat expansive, and quite well demarcated are usually unicameral bone cysts. Care should be

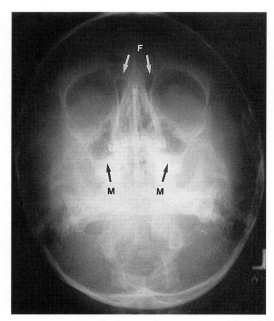

FIGURE 8–89. **Normal sinuses in a 5-year-old child.** The maxillary sinuses (M) are poorly developed at this age and only partially pneumatized, and the frontal sinuses (F) are only beginning to develop.

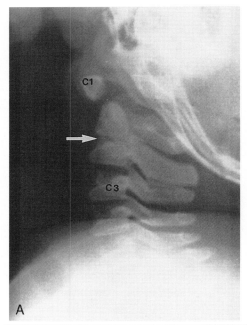

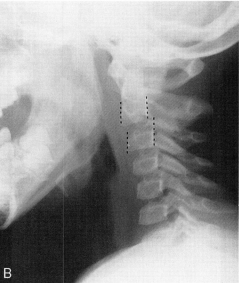

FIGURE 8–90. **Normal variations of the cervical spine in children.** *A,* A lateral view in a newborn child shows a cleft where the odontoid *(arrow)* is not yet completely fused to the body of C2. This is normal. *B,* Pseudosubluxation of C2 on C3 is a common normal variant in children; it occurs only at this level, particularly when the neck is straight or slightly flexed.

taken, however, in the diagnosis because the third most common site of osteogenic sarcoma is the proximal humerus.

ELBOW

The pediatric elbow can cause difficulties in interpretation owing to the development of various ossification centers. The epiphysis of the radial head initially appears at approximately 3 to 5 years of age, and the olecranon apophysis appears be-

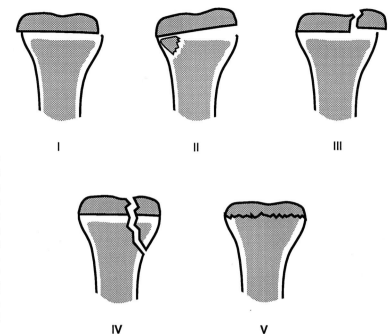

I   II   III

IV   V

FIGURE 8–91. **Salter-Harris classification of epiphyseal fractures in children.** A type I fracture is straight across the epiphyseal plate and may have some lateral displacement of the epiphysis. This occurs 5% of the time. A type II fracture involves a portion of the epiphyseal plate and a corner fracture through the metaphysis. This occurs 75% of the time. A type III fracture involving part of the epiphysis occurs only about 10% of the time. A type IV fracture involving part of the epiphysis and part of the metaphysis occurs about 10% of the time. A type V fracture is direct impaction and has the most serious consequences for further growth.

tween 8 and 11 years. The capitulum of the distal humerus appears at less than 1 year of age, the medial epicondyle at 3 to 6 years of age, the trochlea at 7 to 9 years of age, and the lateral epicondyle at 12 to 14 years of age. The development may even be asymmetric between right and left depending on which arm is dominant (Fig. 8–92). The asymmetric appearance of the lateral condylar ossification cen-

ter can often be mistaken for a fracture, and clinical correlation is essential. Avulsion fractures of the lateral condyle are quite rare, whereas avulsion fractures of the medial condyle are much more common. When this occurs, it is sometimes called *Little Leaguer's elbow* (Fig. 8–93).

In examining the elbow for fracture, remember that visualization of the anterior fat pad lying up

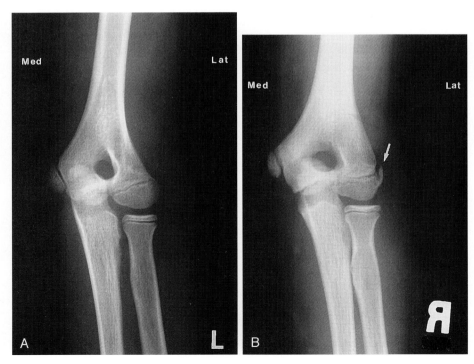

FIGURE 8–92. **Normal variation and development of the elbow in children.** *A,* On an anteroposterior view of the left elbow, the medial epicondyle is visualized, but the lateral is not. *B,* On the right side, the lateral epicondyle *(arrow)* is seen. This asymmetric development from one side to the other can occur normally. Because lateral epicondyle fractures are rare, an apophysis should be suspected.

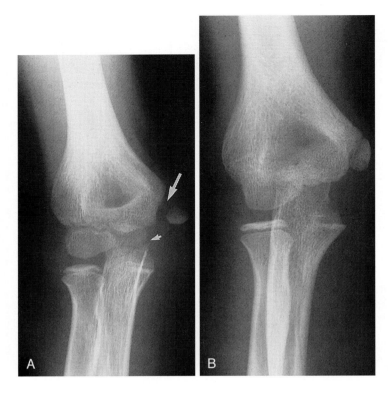

FIGURE 8–93. **Little Leaguer's elbow.** *A,* An anteroposterior view of the elbow shows an abnormally wide space between the medial epicondyle and the distal humerus *(large arrow).* An olecranon fracture is also seen *(small arrow).* B, The opposite elbow is shown for comparison with the normal position of the medial epicondyle.

against the anterior aspect of the distal humerus is a normal finding. A posterior fat pad should never be seen, and the anterior fat pad should not be displaced or bowed forward (Fig. 8–94). In addition, the apophysis of the olecranon should not be mistaken for a fracture.

A relatively common fracture in children is a supracondylar fracture that extends across the distal aspect of the humerus. When this occurs, there is almost always a bowing forward of the anterior fat pad and visualization of the posterior fat pad. One should evaluate the line formed by the anterior humeral cortex. This line should extend down into the middle third of the capitellum.

Destructive changes involving a joint space usually are produced by inflammatory lesions. They

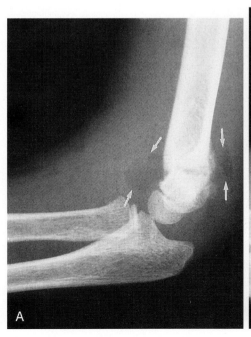
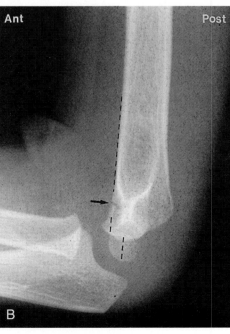

FIGURE 8–94. **Supracondylar fractures.** This is the most common elbow fracture in children. *A,* A lateral view of the elbow shows marked anterior displacement of the anterior fat and visualization of the posterior fat pad *(arrows),* a sign that a fracture is almost certainly present. *B,* In a younger child, a fracture is seen because of the posterior displacement of the capitellum from the anterior humeral line. An incomplete cortical fracture is also seen *(arrow).*

may be the result of infection in the joint space (septic arthritis) or of other chronic inflammatory processes, such as inflammation due to intermittent bleeding within the joint in patients with hemophilia. Significant joint involvement also occurs in children who have juvenile RA.

FOREARM, WRIST, AND HAND

Fractures of the forearm and wrist are quite common in children; a number of the types that occur in adults have already been discussed. Whenever there are multiple fractures, especially those that appear to be in different stages of healing, child abuse should be suspected. The fact that the fractures are of different ages can be ascertained by periosteal reaction or callus around some, but not around other, fracture sites. If child abuse is suspected, additional views of the skull, ribs, pelvis, and both upper and lower extremities should be obtained (Fig. 8–95).

Young children have bones that are relatively plastic, and two unique childhood fractures occur as a result of this plasticity. The first is a *buckle* or *torus fracture.* Sometimes, on a single view, all that can be identified is a slight outward bulge of the cortex, whereas on other views, one may actually see a buckling of the cortex (Fig. 8–96). The other fracture is the so-called *greenstick fracture.* In this fracture, the bone is bent but typically fractured only on one side of the cortex, similar to breaking a green twig (Fig. 8–97).

At the end of any long bone, there can be a number of the Salter-Harris type fractures described earlier. One of the most difficult fractures to see is a nondisplaced, or extremely minimally displaced, Salter-Harris type I fracture through the epiphyseal plate. Often the radiograph at the time of injury is normal; however, a repeat examination 1 to 2 weeks later reveals increasing sclerosis (white lines) across the epiphyseal plate, indicating a healing fracture (Fig. 8–98). Fortunately, nondisplaced Salter-Harris type I fractures are not clinically important.

In a child younger than 10 years, it is quite rare to have fractures of the carpal bones. Occasionally, it is necessary to assess the growth of a child and compare chronologic age with bone age. Bone age is assessed by obtaining a single view of the hands (Fig. 8–99). Typical hand fractures in children involve either Salter-Harris fractures of the fingers or fractures of the terminal phalanges (because children usually get their fingers caught in doors).

Osteomyelitis in young children often involves both the distal metaphysis and the epiphysis of a bone. This is because the epiphysis receives its blood supply from the shaft of the bone. In older children, the epiphysis has its own separate blood supply, and osteomyelitis usually involves the metaphysis just proximal to the epiphyseal plate. With hematogenous spread of bacteria, multiple bones can be involved. The radiographic findings of osteomyelitis include soft tissue swelling, bone destruc-

FIGURE 8–95. **Child abuse.** *A,* A view of the forearm in this child shows extensive periosteal reaction *(small arrows)* and transverse fracture lines *(large arrows).* Fractures of long bones in children, particularly with different stages of healing, are quite suggestive of a battered child. *B,* A lateral view of the lower extremity in the same child also reveals fractures of the distal fibula and tibia *(small arrows)* as well as a metaphyseal corner fracture *(large arrow)* of the distal femur. This latter fracture is also typical of child abuse.

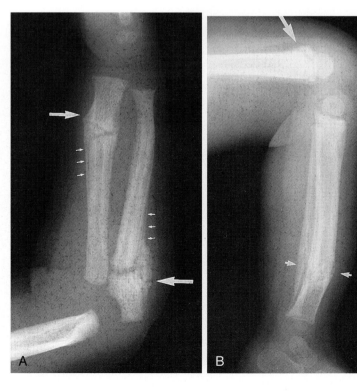

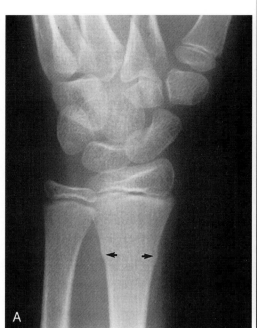

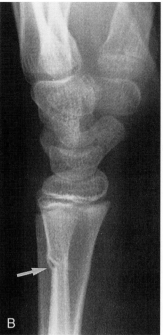

FIGURE 8–96. **Torus or buckle fracture.** *A,* An anteroposterior view of the wrist shows slight bulging of the cortex in the metaphyseal region *(arrows). B,* A lateral view of the wrist shows buckling *(arrow)* of the dorsal cortex. (Case courtesy of L. Mettler.)

tion, and periosteal reaction. As with adults, if a clinical question remains about the presence of osteomyelitis or even septic arthritis, a radionuclide bone scan is often helpful.

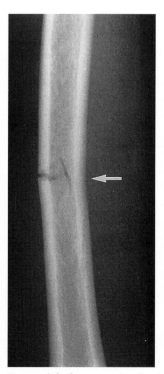

FIGURE 8–97. **Greenstick fracture.** In the humerus of this elementary school child, a direct blow from the direction of the arrow has caused an incomplete transverse fracture *(arrow).*

Pelvis and Hips

Dislocation of the hip in children is usually congenital and occurs more often in girls than in boys. There are a number of ways to make the radiographic diagnosis. Radiographic diagnosis of a congenital hip dislocation is unreliable in the neonate because the ossification center for the femoral head is not developed. Perhaps the simplest radiographic method is evaluation of Shenton's line, which is formed by the medial aspect of the obturator foramen and the medial aspect of the femoral neck. Together, these should form a nice smooth curved arc. A frog-leg view with the legs abducted is useless, because in this position any hip dislocation is reduced. Radiographic diagnosis of congenital hip dislocation should be done rarely, if ever, because the clinical finding of an audible click when the hips are abducted should be sufficient to make the diagnosis. If there is any doubt, ultrasound examination may be useful.

Occasionally, children can develop aseptic necrosis of the epiphysis of the femoral head (Legg-Perthes disease). Boys are more commonly affected than girls. Clinical signs are a limp and pain with limitation in motion of the hip. The radiographic findings are irregularity, sclerosis (increased density), and fragmentation of the epiphysis. There is often a resulting deformity that is followed by a disabling osteoarthritis decades later (Fig. 8–100).

Another pediatric hip abnormality is slipping of the epiphysis of the femoral head. The cause of this is unknown, and it usually does not happen in

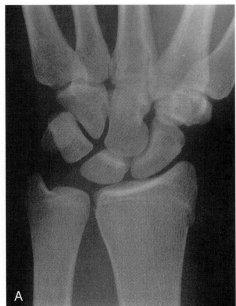

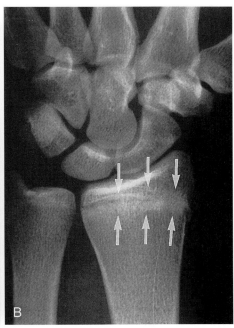

FIGURE 8–98. **Occult Salter-Harris fracture of the distal radius.** *A,* An anteroposterior view of the wrist at the time of the injury does not show any cortical disruption or displacement. *B,* A repeat examination 10 days later shows sclerosis across the epiphyseal plate *(arrows),* indicating healing of an occult Salter-Harris type I fracture.

FIGURE 8–99. **Normal development anatomy of the hand during childhood.** A 2-year-old male *(A),* 5-year-old male *(B),* 7-year-old male *(C),* and 15-year-old male *(D).* In general, the approximate age can be guessed, because the number of carpal bones is usually close to the child's age in years until about 7 years.

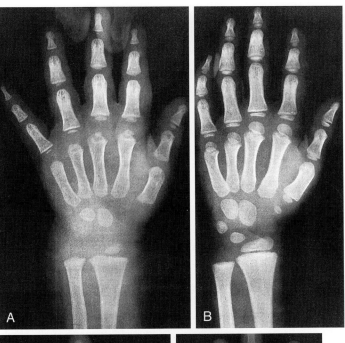

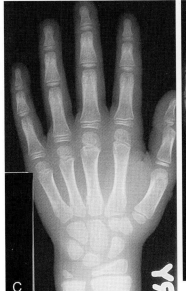

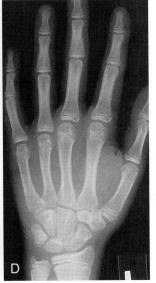

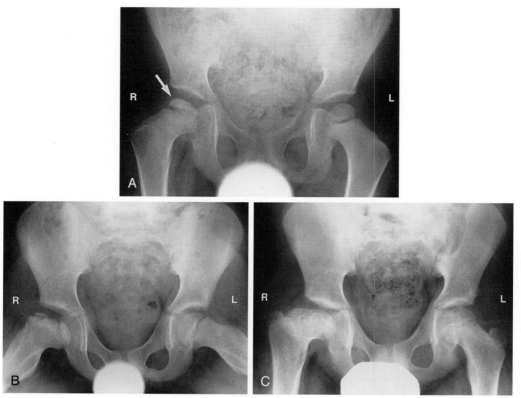

FIGURE 8–100. **Legg-Perthes disease.** *A,* An anteroposterior view of the pelvis demonstrates fragmentation and sclerosis of the right femoral epiphysis *(arrow)* in this 6-year-old male. *B,* A follow-up film obtained 8 years later shows continuing deformity due to the osteonecrosis. The patient developed significant degenerative arthritis *(C)* by the age of 12 years.

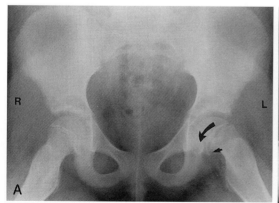

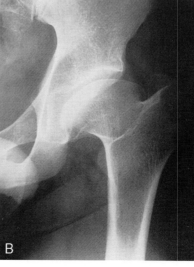

FIGURE 8–101. **Slipped capital femoral epiphysis.** *A,* An antero-posterior view of the pelvis in this overweight teenage male shows slipping of the left femoral epiphysis relative to the femoral neck *(arrows).* This essentially is a Salter-Harris type I fracture. *B,* Follow-up film of the left hip 10 years later shows significant deformity, which will result in degenerative arthritis.

children younger than 9 years. The diagnosis is made radiographically by noting a thickened epiphyseal plate and medial displacement of the femoral head relative to the femoral neck (Fig. 8–101). The lateral or abducted frog-leg view of the hip offers the best view of these findings. When the epiphysis fuses, there is no more slippage, but the deformity that has occurred is permanent, and later degenerative disease is a common result.

Arthritic changes in children are quite rare with the exception of juvenile RA and hemophilia. Both these diseases can cause fluid collections within the joint, resulting in destruction of the cartilage, followed by degenerative change. There may also be hyperemia, which results in overgrowth of the epiphyseal region of the bone. The joint effusions, irregularity of the articular surface, and subsequent degenerative changes are easily visualized on radiographs.

Ewing's tumor typically occurs in the shaft of the long bones or in flat bones, such as the pelvis, scapula, and ribs. In contrast, osteogenic sarcomas occur most commonly in the distal femur, less commonly in the proximal tibia and proximal humerus, and rarely elsewhere. An osteogenic sarcoma may present as a destructive lesion in the central portion of the bone or with periosteal reaction and soft tissue swelling. Often, an MRI scan is useful to show the soft tissue extent of the tumor.

A number of characteristic traumatic tibial lesions occur in children. As mentioned earlier, the proximal tibial epiphysis normally has an anterior projection that slopes down over the front of the tibia. Radiographically, this is best seen on the lateral view (see Fig. 8–64). This appearance can look a little bit irregular, however, if a small fragment is pulled off, and if the patient has pain, this is consistent with the diagnosis of Osgood-Schlatter injury. This is relatively frequent in children 10 to 15 years of age, particularly in boys who participate in active sports. It probably represents a partial avulsion of the anterior tubercle by the inferior patellar tendon, and it heals with rest (Fig. 8–102).

In children between the ages of 3 and 5 years, a spiral or oblique fracture of the middle or distal tibia may occur. This is usually referred to as *toddler's fracture*. Sometimes there is a history of twisting the leg or jumping off a chair, but often these injuries are found in children who simply refuse to bear weight on the extremity. If this particular entity is suspected, AP, lateral, and oblique views of the tibia should be obtained (Fig. 8–103).

Salter-Harris type fractures are common in the ankle. As mentioned in the discussion of the wrist, the Salter-Harris type I fractures may not be displaced and may be seen only as increased density about the epiphyseal plate 1 or 2 weeks after injury. If there is significant displacement and disruption of the epiphyseal plate, the radiographic diagnosis is usually not a problem. Sometimes even a Salter-Harris type III fracture can be subtle (Fig. 8–104). The fractures with the worst prognosis are the impacted Salter-Harris type V.

Occasionally, in a patient who has a history of foot trauma or pain, irregularity and increased density or sclerosis of the tarsal navicular (Fig. 8–105)

FIGURE 8–102. **Osgood-Schlatter disease.** A lateral view of the knee demonstrates a tiny avulsion fracture *(arrow)* of the anterior tibial tuberosity in this young male athlete. This disease is quite common and is usually self-limited.

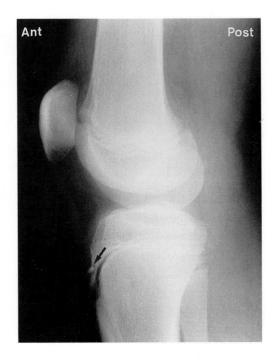

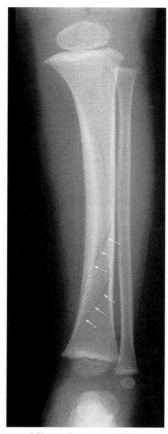

FIGURE 8–103. **Toddler's fracture.** This 3-year-old child refused to walk because of leg pain. A radiograph of the lower leg shows an oblique fracture *(arrows)* of the distal tibia. This fracture may be the result of weight bearing and should not be confused with the fractures of child abuse.

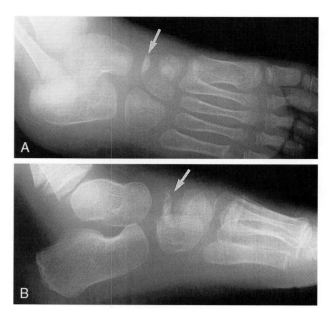

FIGURE 8–105. **Aseptic necrosis of the tarsal navicular.** This usually occurs between the ages of 4 and 8 years and most commonly is recognized incidentally. There may be *(A)* increased density *(arrow)* or *(B)* irregularity *(arrow)* of the tarsal navicular. This is also called *Köhler's osteonecrosis.* The abnormality is almost always self-limited and requires no therapy.

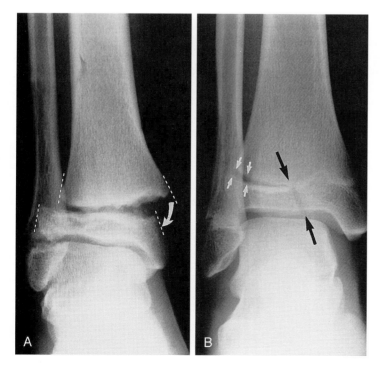

FIGURE 8–104. **Salter-Harris fractures of the ankle.** *A,* A Salter type I fracture is seen with marked lateral displacement *(arrow)* of the epiphysis relative to the tibial metaphysis. *B,* A Salter type III fracture *(arrows)* of the lateral tibial epiphysis. This is also called a Tillaux fracture and probably occurs because the growth plate fuses from medial to lateral, making the medial side stronger.

may be noticeable. This is referred to as *Köhler's disease*. Whether this condition is a result of trauma or aseptic necrosis is uncertain; it is often seen incidentally in a child with a twisted ankle. The patient occasionally may have pain over the navicular. This condition essentially always heals without any intervention. For some reason, the other tarsal bones are rarely, if ever, involved in this process. This finding should almost be regarded as a normal variant.

GENERAL SUGGESTED READINGS

Greenspan R: Orthopaedic Radiology: A Practical Approach, 2nd ed. Philadelphia, Lippincott Williams & Wilkins, 1992.

Helms CA: Fundamentals of Skeletal Radiology, 2nd ed. Philadelphia, WB Saunders, 1994.

Resnick D: Diagnosis of Bone and Joint Disorders, 3rd ed. Philadelphia, WB Saunders, 1994.

Rogers LF: Radiology of Skeletal Trauma, 2nd ed. Philadelphia, WB Saunders, 1992.

9

NONSKELETAL PEDIATRIC IMAGING

Most of the pediatric bone lesions have been discussed in a special section at the end of Chapter 8. Congenital cardiac lesions have been detailed in Chapter 5. This chapter discusses imaging techniques for other commonly encountered pediatric problems (Table 9–1).

HEAD

Normal Anatomy and Imaging

Imaging of the fetal and infant brain can be done using ultrasonography, as long as the fontanelles remain open. Structures that can normally be visualized include the lateral ventricles, choroid plexus, thalamus, temporal lobes, and posterior fossa. The two most common indications for ultrasound imaging of the head of an infant are (1) evaluation of ventricular enlargement (hydrocephalus) and (2) assessment of suspected brain hemorrhage. The major advantages of ultrasound imaging in this application are that it can be done portably in the neonatal intensive care unit and that ionizing radiation is not used. This is important because these studies are often repeated multiple times for continuing evaluation.

Brain tumors in children are evaluated by computed tomography (CT) or magnetic resonance imaging (MRI). With MRI, there is need for sedation;

monitoring of respiration and other functions of the pediatric patient in a high magnetic field is difficult. CT scanning is easier to perform. About half of brain tumors in children are astrocytomas; medulloblastomas (20%), ependymomas (10%), and craniopharyngiomas (5%) are less common.

Childhood Seizures

Seizures may be provoked by infection, trauma, toxins, metabolic abnormality, tumor, hypoxia, cerebrovascular disease, cerebral malformation, or congenital abnormality. They may also occur without obvious cause. Febrile seizures usually occur between the ages of 6 months and 4 years, and most are generalized tonic-clonic seizures.

Imaging is recommended for children with new-onset seizures who have experienced head trauma or partial seizures and for those who have an abnormal neurologic examination or an abnormal electroencephalogram. Imaging is not necessary for uncomplicated febrile seizures or in a patient with an obvious provoking cause. MRI is the usual imaging modality of choice, although noncontrasted CT is used initially if intracranial hemorrhage or recent trauma is suspected. For those children with a prior history of seizures, imaging is usually only done if the seizures are poorly controlled, or associated with a new neurologic deficit, or to follow known abnormalities such as a tumor.

TABLE 9–1 Imaging of Pediatric Problems

Suspected Problems	Imaging Test of Choice
Neonatal hydrocephalus or intracranial hemorrhage	Cranial ultrasound
Uncomplicated febrile seizure	No imaging needed
Seizure (neurologic deficit, partially unresponsive to therapy, new without obvious provoking factor)	MRI
Seizure (post-trauma)	Noncontrast CT
Croup or epiglottitis	Lateral soft tissue view of neck
Suspected inhaled foreign body	Inspiration/expiration or decubitus chest
Difficulty breathing	Chest radiograph
Esophageal atresia or tracheoesophageal fistula	Lateral radiograph with soft feeding tube in place
Asthma (uncomplicated)	No imaging needed
Asthma (poor response to therapy, complicated)	Chest radiograph
Suspected pneumonia	Chest radiograph
Congenital heart disease or congestive heart failure	Chest radiograph, echocardiogram
Gastroesophageal reflux	Barium swallow or nuclear medicine reflux study
Pyloric stenosis	Ultrasound
Duodenal atresia, stenosis, or midgut volvulus	Plain radiograph (use air as contrast)
Meconium ileus	Plain film and Gastrografin enema
Intussusception	Plain film followed by reduction utilizing air or Gastrografin enema
Necrotizing enterocolitis	Plain film of the abdomen and possible left lateral decubitus views (to look for free air)
Hirschsprung's disease	Barium or Gastrografin enema
Biliary atresia or neonatal hepatitis	Nuclear medicine hepatobiliary scan
Abdominal mass	Plain film of abdomen and ultrasound or CT
Meckel's diverticulum	Nuclear medicine Meckel's scan
Rectal bleeding	See text
Child abuse	Radiographic bone survey and possibly nuclear medicine bone scan
Osteomyelitis, cellulitis, or septic arthritis	Plain radiograph, MRI or three-phase nuclear medicine bone scan

▓ NECK

Croup and Epiglottitis

In cases of suspected croup or epiglottitis, lateral soft tissue views of the neck are often done for evaluation of the pediatric airway. The child's neck should be extended. In a young child, when the neck is flexed, the trachea can buckle forward, causing the appearance of a retropharyngeal mass (Fig. 9–1).

Acute epiglottitis usually occurs in older children (between 2 and 7 years of age) and most commonly is due to *Haemophilus influenzae*. This can be a life-threatening disease, and the clinical findings are severe sore throat, high fever, a muffled voice, and stridor. The patients can often breathe easier sitting up, and they drool. This is a true pediatric emergency. Because intubation can be necessary on extremely short notice, a physician should accompany the child to the x-ray department. The lateral soft tissue view of the neck shows a thickened epiglottis, often appearing bulbous (in the shape of a thumb) (Fig. 9–2). The normal epiglottis is a delicate, thin, curved structure. Other findings include ballooning of the hypopharynx and subglottic edema in about one fourth of cases.

Croup typically occurs in young children (between 6 months and 3 years of age), and it usually has a respiratory syncytial viral (RSV) origin. The children often have a brassy cough (like the barking of a seal) and inspiratory stridor. Occasionally, the airway may be edematous enough to require an artificial airway. The radiographic findings on the lateral view are marked ballooning of the pharynx and hypopharynx. On the anteroposterior (AP) view, the upper portion of the trachea is shaped like a steeple (Fig. 9–3). The *steeple sign*, caused by subglottic edema, is not pathognomonic because it can also occur in some children who have epiglottitis.

▓ CHEST

Normal Anatomy and Imaging

One of the major differences between the normal chest of an adult or child and that of a neonate is

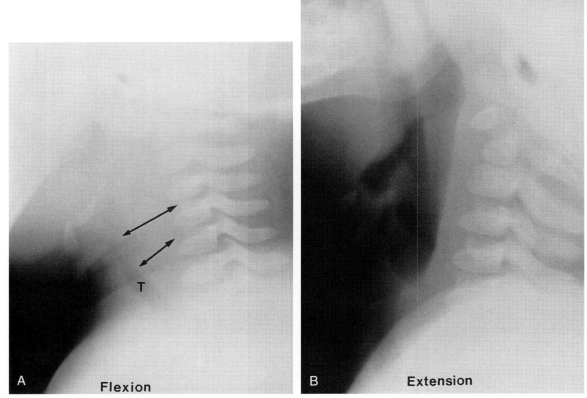

FIGURE 9–1. **Pseudoretropharyngeal abscess.** *A,* A lateral soft tissue view of a child's slightly flexed neck shows the trachea (T) bowed forward, which suggests the presence of a retropharyngeal soft tissue mass *(arrows).* *B,* A lateral view done a few minutes later of the same child with the neck extended shows a normal prevertebral soft tissue pattern.

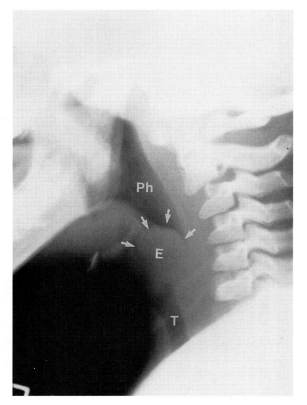

FIGURE 9–2. **Epiglottitis.** A lateral soft tissue view of the neck shows a ballooned pharynx (Ph) with a swollen epiglottis (E) in the shape of a large thumbprint *(arrows).* T = trachea.

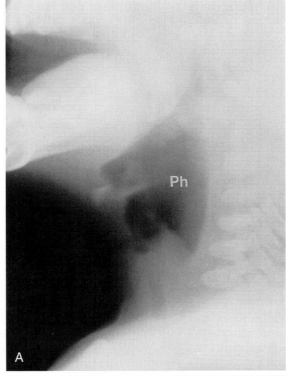

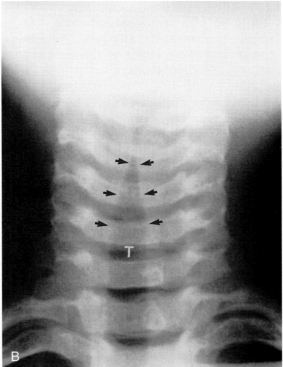

FIGURE 9–3. **Croup.** In a child with a barking cough, a lateral soft tissue view of the neck *(A)* demonstrates a markedly ballooned pharynx (Ph). An anteroposterior view of the neck *(B)* shows a steeple-shaped trachea *(arrows)* caused by subglottic edema.

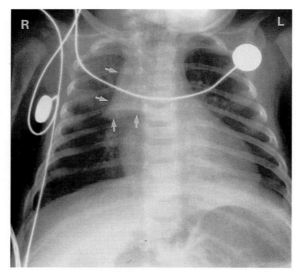

FIGURE 9–4. **Normal thymic shadow.** A posteroanterior view of the chest shows a prominent thymic shadow (arrows). Sometimes referred to as the sail sign, this is a normal finding.

the presence of the thymus. The thymus is routinely identified on chest films from birth to approximately 2 years of age. The thymus is usually seen as a widening of the soft tissues of the upper mediastinum, although occasionally it may appear to project out into the lung (the *sail sign*) (Fig. 9–4). The sail sign is normal and not an indication of an accompanying pneumothorax.

Children with pneumonias, bronchiolitis, or reactive airway disease usually have hyperinflation. In most normal young children, the most superior portion of the hemidiaphragm is at the level of the posterior eighth rib. If the diaphragms are lower than this, hyperinflation should be considered, and pathology may well be present. On a chest radiograph, rotation of the patient can cause problems in interpretation. As the patient is rotated to the left, the right cardiac border projects over the spine, and the right lower lobe pulmonary vessels can become emphasized, mimicking an infiltrate.

A favorite x-ray examination is the "babygram." This is an AP view of both the chest and the abdomen. In extremely small infants, the x-ray exposure can be adequate to visualize pulmonary vasculature, bowel gas, and skeletal structures. However, if you are only interested in the chest, a plain chest radiograph should be ordered to avoid unnecessary radiation exposure.

Foreign Bodies

Foreign bodies can be either aspirated or ingested. Most foreign bodies consist of vegetable material (such as peanuts) or plastic. Vegetable and plastic items are usually not visible on a radio-

graph. When a foreign body is aspirated into a bronchus, there are two possibilities. The first is that the object becomes completely impacted and does not allow air to pass during either inspiration or expiration. In this case, the air distally becomes resorbed, and postobstructive atelectasis or a focal infiltrate with associated volume loss occurs.

The second possibility is that the object only incompletely obstructs the bronchus and acts as a ball-valve. Thus, if there is suspicion of an inhaled foreign body, an inspiration and expiration film should be obtained. On the inspiration film, there may be postobstructive atelectasis, or the film may be normal. If the film is normal, there still may be a ball-valve phenomenon. On the expiration view, air is trapped on the affected side, while the unaffected lung decreases in volume. When this happens, there is a resultant shift of the mediastinum toward the normal, unaffected side (Fig. 9–5). If the child is too young to cooperate, right and left lateral decubitus chest radiographs give the same information. The dependent lung should normally get smaller.

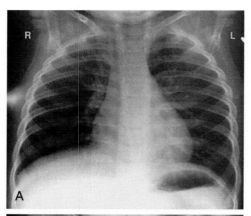

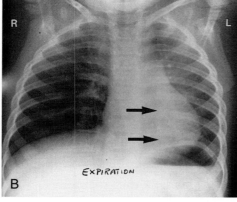

FIGURE 9–5. **Foreign body in right mainstem bronchus.** In this case, the mother thought the child inhaled a peanut. *A,* An inspiration view of the chest looks essentially normal. *B,* An expiration view shows that the left lung has decreased in volume (as expected) but that there is a shift of the heart to the left (arrows). The right lung remains hyperinflated because of the inability of the air to escape the ball-valve phenomenon caused by the foreign body.

Swallowed objects may be caught within the esophagus. In children, the objects that are large enough to remain in the esophagus are typically coins. These may be lodged at the level of the thoracic inlet or just above the level of the aortic arch (Fig. 9–6). Another common foreign object that may lodge in either the hypopharynx or the esophagus is a fish bone or chicken bone. Chicken bones are sometimes visualized on radiographs, but most fish bones are composed of cartilage and are essentially invisible on x-ray examination.

Tubes and Lines

A discussion of central venous catheters, jugular catheters, and pleural tubes has been included in Chapter 3. The tubes and catheters that are of specific interest in children are endotracheal tubes and umbilical artery (UAC) and umbilical vein (UVC) catheters. The tip of an endotracheal tube should be at least as far down as the level of the medial clavicles or at the level of the vertebral body of T1 or T2. The endotracheal tube should also have its tip located 1 or 2 cm above the carina. If the carina cannot be easily visualized, you should remember that on an AP or a posteroanterior chest radiograph, a tube with its tip projecting over the vertebral body of T5 is probably too low. Endotracheal tubes that are too low usually go down the right mainstem bronchus because this is more vertical in orientation than the left mainstem bronchus. Initially, an endotracheal tube positioned in the right mainstem bronchus may demonstrate a relatively normal-appearing lung. With time, however, because only the lower lobe and middle lobe bronchi are being ventilated, the selective obstruction of the right upper lobe bronchus causes right upper lobe atelectasis with progressive collapse (Fig. 9–7) or generalized left lung collapse.

UACs and UVCs are easily differentiated on the lateral view of the abdomen and chest. The UAC proceeds inferiorly from the umbilicus down into the pelvis and then turns and comes up the aorta (Fig. 9–8). Usually, the tip of a UAC is positioned at approximately the level of the vertebral body of T8. If a UAC is advanced too far, it can either proceed up into the great vessels of the head and neck or go anteriorly in the aortic arch. A UVC is also best identified on the lateral view. It can be seen progressing immediately superiorly from the umbilicus and then posteriorly along the liver and into the inferior vena cava and right atrium. If both a UAC and a UVC are present on an AP view it is

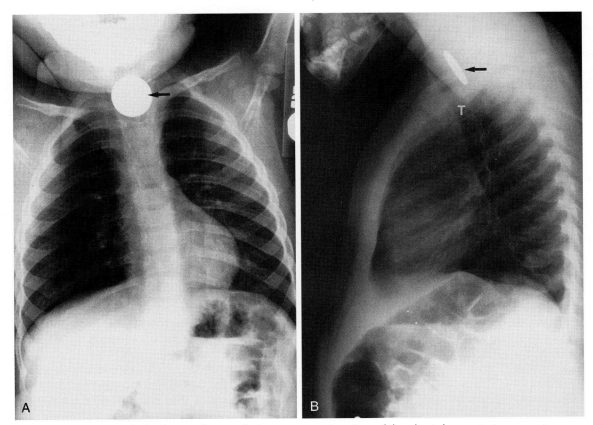

FIGURE 9–6. **Coin in the esophagus.** *A,* A posteroanterior view of the chest demonstrates a quarter *(arrow)* that is lodged in the esophagus just at the thoracic inlet. *B,* The lateral view also shows the coin *(arrow)* behind the trachea in the esophagus.

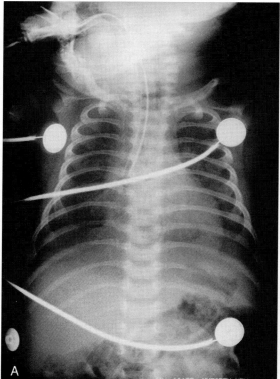

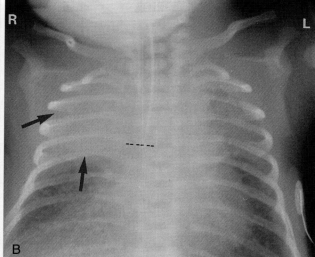

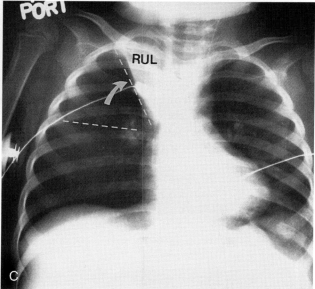

FIGURE 9–7. **Progressive right upper lobe atelectasis.** *A,* A posteroanterior view of the chest demonstrates an endotracheal tube with the tip down in the right mainstem bronchus. This often obstructs the right upper lobe (RUL) bronchus. *B,* Early atelectasis of the RUL occurs with resorption of air, causing consolidation *(arrows)* and slight upward bowing of the minor fissure. *C,* As collapse of the RUL becomes complete, the minor fissure rotates upward and medially *(curved arrow),* and the completely collapsed RUL remains as a small density along the right paratracheal region.

often not easy to tell them apart. Imagine where the umbilicus should be. A catheter that goes straight up and slightly to the right of the midline is a UVC, and one that goes down toward the pelvis and then toward the head is a UAC.

Another catheter that can sometimes be confusing is a ventriculoperitoneal shunt catheter. These shunts, which are placed for relief of hydrocephalus, extend from the lateral ventricle of the brain, down along the soft tissues of the neck and anterior chest wall, and then into the peritoneal cavity. Less commonly, the distal shunt tip may be placed in the right atrium.

Respiratory Diseases in the Newborn

A number of entities can cause neonatal respiratory difficulty (Table 9–2). It is important to be able to recognize a congenital diaphragmatic hernia, because it is a cause of respiratory distress in the neonatal period; it carries a mortality rate well in excess of 50%. Clinical manifestations are a scaphoid abdomen and bowel sounds in the chest. There can also be cyanosis caused by pulmonary hypoplasia and pulmonary hypertension. These hernias occur more commonly on the left and displace the heart and tracheal structures to the right. There is an opacity within the chest, which has air-filled spaces within it, often recognizable as bowel (Fig. 9–9).

At birth, there can be meconium aspiration. *Meconium* is the term used for the first stool evacuated after birth, and it is composed of mucus, epithelial cells, bile, and debris. In fetal distress there may be evacuation of meconium into the amniotic fluid. About 10% of the time this causes respiratory problems. At birth, as a result, there may be coarse

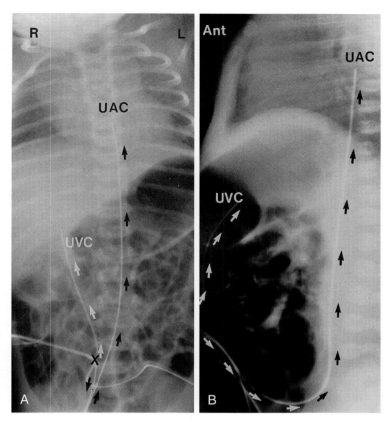

FIGURE 9–8. **Differentiation of umbilical artery (UAC) and umbilical vein (UVC) catheters.** *A,* On the anteroposterior view "babygram," if you imagine the position of the umbilicus (at the position of the *X*), the catheter that initially goes inferiorly and then turns and goes superiorly just to the left of midline is the UAC *(black arrows).* The catheter that goes into the umbilical region and immediately progresses cephalad and slightly to the right of the midline *(white arrows)* is the UVC. *B,* A lateral view on the same infant demonstrates the inferior, then the posterior and superior, course of the UAC, as well as the immediate superior course of the UVC progressing toward the inferior portion of the liver.

patchy infiltrates and hyperinflation of the lungs, which clears in about 3 to 5 days. Pneumothorax or pneumomediastinum occurs in about 25% of cases.

Another cause of respiratory distress within 48 hours of birth is transient tachypnea of the newborn (TTN). Lung volumes may be larger than normal, and there may be linear or streaky opacities that clear within 2 days. TTN is really a clinical, not a radiographic, diagnosis; it is due to delayed resorption of amniotic pulmonary liquid.

Hyaline membrane disease (HMD) is caused by surfactant deficiency and results in low lung volumes (unless the infant is intubated) with granular or ground-glass opacities of both lungs on radio-graphs. Any opacity in the lungs of a premature infant should be considered to be HMD until another cause is established. Air bronchograms (dark, branching tubular shadows) are often present; rarely, there is a pleural effusion. HMD typically becomes radiographically apparent at 4 to 6 hours after birth.

With HMD or pneumonia, infants may need positive-pressure ventilation. The complications of this respiratory therapy include *bronchopulmonary dysplasia* (BPD) and *pulmonary interstitial emphysema* (PIE). PIE refers to accumulation of air outside of alveoli in the interstitial or perivascular spaces. The imaging features include tortuous linear lucency

TABLE 9–2 X-ray Findings of Respiratory Distress in the Newborn

Entity	Time	Lung Volume	Lung Findings
Diaphragmatic hernia	At birth	Compressed	Bowel in chest
Meconium aspiration	At birth	Increased	Coarse, patchy infiltrates
Transient tachypnea	0–2 days	Normal or increased	Homogeneous diffuse or linear infiltrates
Hyaline membrane disease	0–7 days	Decreased*	Granular infiltrates
Neonatal pneumonia	Variable	Variable	Granular or patchy infiltrates
Pneumothorax	Variable	Decreased	Lucent dark area at lung edge†

* Can be increased if the patient is on positive-pressure ventilation (PEEP).
† Pneumothorax is much more common in children who are on PEEP.
You should look carefully for a basilar, medial, or anterior pneumothorax, because the films are usually done supine.

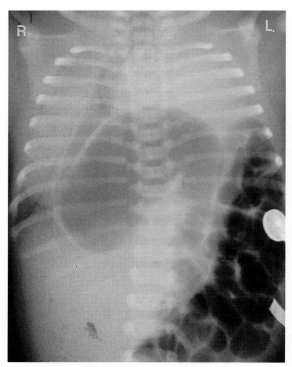

FIGURE 9–9. **Diaphragmatic hernia.** This newborn had significant respiratory difficulty. An anteroposterior view of the chest and abdomen demonstrates opacification of the left hemithorax, with bowel loops pushing up into the opacified left hemithorax. This condition carries a high fatality rate and should be recognized immediately.

that radiates outward from the hilum and may extend all the way to the periphery of the lung. These do not resemble the typical branching pattern of the bronchial tree but are more irregular (Fig. 9–10). PIE may rapidly result in life-threatening complications, such as pneumothorax, pneumomediastinum, or pneumopericardium.

Because the AP chest x-ray examinations of newborns or neonates are usually obtained with the infant in a supine position, a pneumothorax may be difficult to appreciate. This is because the air is usually located anteriorly (and not superiorly or laterally) in the pleural space. Sometimes the only signs may be lucency at the base of the lung or along the medial aspect of the lung. Often, a lateral radiograph taken with the child lying supine is necessary to demonstrate an anterior pneumothorax (Fig. 9–11).

BPD is thought to be the result of oxygen toxicity or barotrauma associated with respiratory therapy. BPD usually progresses as either HMD or neonatal pneumonia is resolving. It typically worsens from approximately 1 week to 1 month of life. The lungs characteristically become hyperinflated, in spite of the fact that they may have diffuse opacity with linear densities caused by fibrosis. There may also be areas of rounded lucency within the lung.

Bronchiolitis, Reactive Airways Disease, and Pneumonia

Neonatal pneumonia may result in a lung that is low in volume, normal, or hyperinflated. The lung opacities are typically granular, and the time course is variable. Neonatal pneumonias are due to transplacental infection from TORCH (*to*xoplasmosis, *ru*bella, *c*ytomegalovirus, *h*erpes) or from perineal flora acquired as a result of premature rupture of the membranes or while passing through the birth canal.

Infants and young children (several weeks to 1 year of age) may have a viral pneumonia caused either by RSV or by *H. influenzae*. With these, the early stage is bronchiolitis. About 15% of children younger than 2 years develop bronchiolitis and present with rhinorrhea, sneezing, cough, and low-grade fever followed by the rapid onset of tachypnea and wheezing. Most cases occur during winter and early spring. Many patients do not need imaging. Usually chest x-ray examinations are performed if the child is sick enough to require hospitalization, or if there is a suspicion of underlying pneumonia, unexpected deterioration in the patients condition or underlying heart or lung disease. Many patients do not have infiltrates on the chest radiograph, and hyperinflation may be the only radiographic finding. Bronchiolitis is most commonly due to RSV. As these viral pneumonias progress, children may also develop perihilar or peribronchial opacities. This can be seen as peribronchial cuffing or hilar adenop-

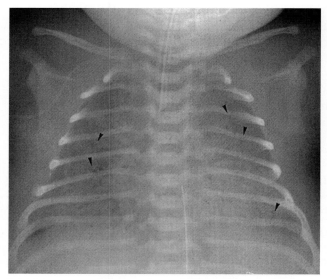

FIGURE 9–10. **Pulmonary interstitial emphysema (PIE).** This anteroposterior view of the chest shows generalized opacification of both lungs in a child with hyaline membrane disease. The *arrowheads* indicate linear air collections that do not follow the normal branching bronchial pattern and represent air in the interstitium. These patients often quickly progress to having a pneumothorax.

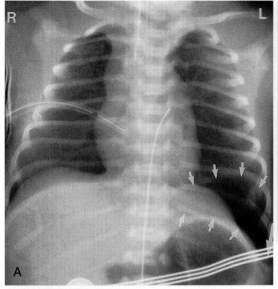

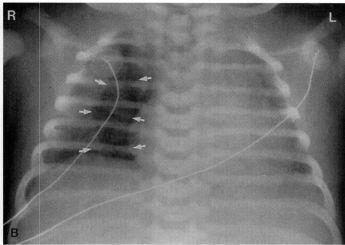

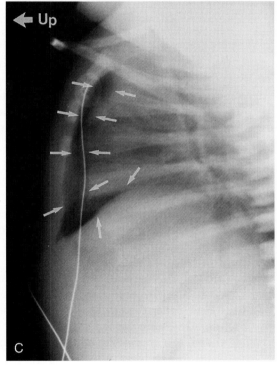

FIGURE 9–11. **Pneumothorax on supine chest radiograph.** *A,* In this infant, a right chest tube has already been placed because a pneumothorax is present. There is, however, a lucency at the left lung base *(small arrows)* representing a loculated pneumothorax. Note, in addition, a deep sulcus sign *(large arrow). B,* An antero-posterior view of the chest in another infant demonstrates a lucency or dark area overlying the medial aspect of the right lung and outlining the right cardiac border *(arrows).* This represents an anterior medial right pneumothorax. *C,* A lateral view of the chest with this patient supine is the best way to see an anterior pneumothorax. This is seen as a dark collection of air in the retrosternal region and in the anterior costophrenic angle *(arrows).*

athy. The peribronchial cuffing can be seen by looking for an outline of a bronchus in the region of the hilum and noting that the bronchial wall (seen on end as a circle) is thicker than a line traced by a fine lead pencil.

As children get somewhat older (age 1 to 3 years), they develop bacterial pneumonias. Pneumococcus is a common pathogen at age 1 to 3 years, whereas *Staphylococcus aureus* and *H. influenzae* are usually seen during infancy. Bacterial pneumonias typically cause alveolar infiltrates with lobar or segmental consolidations, often with effusion. Staphylococcal pneumonias may cause pneumothorax and also may cavitate. Most of the bacterial pneumonias

have appearances similar to those already described for adults. The two exceptions are the cavitating staphylococcal pneumonias and, occasionally, the descriptively termed *round pneumonia*. A round pneumonia is usually a bacterial pneumonia in an early stage, and later, typical lobar consolidations may develop.

Asthma

Asthma is one of the most common pulmonary disorders in children. Reversible airway obstruction can range from mild to life threatening. Asthma and wheezing (easy inspiration and difficult expiration) should be differentiated from stridor (difficult inspiration and easier expiration). The latter indicates an upper airway obstruction. The initial work-up of asthma includes history, physical examination, and pulmonary function tests (particularly forced expiratory volume in one second [FEV_1]). In young children, it is important to exclude inhaled foreign bodies, cystic fibrosis, enlarged lymph nodes, or neoplasms obstructing the bronchi. For patients with known asthma and a simple attack, a chest radiograph is not indicated. If there is suspicion of a complicating factor (fever or pneumonia) or a poor response to therapy, a chest radiograph is indicated.

Cystic Fibrosis

Cystic fibrosis is caused by a dysfunction of the exocrine glands, resulting in the production of thick mucus that accumulates in the lungs, leading to bronchitis and recurrent pneumonias. It is an autosomal recessive disorder and is the most common lethal genetic disease affecting whites. Pulmonary findings are present in essentially all cases by the time a child is 10 years of age or more. The most obvious finding is hyperinflation. Essentially, the chest radiograph looks like that of an adult with chronic obstructive pulmonary disease. There is an increased AP diameter and flattening of the hemidiaphragms. In addition, the lungs generally appear "dirty." There is peribronchial thickening and bronchiectasis with increased pulmonary markings at the lung bases (Fig. 9–12). These are not lobar or segmental infiltrates.

Children with cystic fibrosis are also prone to a wide variety of gastrointestinal problems, including meconium ileus, meconium peritonitis, rectal prolapse, volvulus, intussusception, pancreatitis, jaundice, growth failure, and vitamin deficiencies. One should suspect cystic fibrosis in any child with recurrent respiratory or gastrointestinal symptoms.

■ ABDOMINAL REGION

Tracheoesophageal Fistula

Tracheoesophageal fistula (TEF) may be suspected in an infant born of a gestation with polyhydramnios. TEF is usually clinically apparent, presenting as excessive salivation as well as the onset of aspiration, coughing, and choking as soon as an attempt to feed the child is made. Ninety-five percent of patients with a TEF have a blind-ending esophagus. The diagnosis is usually made by passing a small, soft feeding tube down the esophagus to the blind end and taking a lateral radiograph. If

necessary, air can be injected to help visualization. Instillation of barium or other contrast material is rarely, if ever, indicated. In those few patients with an H-type fistula and a patent esophagus, it may take months to arrive at the diagnosis, but the disorder should be suspected in a child with recurrent pneumonias or chronic cough. Forty percent of patients with TEF have associated cardiac and other gastrointestinal anomalies. The VATER syndrome describes the association between *v*ertebral anomalies (hemivertebra), *a*nal atresia, *T*EF, and *r*adial limb dysplasia.

Acute Gastroenteritis

The usual clinical presentation is acute onset of diarrhea, vomiting, or both. Dehydration is the major complication. Acute gastroenteritis is usually due to viruses (*Rotavirus* or Norwalk agent). In extremely ill patients, a stool culture or toxin assay is indicated. If the patient has abdominal pain or distension, the differential diagnosis includes appendicitis, intussusception, or bowel obstruction. In these circumstances, a plain and upright film of the abdomen or a CT scan may be helpful. These are discussed in more detail in Chapter 6. For simple gastroenteritis, no imaging studies are indicated.

Bowel Obstruction

Air should normally be seen in the abdomen of the neonate in the following temporal progression: the stomach 2 hours after birth, the small bowel at 6 hours, and the rectum by 24 hours.

Hypertrophic pyloric stenosis is the second most common gastrointestinal condition and requires surgery in the first 2 months of life. Pyloric stenosis is more common in male infants and should be suspected if there is a maternal or sibling history of the condition. The typical clinical symptom is nonbilious vomiting during the second to fourth week of life. There may be a palpable olive-shaped mass to the right of the umbilicus. A plain film of the abdomen shows a stomach that is dilated to greater than 7 cm, and peristaltic waves can sometimes be seen, giving the stomach a caterpillar appearance. The diagnosis is confirmed by using abdominal ultrasound imaging to visualize the thickened pyloric muscle. The pyloric muscle should not be more than 4 mm in thickness (mucosa to outside wall) or greater than 18 mm in length (Fig. 9–13).

Duodenal atresias, midgut volvulus, and pyloric stenosis are apparent because they produce obstruction and vomiting. Under these circumstances, you should consult the radiologist as to what imaging

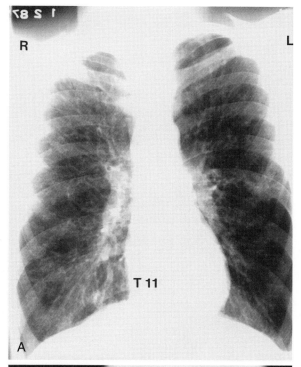

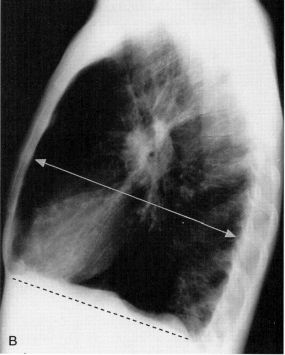

FIGURE 9–12. **Cystic fibrosis.** *A,* The posteroanterior view of the chest in this young teenager demonstrates marked hyperinflation, with the hemidiaphragms being flattened and pushed down to the level of the posterior 11th ribs (T11). There is also diffuse bronchial thickening throughout both lungs. *B,* The lateral view of the chest shows an increase in anteroposterior diameter *(double-sided arrow)* and flattening of the hemidiaphragms *(dotted line).* These findings in an adult would normally be associated with chronic obstructive pulmonary disease. However, in a teenager or child, they are almost certainly due to cystic fibrosis.

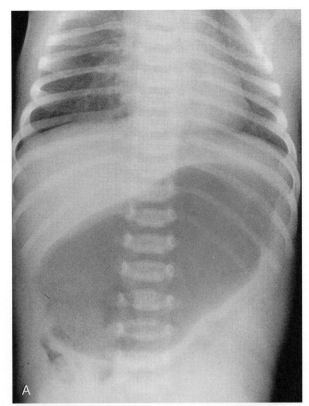

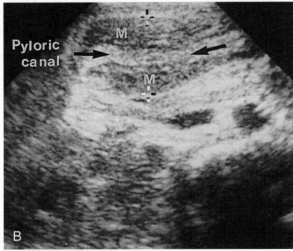

FIGURE 9–13. **Pyloric stenosis.** *A,* A supine film of the abdomen shows a markedly dilated, gas-filled stomach. *B,* A transverse ultrasound study of the upper abdomen shows the thickened pyloric muscle (M) on both sides of the pyloric canal *(arrows).*

procedure would be best. The approximate level of obstruction in the bowel is typically determined on the plain film by seeing how far bowel gas has progressed through the gastrointestinal tract. If gas is seen only in the stomach or the stomach and duodenum (the *double-bubble sign*), a proximal obstruction is likely. Duodenal atresia or midgut volvulus should be suspected in a birth with polyhydramnios and an infant who has bile-stained

vomiting. Duodenal atresia is the most common cause of the double-bubble sign, with annular pancreas being next most common. Duodenal bands, webs, and midgut volvulus are less frequent. Duodenal atresia has been associated with Down syndrome. Midgut volvulus, although less common, is important to consider, because there is a high mortality rate without intervention. A midgut volvulus occurs when the small bowel and proximal colon rotate about the axis of the superior mesenteric artery. This can cause arterial compromise and gangrene.

If air is seen beyond the duodenum but not into the distal small bowel or colon, one should think of midlevel lesions. Atresias can occur in the jejunum and ileum. With any of these entities, even with x-ray contrast studies, it is not possible to tell with certainty either the site or the length of the atresia or even to differentiate an atresia from a midgut volvulus. As a result, most pediatric surgeons are content with the plain x-ray findings before proceeding to surgery. Occasionally, some request a barium enema to look for a microcolon before surgery.

If gas is seen throughout most of the abdomen of a neonate but not in the region of the rectum, a distal small bowel or colon obstruction should be suspected. This may be the result of either a meconium ileus or Hirschsprung's disease. A note of caution should be entered here relative to the appearance of bowel gas in a neonate or very young child. In this age group, gas in the small bowel and colon look exactly the same. Rather, differential diagnoses are made on the basis of whether there is gas in the proximal or distal bowel.

Meconium ileus is seen in 50% of patients with cystic fibrosis. On an enema performed with water-soluble contrast, the colon is seen to be quite small (microcolon), because it was unused during fetal life (Fig. 9–14). Hirschsprung's disease is due to the absence of neural cells in the distal segment of the colon; in the first 6 weeks of life, these children present with obstruction or constipation. The disorder should be suspected in any infant who fails to pass meconium in the first 24 hours of life. In about 75% of patients, the abnormal segment is restricted to the rectosigmoid colon. On a barium enema, a narrowed segment may be identified (Fig. 9–15).

Intussusception is invagination of a segment of bowel into more distal bowel and usually occurs with ileum telescoping into colon. Forty percent of patients present between 3 and 18 months of age, most with pain and vomiting. A lesser number have an associated abdominal mass or rectal bleeding. Intussusception is rarely seen in neonates. Clinically, the children have an acute onset of colicky pain, and they may cry, draw up their knees, and vomit. Sometimes a sausage-shaped mass can be

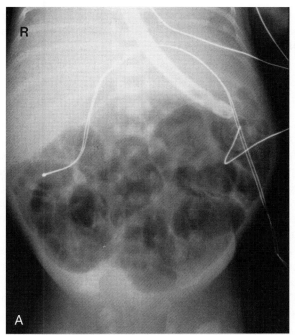

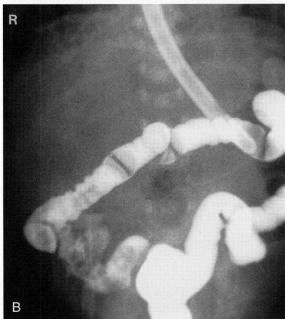

FIGURE 9–14. **Meconium ileus.** *A,* An anteroposterior view of the abdomen demonstrates dilated bowel. In a child of this age it is not possible to differentiate the colon from the small bowel. There is, however, no gas seen within the rectum. *B,* A Gastrografin enema has been performed, and the colon is noted to be quite small (a microcolon). There are intraluminal defects seen in the colon at the level of the ileocecal valve, because there is usually obstruction at this level resulting from the thick tenacious meconium adhering to small bowel.

felt in the upper abdomen. Radiographically, plain films are often normal. If the intussusception has occurred within 24 hours before patient presentation, there is a good chance that a radiologist can reduce it with a water-soluble contrast enema. Cur-

rently, however, most radiologists prefer to reduce intussusception simply using air (Fig. 9–16). If this fails, surgery is necessary. Reduction by a radiologist should not be attempted if there are clinical signs of peritonitis or shock. Other relatively common lesions to bear in mind when a proximal bowel obstruction is suspected in a child 6 to 30 months of age are an incarcerated inguinal hernia and appendicitis.

Necrotizing Enterocolitis

This is the most common gastrointestinal emergency in premature infants. It usually develops within the first week after birth but can be seen up to 2 months after birth. Clinical signs are abdominal tenderness, rectal bleeding, and a septic shock-like appearance. The earliest radiographic sign is air within the wall of the bowel (pneumatosis) or a bubbly appearance of the bowel. Another early finding is small bowel dilatation due to an adynamic ileus (Fig. 9–17). A common complication and indication for surgery includes free air within the peritoneal cavity, which indicates a bowel perforation. Gas in the portal vein may also be identified. In contrast to adults, in whom this condition generally portends a fatal outcome, the outcome in children with portal venous air is not as severe.

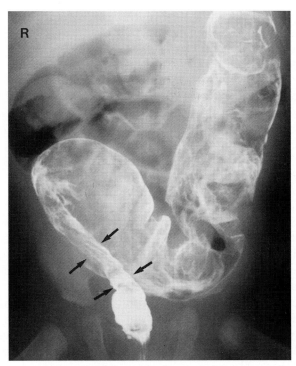

FIGURE 9–15. **Hirschsprung's disease.** This abnormality is due to an absence of myenteric plexus cells in the distal colon. A barium enema demonstrates a narrowed segment in the rectum and a markedly dilated sigmoid and descending colon.

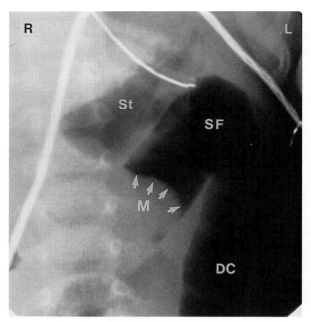

FIGURE 9–16. **Intussusception.** This 3-year-old had colicky abdominal pain and rectal bleeding. There is invagination of a segment of bowel into more distal bowel. Ileocolic and ileoileocolic intussusceptions represent 90% of occurrences. Here, a film has been obtained while the radiologist is reducing the intussusception with air. Air is seen in the distal colon (DC) and the splenic flexure (SF); the mass (M) representing the leading portion of the intussuscepted segment is clearly identified *(arrows)*. St = stomach; L = left; R = right.

On a supine view, if there is a large amount of free air within the peritoneal cavity, the air outlines the falciform ligament of the liver (the *football sign*). This is a fairly subtle sign; a large amount of air may be present in the peritoneal cavity, and it may easily be overlooked on a supine film. For this reason, a left lateral decubitus view, which will show air over the lateral margin of the liver, is often recommended.

Meckel's Diverticulum

This is a vestigial remnant of the omphalomes-enteric duct, and it may contain gastric mucosa. Clinical signs are painless rectal bleeding and, occasionally, intestinal obstruction. Meckel's diverticulum follows what is known as "the rule of twos." It occurs in 2% of the population; it usually presents before 2 years of age; and the diverticulum is usually located in the ileum within 2 feet of the ileocecal valve. If gastric mucosa is present in the diverticulum, there may be resultant ulceration and hemorrhage. In patients with rectal bleeding before 2 years of age, Meckel's diverticulum should be considered. The imaging study of choice is a nuclear medicine scan done with technetium-99m pertech-

netate. This concentrates in the normal and ectopic gastric mucosa and allows identification of Meckel's diverticulum (Fig. 9–18).

Neonatal Jaundice

In some young infants (2 to 3 weeks old), jaundice can develop. The usual diagnostic dilemma is whether the infant has neonatal hepatitis or biliary atresia. The imaging test of choice is a nuclear medicine hepatobiliary scan. This involves giving a small amount of radioactive tracer that is concentrated by the liver and then excreted via the biliary system. If any excretion into the small bowel is detected on the images, biliary atresia is excluded. Occasionally in patients with severe hepatitis and slow hepatic excretion, follow-up images are needed at 24 hours postinjection to be certain of the diagnosis.

Abdominal Masses

Abdominal masses in children are usually initially worked up by clinical examination. Because the information is usually limited, a plain film of the abdomen and a CT or ultrasound are usually

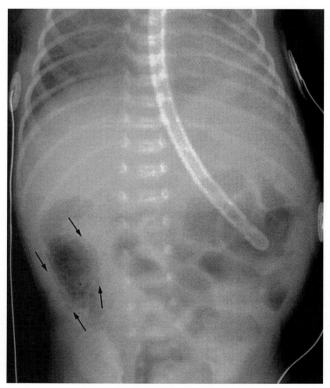

FIGURE 9–17. **Necrotizing enterocolitis.** This represents the most common gastrointestinal emergency in premature infants. A film of this 5-day-old infant shows abnormal collections of air within the bowel wall *(arrows)*.

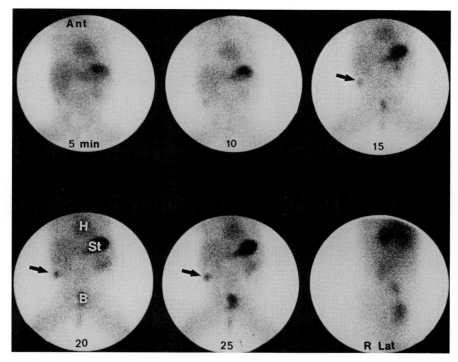

FIGURE 9–18. **Meckel's diverticulum.** In this 2-year-old child who had unexplained rectal bleeding, a nuclear medicine study was performed using radioactive material that concentrates in gastric mucosa (technetium-99m pertechnetate). Sequential 5-minute images of the abdomen are obtained. On the 20 minute image, the heart (H), stomach (St), and bladder (B) are clearly seen, in addition to an ectopic focus of activity (arrow) representing a Meckel diverticulum.

done. The differential diagnosis of an abdominal mass varies with the child's age. A mass in the abdomen of a child of any age most likely arises from the kidneys. In a neonate, 55% of masses are renal in origin (hydronephrosis or multicystic dysplastic kidney), and the remainder are usually gastrointestinal duplications, cysts, and hemangioendotheliomas of the liver.

If a mass appears to be in the flank in an older infant or child, Wilms' tumor, neuroblastoma, and hydronephrosis account for about 80% of the lesions. Other possibilities include abscesses, cysts, and hepatoblastomas. Neuroblastomas have calcification approximately 90% of the time (Fig. 9–19) and are usually seen in patients younger than 2 years. They present as masses external to the kidney and tend to displace the kidney rather than deform it. Because neuroblastomas arise from neural tissue, they are also relatively common in the region of the adrenal glands, along the sympathetic chain, and in the posterior mediastinum. Wilms' tumor begins within the kidney; on an intravenous pyelogram, it is seen as a renal mass, deforming the normal collecting system (Fig. 9–20). Wilms' tumors are bilateral 10% of the time and are rarely calcified. The average age of presentation is 2 to 3 years, which is older than the usual age for neuroblastomas.

Rectal Bleeding

Rectal bleeding in children should be classified as dark or bright red and painless or painful. Dark red blood usually indicates upper GI origin and the differential diagnosis includes foreign body, varices, peptic ulcer, and bowel duplication. Painful dark or bright rectal bleeding is associated with volvulus, mesenteric thrombosis, and Meckel's diverticulum. Bright red painless bleeding may be due to a polyp, neoplasm, colitis, or sigmoid intussusception. Painful bright red bleeding is most commonly due to an anal fissure, hemorrhoids, or rectal prolapse; for these, no imaging studies are usually needed. Rectal bleeding in young children can also be due to an allergy to formula.

The work-up of any rectal bleeding should begin with a rectal examination. If an obvious cause is not identified and particularly if there is associated pain, vomiting, guarding, rebound, or abdominal distension, a surgical consultation should be obtained. The imaging work-up depends on which of the causes is felt to be most likely, although either endoscopy or a plain film of the abdomen with an air or barium enema is often obtained.

Urinary Abnormalities

There are two relatively common urinary problems in children—hydronephrosis and ureterovesicular reflux. The most common cause of hydronephrosis in a child is an obstruction at the junction of the lower portion of the renal pelvis and the upper ureter. The entity is bilateral in 20% of cases. The initial imaging test of choice is an intravenous pyelogram. Although the dilated collecting system can be visualized with ultrasonography, there is

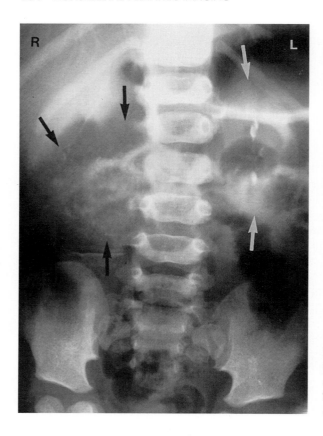

FIGURE 9–19. **Retroperitoneal neuroblastoma.** On this intravenous pyelogram, the left kidney appears to be functioning well *(white arrows).* On the right side, no functional kidney is identified, but there are multiple scattered tiny amorphous calcifications *(black arrows),* which are often seen with this tumor.

usually not enough anatomic detail of the ureter and not enough information about the renal function. Postoperative follow-up functional studies in these children are usually done with a nuclear medicine Lasix renogram. The radiation dose is lower, and there is no risk of a contrast agent reaction. If only information about the degree of dilatation of

the collecting system is desired, ultrasound imaging is the test of choice.

Ureterovesicular reflux is due to maldevelopment of the flap valve that is created as the ureter crosses obliquely through the bladder wall. Less commonly, it can be due to ectopic insertion of a ureter or to a ureterocele. On a contrast study, any visible reflux

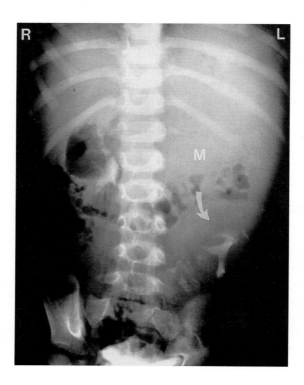

FIGURE 9–20. **Wilms' tumor.** On this intravenous pyelogram, the collecting system of the right kidney is identified along the lateral border of L1, L2, and L3. The collecting system of the left kidney has been displaced inferiorly *(curved arrow)* by a mass (M), and the collecting system has been distorted, suggesting that the M is intrarenal in origin. This is a common way of differentiating an intraparenchymal Wilms tumor from an extrarenal neuroblastoma.

of urine from the bladder into a ureter is abnormal. If severe, it is surgically repaired because of the increased risk of infection. The most common imaging method is a cystogram. The patient is catheterized, contrast material is put into the bladder, and the radiologist looks for contrast material in the ureters. This involves a relatively high radiation dose to the child's gonads, but the anatomic resolution is good. If repeated evaluations of reflux are necessary, a nuclear medicine cystogram can provide good quantitative information with a much lower dose.

Multicystic dysplastic kidney is a unilateral process resulting from a severe ureteropelvic junction obstruction in utero. As a result, there is no functional renal parenchyma, and the kidney is represented by a large number of noncommunicating cysts. Calcification may be present. Renal vessels are absent or quite small. A retrograde pyelogram shows a blind-ending ureter. Surgery is not immediately necessary. There is another congenital condition called *multilocular cystic nephroma*, which has large cystic areas. Calcifications in this entity are rare.

Neonatal or infantile polycystic disease does not present with a dominant abdominal mass. Each has ectasia of renal tubules, but there are no obvious cysts that are visible by imaging methods. Ultrasonography is the test of choice in the neonatal form and demonstrates extensive tubular ectasia. Death usually occurs in months or years. There is little associated hepatic fibrosis. In the infantile form, only about 20% of the tubules are ectatic, and symptoms do not appear for 3 to 6 months. There is moderate hepatic fibrosis. In the juvenile form, fewer tubules are ectatic, and symptoms appear at 1 to 5 years of age. The liver fibrosis is severe in this form, and death results from portal hypertension.

GENERAL SUGGESTED READINGS

Swischuk L: Imaging of the Newborn, Infant, and Young Child, 4th ed. Philadelphia, Lippincott Williams & Wilkins, 1997.

TYPICAL PRICE RANGE OF SOME IMAGING PROCEDURES*

Diagnostic Radiology

Chest	$30–130
Abdomen	30–130
Pelvis	30–140
Hand	24–104
Ankle	24–110
Barium enema	90–300
Intravenous pyelogram	100–240
Mammogram	45–200

Computed Tomography

Brain with contrast only	240–700
with and without contrast	290–950

Magnetic Resonance Scan

Brain with contrast	525–1600
with and without contrast	880–1700

Nuclear Medicine

Bone scan	190–460
Myocardial perfusion	455–710

Ultrasound

Fetal	120–500
Right upper quadrant	70–300

* Price includes hospital and physician charges. Lower end of range is the fee paid by Medicare, and the upper end is the total fee charged (as compared with paid). Many contracted imaging services offer 20 to 40% discounts on charged fees.

2

RADIATION DOSES FROM VARIOUS EXAMINATIONS*

Examination	Effective Dose (mrem)	Gonadal Dose (mrem)
Extremities	1	<1
Skull	22	<1
Chest (two views)	10	1
KUB (abdomen, one view)	60	97/221†
Lumbar spine	130	218/721
CT (head and body)	110	—
Barium enema	410	175/900
Hip and pelvis	50	210/600
Nuclear Medicine		
Bone scan	440	320/440
Lung scan	150	228/30
Cardiac (thallium)	710	1900/560
Hepatobiliary	370	19/50
All Ultrasound	None	None
All Magnetic Resonance Scans	None	None

* The effective dose from natural background radiation in the United States is 300 mrem per year.
† Refers to male/female. Gonadal dose in the female approximates dose to the fetus in a pregnant female.

INDEX

Note: Page numbers in *italics* indicate figures; those followed by t indicate tables.